Paramedic Care

Principles & Practice

Paramedicine Fundamentals

Workbook

Fourth Edition

Paramedic Care

Principles & Practice

Paramedicine Fundamentals

Workbook

Fourth Edition

ROBERT S. PORTER

REVISED BY

TONY CRYSTAL, Sc.D., EMT-P

EMS Program Coordinator
Richland Community College
Decatur, Illinois

BRYAN E. BLEDSOE, DO, FACEP, FAAEM, EMT-P

Professor of Emergency Medicine
Director, Prehospital and Disaster Medicine Fellowship
University of Nevada School of Medicine
Attending Emergency Physician
University Medical Center of Southern Nevada
Medical Director, MedicWest Ambulance
Las Vegas, Nevada

ROBERT S. PORTER, MA, EMT-P

Senior Advanced Life Support Educator
Madison County Emergency Medical Services
Canastota, New York

RICHARD A. CHERRY, MS, NREMT-P

Director of Training
Northern Onondaga Volunteer Ambulance
Liverpool, New York

PEARSON

Boston Columbus Indianapolis New York San Francisco Upper Saddle River
Amsterdam Cape Town Dubai London Madrid Milan Munich Paris Montréal Toronto
Delhi Mexico City São Paulo Sydney Hong Kong Seoul Singapore Taipei Tokyo

Publisher: *Julie Levin Alexander*
Publisher's Assistant: *Regina Bruno*
Editor-in-Chief: *Marlene McHugh Pratt*
Senior Managing Editor for Development: *Lois Berlowitz*
Editorial Project Manager: *Triple SSS Press Media Development, Inc.*
Assistant Editor: *Jonathan Cheung*
Director of Marketing: *David Gesell*
Marketing Manager: *Brian Hoehl*
Marketing Specialist: *Michael Sirinides*
Managing Editor for Production: *Patrick Walsh*
Production Liaison: *Faye Gemmellaro*
Production Editor: *Muralidharan Krishnamurthy/S4Carlisle Publishing Services*
Manufacturing Manager: *Ilene Sanford*
Cover Design: *Kathryn Foot*
Cover Image: *© corepics/Shutterstock*
Composition: *S4Carlisle Publishing Services*
Cover and Interior Printer/Binder: *Edwards Brothers Malloy*

NOTICE ON CPR AND ECC

The national standards for cardiopulmonary resuscitation (CPR) and emergency cardiovascular care (ECC) are reviewed and revised on a regular basis and may change slightly after this manual is printed. It is important that you know the most current procedures for CPR and ECC, both for the classroom and your patients. The most current information may always be downloaded from www.bradybooks.com or obtained from the appropriate credentialing agency.

NOTICE ON CARE PROCEDURES

It is the intent of the authors and publisher that this Workbook be used as part of a formal Paramedic program taught by qualified instructors and supervised by a licensed physician. The procedures described in this Workbook are based upon consultation with EMS and medical authorities. The authors and publisher have taken care to make certain that these procedures reflect currently accepted clinical practice; however, they cannot be considered absolute recommendations.

The material in this Workbook contains the most current information available at the time of publication. However, federal, state, and local guidelines concerning clinical practices, including, without limitation, those governing infection control and universal precautions, change rapidly. The reader should note, therefore, that the new regulations may require changes in some procedures.

It is the responsibility of the reader to familiarize himself or herself with the policies and procedures set by federal, state, and local agencies as well as the institution or agency where the reader is employed. The authors and the publisher of this Workbook disclaim any liability, loss, or risk resulting directly or indirectly from the suggested procedures and theory, from any undetected errors, or from the reader's misunderstanding of the text. It is the reader's responsibility to stay informed of any new changes or recommendations made by any federal, state, and local agency as well as by his or her employing institution or agency.

Brady
is an imprint of

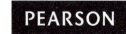

www.bradybooks.com

10 9 8 7 6 5 4 3 2 1
ISBN 10: 0-13-211237-X
ISBN 13: 978-0-13-211237-6

Dedication

This workbook is dedicated to the important people in your life: your wife/husband, mother, father, sister, brother . . . and friends who support you and the time and passion you devote to Emergency Medical Service.
Without them, this endeavor would be lonely and much less rewarding.

–ROBERT S. PORTER

CONTENTS

INTRODUCTION

Welcome to the self-instructional Workbook for *Paramedic Care: Principles & Practice*. This Workbook is designed to help guide you through an educational program for initial or refresher training that follows the guidelines of the 2009 *National EMS Education Standards*. The Workbook is designed to be used either in conjunction with your instructor or as a self-study guide you use on your own.

This Workbook features many different ways to help you learn the material necessary to become a paramedic, as described next.

Features

Review of Chapter Objectives

Each chapter of *Paramedic Care: Principles & Practice* begins with objectives that identify the important information and principles addressed in the chapter reading. To help you identify and learn this material, each Workbook chapter reviews the important content elements addressed by these objectives as presented in the text.

Case Study Review

Each chapter of *Paramedic Care: Principles & Practice* includes a case study, introducing and highlighting important principles presented in the chapter. The Workbook reviews these case studies and points out much of the essential information and many of the applied principles they describe.

Content Self-Evaluation

Each chapter of *Paramedic Care: Principles & Practice* presents an extensive narrative explanation of the principles of paramedic practice. The Workbook chapter (or chapter section) contains between 10 and 50 multiple-choice questions to test your reading comprehension of the textbook material and to give you experience taking typical emergency medical service examinations.

Special Projects

The Workbook contains several projects that are special learning experiences designed to help you remember the information and principles necessary to perform as a paramedic. Special projects include crossword puzzles, fill-in-the-blank exercises, and a variety of other activities.

Chapter Sections

Several chapters in *Paramedic Care: Principles & Practice* are extensive and contain a great deal of subject matter. To help you grasp this material more efficiently, the Workbook breaks these chapters into sections with their own objectives, content review, and special projects.

Content Review

The Workbook provides a comprehensive review of the material presented in Volume 2 of *Paramedic Care: Principles & Practice*. After the last text chapter has been covered, the Workbook presents an extensive content self-evaluation component that helps you recall and build upon the knowledge you have gained by reading the text, attending class, and completing the earlier Workbook chapters.

Emergency Drug Cards

At the end of this Workbook are Emergency Drug Cards. These alphabetized 3" x 5" cards present the names/classes, descriptions, indications, contraindications, precautions, and routes and dosages of drugs the paramedic is most likely to encounter in prehospital care. Detach the cards and use them in flash card fashion. Practice until you can give the correct route, dosage, indications, and contraindications for each drug.

HOW TO USE THIS SELF-INSTRUCTIONAL WORKBOOK

The self-instructional Workbook accompanying *Paramedic Care: Principles & Practice* may be used as directed by your instructor or independently by you during your course of instruction. The following recommendations are intended to guide you in using the Workbook independently.

- Examine your course schedule and identify the appropriate text chapter or other assigned reading.

- Read the assigned chapter in *Paramedic Care: Principles & Practice* carefully. Do this in a relaxed environment, free of distractions, and give yourself adequate time to read and digest the material. The information presented in *Paramedic Care: Principles & Practice* is often technically complex and demanding, but it is very important that you comprehend it. Be sure that you read the chapter carefully enough to understand and remember what you have read.

- Carefully read the Review of Chapter Objectives at the beginning of each Workbook chapter (or section). This material includes both the objectives listed in *Paramedic Care: Principles & Practice* and narrative descriptions of their content. If you do not understand or remember what is discussed from your reading, refer to the referenced pages and reread them carefully. If you still do not feel comfortable with your understanding of any objective, consider asking your instructor about it.

- Reread the case study in *Paramedic Care: Principles & Practice*, and then read the Case Study Review in the Workbook. Note the important points regarding assessment and care that the Case Study Review highlights and be sure that you understand and agree with the analysis of the call. If you have any questions or concerns, ask your instructor to clarify the information.

- Take the Content Self-Evaluation at the end of each Workbook chapter (or section), answering each question carefully. Do this in a quiet environment, free from distractions, and allow yourself adequate time to complete the exercise. Correct your self-evaluation by consulting the answers at the back of the Workbook, and determine the percentage you have answered correctly (the number you got right divided by the total number of questions). If you have answered most of the questions correctly (85 to 90 percent), review those that you missed by rereading the material on the pages listed in the answer key and be sure you understand which answer is correct and why. If you have more than a few questions wrong (less than 85 percent correct), look for incorrect answers that are grouped together. This suggests that you did not understand a particular topic in the reading. Reread the text dealing with that topic carefully, and then retest yourself on the questions you got wrong. If incorrect answers are spread throughout the chapter content, reread the chapter and retake the Content Self-Evaluation to ensure that you understand the material. If you don't understand why your answer to a question is incorrect after reviewing the text, consult with your instructor.

- In a similar fashion, complete the exercises in the Special Projects section of the Workbook chapters (or sections). These exercises are specifically designed to help you learn and remember the essential principles and information presented in *Paramedic Care: Principles & Practice*.

- When you have completed this volume of *Paramedic Care: Principles & Practice* and its accompanying Workbook, prepare for a course test by reviewing both the text in its entirety and your class notes. Then take the Content Review examination in the Workbook. Again, review your score and any questions you have answered incorrectly by referring to the text and rereading the page or pages where the material is presented. If you note groupings of wrong answers, review the entire range of pages or the full chapter they represent.

If, during your completion of the Workbook exercises, you have any questions that either the textbook or Workbook doesn't answer, write them down and ask your instructor about them. Prehospital emergency medicine is a complex and complicated subject, and answers are not always black and white. It is also common for different EMS systems to use differing methods of care. The questions you bring up in class, and your instructor's answers to them, will help you expand and complete your knowledge of prehospital emergency medical care.

GUIDELINES TO BETTER TEST-TAKING

The knowledge you will gain from reading the textbook, completing the exercises in the Workbook, listening in your paramedic class, and participating in your clinical and field experience will prepare you to care for patients who are seriously ill or injured. However, before you can practice these skills, you will have to pass several classroom written exams and your state's certification exam. Your performance on these exams will depend not only on your knowledge but also on your ability to answer test questions correctly. The following guidelines are designed to help your performance on tests and to better demonstrate your knowledge of prehospital emergency care.

1. Relax and be calm during the test.

A test is designed to measure what you have learned and to tell you and your instructor how well you are doing. An exam is not designed to intimidate or punish you. Consider it a challenge, and just try to do your best. Get plenty of sleep before the examination. Avoid coffee or other stimulants for a few hours before the exam, and be prepared.

Reread the text chapters, review the objectives in the Workbook, and review your class notes. It might be helpful to work with one or two other students and ask each other questions. This type of practice helps everyone better understand the knowledge presented in your course of study.

2. Read the questions carefully.

Read each word of the question and all the answers slowly. Words such as "except" or "not" may change the entire meaning of the question. If you miss such words, you may answer the question incorrectly even though you know the right answer.

Example:
The art and science of emergency medical services involves all of the following EXCEPT

   A. sincerity and compassion.
   B. respect for human dignity.
   C. placing patient care before personal safety.
   D. delivery of sophisticated emergency medical care.
   E. none of the above.

The correct answer is C, unless you miss the "EXCEPT."

3. Read each answer carefully.

Read each and every answer carefully. Although the first answer may be absolutely correct, so may the rest, and thus the best answer might be "all of the above."

Example:
Indirect medical direction is considered to be

   A. treatment protocols.
   B. training and education.
   C. quality assurance.
   D. chart review.
   E. all of the above.

Although answers A, B, C, and D are each correct, the best and only acceptable answer is "all of the above," E.

4. Delay answering questions you don't understand and look for clues.

When a question seems confusing or you don't know the answer, note it on your answer sheet and come back to it later. This will ensure that you have time to complete the test. You will also find that other questions on the test may give you hints to answer the one you've skipped over. It will also prevent you from being frustrated with an early question and letting it affect your performance.

Example:
Upon successful completion of a course of training as an EMT-P, most states will

    A.   certify you. (correct)
    B.   license you.
    C.   register you.
    D.   recognize you as a paramedic.
    E.   issue you a permit.

Another question, later in the exam, may suggest the right answer:

The action of one state in recognizing the certification of another is called

    A.   reciprocity. (correct)
    B.   national registration.
    C.   licensure.
    D.   registration.
    E.   extended practice.

5. Answer all questions.

Even if you do not know the right answer, do not leave a question blank. A blank question is always wrong, whereas a guess might be correct. If you can eliminate some of the answers as wrong, do so. It will increase the chances of a correct guess.

A multiple-choice question with five answers gives a 20 percent chance of a correct guess. If you can eliminate one or more incorrect answers, you increase your odds of a correct guess to 25 percent, 33 percent, and so on. An unanswered question has a 0 percent chance of being correct.

Just before turning in your answer sheet, check to be sure that you have not left any items blank.

Example:
When a paramedic is called by the patient (through the dispatcher) to the scene of a medical emergency, the medical direction physician has established a physician/patient relationship.

    A.   True
    B.   False

A true/false question gives you a 50 percent chance of a correct guess.

The hospital health professional(s) responsible for sorting patients as they arrive at the emergency department is/are usually the

    A.   emergency physician.
    B.   ward clerk.
    C.   emergency nurse.
    D.   trauma surgeon.
    E.   both A and C (correct)

Paramedic Care
Principles & Practice
Paramedicine Fundamentals

Workbook

Fourth Edition

Chapter

1

Pathophysiology

Because Chapter 1 is lengthy, it has been divided into parts to aid your study. Read the assigned text-book pages; then, progress through the objectives and self-evaluation materials as you would with other chapters. When you feel secure in your grasp of the content, proceed to the next section.

Review of Chapter Objectives

After reading this chapter, you should be able to:

1. **Define key terms introduced in this chapter.**

   Knowing and being able to apply the key terms in each chapter is critical to understanding chapter concepts. Write the list of key terms. Then write the definition of each one in your own words. Check your understanding by confirming the definitions in the text glossary. Correct any misunderstandings. Create a study aid by writing each key term on the front of an index card and the definition on the back. Use the cards to quiz yourself or to have someone quiz you.

2. **Describe the relationship between homeostasis and health.**   **p. 6**

   The human body normally maintains its internal environment in a steady state of balance that is termed homeostasis. A significant disruption in homeostasis often leads to disease. Disease is an abnormal structural or functional change within the body.

Part 1: Disease, p. 7

Review of Chapter Objectives

After reading this part of the chapter, you should be able to:

3. **Explain how the predisposing factors of age, gender, genetics, lifestyle, and environment impact the development of disease.**   **pp. 7–8**

   Age. Humans at both ends of the age spectrum are especially vulnerable to disease. Infants are vulnerable because their immune systems are immature and they have not developed the necessary defenses. As we age, there is a decline in immune function that places us at increased risk for disease in our later years. This is due to a general decline in homeostatic function.

   Gender. Gender also plays a role in disease development. Often, these differences in disease development are due to the effects of the sex hormones.

Genetics. A major factor in the development of disease is genetics. Certain diseases are more common in certain families. Because our ethnicity and race are also genetically encoded, certain diseases are common in certain races.

Lifestyle. Another major factor in the development of disease is lifestyle. Today, foods are processed, removing many of the healthful ingredients that protected our ancestors from some of the diseases that are common today. In addition, the modern population obtains considerably less exercise than earlier generations because of the availability of cars and other forms of mechanized transportation and the fact that many farm and industry jobs that demanded intense physical labor have been replaced by more sedentary occupations. When you combine a lack of exercise with a diet that is devoid of quality calories (but rather is high in fats and carbohydrates), you end up with obesity. Obesity is one of the biggest health problems in the United States and is quickly becoming as great a problem in other developed countries such as the United Kingdom, Australia, and Canada.

Environment. We now know that numerous environmental factors are associated with the development of disease. For example, exposure to asbestos has been directly linked to the development of an uncommon lung cancer called mesothelioma. Pollutants have been linked to the development of significant birth defects (such as anencephaly) in babies born to Mexican mothers in the lower Rio Grande River valley in south Texas, presumably caused by chemicals dumped into the river upstream. In the Ukraine, the incidence of cancers, specifically thyroid cancer, has increased dramatically following the nuclear disaster in 1986 at Chernobyl. Cumulative exposure to toxic substances also plays a role in disease development.

4. **Explain the basis of infectious, immunologic, inflammatory, ischemic, metabolic, nutritional, genetic, congenital, neoplastic, traumatic, physical, iatrogenic, and idiopathic classifications of diseases.**   pp. 9–11

Infectious. Infectious diseases are those that result from invasion of the body and colonization by a pathogenic organism.

Immunologic. Overreactions of the immune system, commonly called allergies or hypersensitivity, can cause diseases such as anaphylaxis.

Inflammatory. Inflammatory diseases are those that result from the body's response to another disease process (primary disease).

Ischemic. Many diseases are due to diminished blood supply. Thus, the affected tissues may be deprived of oxygen and essential energy substrates, which can lead to cell death.

Metabolic. Metabolic diseases result when there is a disturbance in the biochemical and metabolic processes within the body.

Nutritional. Nutritional diseases primarily result from a deficiency in one or all of the major nutritional sources (carbohydrates, proteins, fats). Vitamin deficiencies can also lead to nutritional diseases, because vitamins are required for normal metabolic processes.

Genetic. Genetic diseases are those that are coded for in a person's genetic material and thus are passed from parent to child.

Congenital. Certain diseases can result from problems that occur during fetal development. Most fetal development occurs during the first trimester of life. It is during this period that the fetus is most susceptible to external factors that can adversely affect development (teratogens).

Neoplastic. On occasion, certain cells will begin abnormal or uncontrolled cell growth. This process is referred to as neoplasia. The result is a tumor, or neoplasm. A neoplasm can be benign (not cancerous, not able to spread to other tissues) or malignant (cancerous, able to spread), depending on the changes present in the cell line.

Trauma. External physical forces can mechanically change or disrupt the structure of the body and, as a result, affect body function. These external forces are referred to as trauma.

Physical agents. Myriad physical agents can adversely affect body structure and function. These include chemicals, poisons, ionizing radiation, extremes in temperature, changes in atmospheric pressure, and electrical shock.

Iatrogenic. Medical treatments for a disease can sometimes result in the development of other diseases or problems. A disease that occurs in this way is referred to as an iatrogenic disease.

Idiopathic. In many instances the specific cause of a disease is unknown. In this case, the disease is classified as idiopathic. Sometimes, a cause may be identified later. However, in many cases a specific cause is never found.

Case Study Review

Reread the case study on pages 5–6 in Paramedic Care: Paramedicine Fundamentals; *then, read the following discussion.*

This case study demonstrates the important link between understanding the disease process (pathophysiology) and the assessment and care of the patient.

Dispatch information gives Armando and his partner Sam a starting point for their patient interaction. While recognizing a particular address or patient gives responding personnel an insight into what they may or may not encounter, the experienced paramedic will use this information combined with appropriate scene size-up and patient assessment to develop an appropriate management plan for the situation found.

Armando and Sam find Bill in a compromised state. They properly position the patient and assure he has a patent airway. The patient's presentation and known history lead Armando to suspect Bill is hypoglycemic. Sam looks for a vein; however, neither he nor his partner is able to find an appropriate site. Armando makes the decision to establish an intraosseous (IO) line as opposed to administering glucagon intramuscularly. The patient responds to the treatment and care is transferred to the hospital without incident.

After the call, Sam and Armando discuss the call. Armando uses this teaching opportunity to discuss the physiology of the liver and how it may be impacted by various conditions and diseases. This type of call review is a valuable tool in an EMS provider's professional development, and ultimately leads to improvement in the quality of care provided.

Content Self-Evaluation

MULTIPLE CHOICE

_____ 1. The human body normally maintains its internal environment in a steady state of balance that is termed
    A. pathology.
    B. pathophysiology.
    C. disease.
    D. homeostatsis.
    E. sequelae.

_____ 2. Which of the following predisposing factors to disease can you change?
    A. Age
    B. Gender
    C. Genetics
    D. Lifestyle
    E. Family history

_____ 3. A defined sequence of events that leads to development of a disease is called
    A. idiopathic.
    B. pathogenesis.
    C. pathology.
    D. etiology.
    E. clinical presentation.

_____ 4. A sign is what the patient tells you about the disease—a subjective complaint.
    A. True
    B. False

_____ 5. An objective finding that you can identify through physical examination is referred to as a symptom.
   A. True
   B. False

_____ 6. Some diseases have a sudden onset and are referred to as
   A. acute.
   B. chronic.
   C. predisposing.
   D. insidious.
   E. metabolite.

_____ 7. Diseases that result from invasion of the body and colonization by a pathogenic organism are classified as
   A. congenital.
   B. metabolic.
   C. ischemic.
   D. pathogenic.
   E. infectious.

_____ 8. Sometimes the immune system fails to recognize certain tissues as belonging to the host and mounts an immune response as if the tissues were foreign. This phenomenon is called
   A. immunologic disease.
   B. autoimmune disease.
   C. inflammatory disease.
   D. ischemic disease.
   E. congenital disease.

_____ 9. Diseases that result from the body's response to another disease process are classified as
   A. infectious.
   B. ischemic.
   C. inflammatory.
   D. ischemic.
   E. metabolic.

_____ 10. Diseases due to diminished blood supply are classified as
   A. congenital.
   B. iatrogenic.
   C. immunologic.
   D. neoplastic.
   E. ischemic.

_____ 11. Diseases that result when there is a disturbance in the biochemical processes within the body are classified as
   A. metabolic.
   B. inflammatory.
   C. trauma.
   D. iatrogenic.
   E. neoplastic.

_____ 12. Diseases that primarily result from a deficiency in carbohydrates, proteins, fats, or vitamin are classified as
   A. metabolic.
   B. congenital.
   C. neoplastic.
   D. iatrogenic.
   E. nutritional.

_____ 13. Diseases that are coded for in a person's DNA material and thus are passed from parent to child are classified as
   A. idiopathic.
   B. congenital.
   C. genetic.
   D. ischemic.
   E. iatrogenic.

_____ 14. Diseases that can result from problems that occur during fetal development are classified as
   A. idiopathic.
   B. congenital.
   C. genetic.
   D. ischemic.
   E. iatrogenic.

_____ 15. Diseases that result from the abnormal or uncontrolled growth of cells are classified as
   A. iatrogenic.
   B. ischemic.
   C. inflammatory.
   D. neoplastic.
   E. congenital.

©2013 Pearson Education, Inc.
Paramedic Care: Principles & Practice, Vol. 2, 4th Ed.

Special Project

MATCHING

Match the classifications of disease with the appropriate example.

A. infectious

B. immunologic

C. inflammatory

D. ischemic

E. metabolic

F. nutritional

G. genetic

H. congenital

I. neoplastic

J. trauma

K. physical agents

L. iatrogenic

_____ 1. Transitional-cell bladder cancer, caused by exposure to chemicals such as ink, and ultraviolet keratitis (welder's flash) that results from looking at a welding arc that is producing ultraviolet radiation.

_____ 2. Hemophilia, Huntington's disease, and color blindness.

_____ 3. Acute coronary syndrome (ACS), ischemic stroke, and ischemic bowel disease.

_____ 4. Diseases that result from vitamin deficiency, such as scurvy and rickets.

_____ 5. A subclavian central intravenous line is placed into a patient. During the line insertion, the dome of the lung is inadvertently punctured, resulting in a pneumothorax.

_____ 6. Cleft lip and palate and Down syndrome.

_____ 7. Fibroid tumors in the uterus, more accurately called uterine leiomyomas, and breast cancer.

_____ 8. Diabetes mellitus, which results from decreased insulin secretion from the endocrine pancreas.

_____ 9. Gonorrhea or chlamydia.

_____ 10. Colonization of prions, viruses, bacteria, and fungi.

_____ 11. Allergies and anaphylaxis.

_____ 12. Blunt injury to a kidney that fractures the kidney into multiple portions.

_____ 13. Tapeworms and liver flukes.

_____ 14. Thyrotoxicosis that results from abnormally elevated levels of thyroid hormones that can markedly increase the basal metabolic rate.

_____ 15. Acquired immune deficiency syndrome (AIDS).

Review of Chapter Objectives

After reading this part of the chapter, you should be able to:

5. Describe the basic chemical structures that make up the body. p. 12

The fundamental chemical unit is the atom. Within the atom are particles, referred to as subatomic particles, which include electrons, protons, and neutrons. Protons and neutrons exist within the nucleus of the atom. Electrons are considerably smaller particles and orbit the nucleus. Protons have a positive electrical charge, neutrons (n) are electrically neutral, and electrons have a negative electrical charge. Opposite charges attract and like charges repel. When the number of protons and the number of electrons are the same, the atomic charge is electrically neutral.

An element is a substance that cannot be separated into simpler substances. The number of protons in the nucleus of an atom (the atomic number) defines the element.

6. Differentiate between covalent, ionic, and hydrogen bonds. pp. 13−15

The equal sharing of electrons results in what is called a covalent bond that tends to hold the atoms together. A substance made up of atoms held together by one or more covalent bonds is referred to as a molecule. Covalent bonds are the strongest of the three types of chemical bonds.

When an atom or molecule gains one or more electrons, there are then more electrons than protons and the atom or molecule has a net negative charge. An atom or molecule with missing electrons and thus a net positive charge is called a cation. An atom or molecule with extra electrons and a net negative charge is called an anion. Because opposite charges attract, bonds form between atoms of opposite (positive/negative) charges. This kind of bond is referred to as an ionic bond.

The equal sharing of electrons forms a covalent bond. However, in selected cases, the sharing of electrons between two atoms is unequal. Thus, different parts of the same molecule can have an unequal charge. An unequal covalent bond is called a polar bond, and the molecule is referred to as a polar molecule. In water (H_2O), two hydrogen (H) atoms share their electrons with a single oxygen (O) molecule. But the electrons spend more time orbiting the oxygen atom compared to the hydrogen atoms. Thus, the oxygen atom has a slightly negative charge and each hydrogen ion has a slight positive charge, thus making the entire water molecule polar. In nature, the hydrogen ions of a water molecule, because they have a slight positive charge, are attracted to the oxygen atom of other water molecules (because they have a slight negative charge). This attraction between a slightly positively charged hydrogen atom and a slightly negatively charged oxygen atom is referred to as a hydrogen bond. Hydrogen bonds are much weaker than either covalent bonds or ionic bonds. Collectively they are important in that they give water its special physical properties.

7. Recognize the six major chemical elements and four major chemical compounds that make up the human body. p. 15

Six elements (carbon, hydrogen, nitrogen, oxygen, phosphorus, and sulfur) make up approximately 98 percent of the body weight of most living organisms. Of these, the four major elements of living systems are carbon (C), hydrogen (H), oxygen (O), and nitrogen (N).

A compound is the chemical union of two or more elements. The four major compounds of living systems are carbohydrates, proteins, nucleic acids, and lipids. Molecules of these compounds are composed mostly of atoms from the four major elements, plus some additional elements, such as phosphorus (P), sulfur (S), iron (Fe), magnesium (Mg), sodium (Na), chlorine (Cl), potassium (K), iodine (I), and calcium (Ca).

8. Describe the nature and roles of carbohydrates, proteins, nucleic acids, lipids, and water in the body. pp. 16–24

Carbohydrates are compounds that contain the elements carbon (C), hydrogen (H), and oxygen (O). Typically, the hydrogen and oxygen atoms occur in a 2:1 ratio. Carbohydrates provide the majority of calories in most diets. They are typically divided into the sugars and the polysaccharides.

Proteins, which are nitrogen-based complex compounds, are the basic building blocks of cells. Proteins are essential for the growth and repair of living tissues. They are the most abundant class of biological chemicals in the body. Proteins consist of smaller building blocks called amino acids.

There are two classes of molecules known as nucleic acids: deoxyribonucleic acid (DNA) and ribonucleic acid (RNA). Deoxyribonucleic acid (DNA) is the nucleic acid that contains the genetic instructions for life. Ribonucleic acid (RNA), a chemical that is similar to DNA, plays a major role in protein synthesis, serving as a template for protein synthesis.

Lipids are chemicals that do not dissolve in water. Lipids are nonpolar, while water is polar. Thus, water is not attracted to lipids, and lipids are not attracted to water. In the human, lipids function in the long-term storage of biochemical energy, insulation, structure, and control. The lipids that pertain to human pathophysiology are triglycerides, phospholipids, and steroids.

Water has been called the "universal solvent." It is abundant in the body and plays a significant role in numerous biological processes. The physical properties of water are essential for life as we know it. Water also plays a major role in the transport of substances throughout the body and plays a significant role in maintaining a constant body temperature.

9. Explain acid-base production, imbalances, and homeostasis in the body. pp. 24–30

A dissociation reaction is any reaction in which a compound or a molecule breaks apart into separate components. Substances that give up protons during chemical reactions are called acids. Likewise, substances that acquire protons during a chemical reaction are called bases. Any chemical reaction that results in the transfer of protons is referred to as an acid-base reaction.

Any significant deviation of pH outside the normal operating parameters (7.35–7.45) can be classified as an acid-base disorder. The two major body systems involved in acid-base balance are the respiratory system and the renal system. There are two classes of acid-base disorders: respiratory acid-base disorders and metabolic acid-base disorders while alkalosis is an excess of base in the body.

Respiratory acidosis occurs when the respiratory system cannot effectively eliminate all the carbon dioxide generated through metabolic activities in the peripheral tissues. Respiratory alkalosis occurs when the respiratory system eliminates too much carbon dioxide through hyperventilation resulting in hypocapnia.

Metabolic acidosis is a deficiency of bicarbonate in the body. It usually results from an increase in metabolic acids—primarily through anaerobic metabolism. Metabolic alkalosis is relatively uncommon and is due to an increase in HCO_3 levels or a decrease in circulating acids. Metabolic alkalosis results from an abnormal loss of hydrogen ions (H^+), an increase in HCO_3 levels, or a decrease in extracellular fluid levels.

Acid-base balance must be tightly controlled. While the buffer systems are effective in binding acids and rendering them harmless, these acids must then be removed from the body. Thus, excess hydrogen ions must be bound to water molecules and removed through the exhalation of carbon dioxide from the lungs or be removed from the body via secretion by the kidneys.

The maintenance of body pH is a constant balance between gains and losses of hydrogen ion that is achieved through the use of the buffer system, the respiratory system, and the kidneys. These systems secrete or absorb hydrogen ions, control the excretion of acids and bases, or create additional buffers when needed.

Content Self-Evaluation

MULTIPLE CHOICE

_____ **1.** The fundamental chemical unit is the
  A. proton.
  B. atom.
  C. neutron.
  D. electron.
  E. element.

_____ 2. Bonds in which atoms share electrons equally are called
   A. hydrogen bonds.
   B. balanced bonds.
   C. ionic bonds.
   D. organic bonds.
   E. covalent bonds.

_____ 3. Bonds formed between atoms of opposite charges are called
   A. hydrogen bonds.
   B. balanced bonds.
   C. ionic bonds.
   D. organic bonds.
   E. covalent bonds.

_____ 4. The attraction between a slightly positively charged hydrogen atom and a slightly negatively charged oxygen atom is referred to as a(n)
   A. hydrogen bond.
   B. balanced bond.
   C. ionic bond.
   D. organic bond.
   E. covalent bond.

_____ 5. Chemicals that contain the element carbon are called organic.
   A. True
   B. False

_____ 6. Sugars include all of the following EXCEPT
   A. lactose.
   B. galactose.
   C. glucose.
   D. amulose.
   E. sucrose.

_____ 7. _____ are essential for the growth and repair of living tissues.
   A. Monosaccharides
   B. Starches
   C. Proteins
   D. Polysaccharides
   E. Disaccharides

_____ 8. Substances that speed up chemical reactions are called
   A. amino acids.
   B. enzymes.
   C. amylopectin.
   D. polymers.
   E. peptides.

_____ 9. Ribonucleic acid (RNA) is the nucleic acid that contains the genetic instructions for life.
   A. True
   B. False

_____ 10. The principal source of energy for most of the energy-utilizing activities of the cells is/are
   A. ribonucleic acid (RNA).
   B. steroids.
   C. deoxyribonucleic acid (DNA).
   D. nucleotides.
   E. adenosine triphosphate (ATP).

_____ 11. _____ function in the long-term storage of biochemical energy, insulation, structure, and control.
   A. Proteins
   B. Amino acids
   C. Lipids
   D. Nucleic acids
   E. Carbohydrates

_____ 12. Substances that give up protons during chemical reactions are called
   A. acids.
   B. bases.
   C. amino acids.
   D. steroids.
   E. ions.

_____ 13. Substances that acquire protons during chemical reactions are called
   A. acids.
   B. bases.
   C. amino acids.
   D. steroids.
   E. ions.

©2013 Pearson Education, Inc.
Paramedic Care: Principles & Practice, Vol. 2, 4th Ed.

14. The most important buffer system in the extracellular fluid is the
   A. protein buffer system.
   B. hydrogen buffer system.
   C. carbonic acid-bicarbonate buffer system.
   D. hemoglobin buffer system.
   E. phosphate buffer system.

15. All of the following are acid-base disorders EXCEPT
   A. respiratory acidosis.
   B. metabolic acidosis.
   C. hydrogen acidosis.
   D. respiratory alkalosis.
   E. metabolic alkalosis.

Special Project

MATCHING

Match the type of acid-base disorder with the characteristic of its presentation.

A. respiratory acidosis

B. respiratory alkalosis

C. metabolic acidosis

D. metabolic alkalosis

_____ **1.** Hypocapnia

_____ **2.** Hypoventilation

_____ **3.** Increased bicarbonate levels

_____ **4.** Anaerobic metabolism

_____ **5.** Hyperventilation

_____ **6.** Decreased bicarbonate levels

_____ **7.** Hypercapnia

_____ **8.** Decrease in circulating acids

Part 3: Disease at the Cellular Level, p. 30

Review of Chapter Objectives

After reading this part of the chapter, you should be able to:

10. Explain the basic structure and function of a typical human cell and each of its components, including the following:

a. plasma membrane   pp. 31−33

Cells are surrounded by a plasma membrane. This membrane consists of several chemicals, of which the phospholipids are among the more important.

The plasma membrane has several functions in addition to the obvious function of separating the extracellular from the intracellular environment. First, the plasma membrane plays a major role in the ability of cells to adhere to each other, or stick together. The plasma membrane helps with cell-cell recognition, the ability of a cell to distinguish one type of cell from another. The plasma membrane maintains the structural integrity of the cell. The plasma membrane also plays a major role in communications between cells. Finally, the cell membrane regulates the movement of substances into and out of the cell.

b. cytoplasm p. 31

Cytoplasm is the thick material surrounding the nucleus that fills the cell.

c. nucleus p. 47

The nucleus is among the largest organelles and contains all of the cell's genetic information. Genetic information is encoded by base sequences on the DNA molecule.

DNA controls cell functions and the production of specific proteins.

d. ribosomes p. 47

Ribosomes are spherical structures that can account for up to 25 percent of the dry weight of a cell. The primary role of the ribosomes is the synthesis of polypeptides and proteins.

e. endoplasmic reticulum pp. 47–48

The endoplasmic reticulum is a network of tubules, vesicles, and sacs that interconnect with the plasma membrane, nuclear envelope, and many of the other organelles in the cell. Certain parts of the endoplasmic reticulum contain ribosomes during protein synthesis and are referred to as rough endoplasmic reticulum (RER). The RER sends the proteins to the Golgi apparatus in vesicles called cisternae or, if they are membrane proteins, insert them into the plasma membrane. The portion of the endoplasmic reticulum without ribosomes is called smooth endoplasmic reticulum (SER). SER has multiple functions, depending on the cell type. The vast network of SER provides an increased surface area for the action or storage of key enzymes and the products of these enzymes. The endoplasmic reticulum also plays a major role in replenishment and maintenance of the plasma membrane. The protein components of the plasma membrane come from the RER, while the lipid components come from the SER.

f. Golgi apparatus p. 48

The Golgi apparatus, also called the Golgi complex, is an important organelle whose function is to process proteins for the cell membrane and other cell organelles.

The Golgi apparatus serves as a sort of "post office" for the cell, as it is essentially a protein-processing and packaging center. The transport vesicles (cisternae) from the endoplasmic reticulum fuse with the face of the Golgi apparatus and empty their protein content into the lumen of the Golgi apparatus. The proteins are then transported to the opposite side of the Golgi apparatus and are modified along the way. They are labeled with a sequence of molecules according to their final destination.

g. lysosomes pp. 48–50

Lysosomes are spherical in shape and surrounded by a single membrane. Lysosomes serve as the "garbage disposal system" of the cells. That is, they degrade and remove products of ingestion (the process called phagocytosis) and worn out parts from the cell. They also play a role in converting complex nutritional molecules to simple nutritional molecules. Lysosomes also process the macro-molecule products needed for cell energy production.

h. vacuoles p. 50

Vacuoles are membrane-bound organelles used for temporary storage or transport of substances such as food sources. The lysosome can fuse with the vacuole membrane and place digestive enzymes into the food vacuole to break down the food source within.

i. peroxisomes p. 50

Peroxisomes are similar to lysosomes in size and the lack of obvious internal structure. Peroxisomes have the ability to generate and degrade hydrogen peroxide (H_2O_2). Hydrogen peroxide is highly toxic to cells. However, it can be degraded to water and oxygen by the enzyme catalase. Peroxisomes are found in virtually all cell types but are more prevalent in the liver and kidneys. They play an important role in detoxifying harmful substances such as alcohols and formaldehyde. Peroxisomes are also important in the breakdown of fatty acids. Because they can produce oxygen, peroxisomes play a role in the regulation of oxygen tension within the cell.

j. mitochondria p. 50

Mitochondria, like the nucleus, are surrounded by a double membrane forming two separate compartments. The inner membrane folds form shelves within the mitochondria, referred to as cristae, where the last phases of cellular respiration occur. The mitochondria also can contain some ribosomes and some of the cell's genetic material. The mitochondria are the "powerhouses" of the cells in that they provide the energy needed for all of a cell's biochemical processes. Cellular

©2013 Pearson Education, Inc.
Paramedic Care: Principles & Practice, Vol. 2, 4th Ed.

respiration, which is the conversion of food to energy, primarily occurs in the mitochondria. The number of mitochondria present varies from cell to cell, depending on the specialized function of the cell.

k. cytoskeleton pp. 50–51

Within eukaryotic cells is a complex system of filaments, microtubules, and intermediate filaments referred to as the cytoskeleton. Microfilaments are made from the protein actin. Microtubules are long, hollow rods made of the protein tubulin. Intermediate filaments are made up of different proteins, depending on the cell type.

The cytoskeleton forms a dynamic three-dimensional structure that fills the cytoplasm and serves as a skeleton for cell stability and as a muscle for cell movement. In addition to stability, the cytoskeleton plays an important role in both intracellular transport and cellular division.

11. Explain the movement of water and solutes into and out of cells under various intracellular and extracellular conditions, including osmosis, diffusion, facilitated diffusion, active transport, endocytosis, and exocytosis. pp. 33–37

Osmosis is a specific type of diffusion. It is the movement of water molecules from an area of high water concentration to an area of low water concentration. Semipermeable membranes, such as the cell membrane, allow the unrestricted movement of water across the membrane, at the same time restricting the movement of solute molecules and ions.

Substances will move across a membrane from an area of higher concentration on one side to an area of lower concentration on the other side until the concentration of the substance is equal in both areas (a state of equilibrium). Even after the concentrations reach equilibrium, because of random movement, the substance continues to move back and forth across the membrane. However, the net rate of movement in each direction now remains the same. This process of passive movement across a membrane is called simple diffusion.

Water-soluble molecules and ionized molecules cannot move through the plasma membrane by simple diffusion. Because of this, their transport must be assisted, or "facilitated," by integral proteins in the plasma membrane through a process called facilitated diffusion. Facilitated diffusion, like simple diffusion, does not require an expenditure of metabolic energy.

Sometimes it is necessary for a cell to move a solute across the plasma membrane against the concentration gradient. As with facilitated diffusion, this process, called active transport, uses a carrier protein but also uses energy in the form of ATP. Thus, with active transport substances are moved from areas of lower solute concentration to higher solute concentration.

Substances can also enter the cell through a process called endocytosis. With endocytosis, large molecules, single-cell organisms (bacteria), and fluid containing dissolved substances can enter the cell. During endocytosis, a section of the plasma membrane encircles the substance to be ingested. Once the substance is completely encircled, the membrane portion is pinched off from the cell membrane, resulting in a sac-like structure called a vesicle. When separated from the cell membrane, the vesicle is released into the cell. Endocytosis is often divided into two categories: phagocytosis, whereby the cell engulfs large particles or bacteria; and pinocytosis, whereby the cell engulfs droplets of fluid carrying dissolved substances.

It is sometimes necessary for large molecules to leave the cells. As with endocytosis, large molecules can leave the cell by becoming encircled in a membrane vesicle. This process, called exocytosis, occurs in a fashion opposite to that of endocytosis. The membrane bound vesicle containing the substance to be released from the cell approaches the cell membrane. There it fuses with the cell membrane, and its contents are released outside the cell.

12. Describe the fluid and electrolyte composition of the cellular environment. pp. 37–41

Water is the most abundant substance in the human body. In fact, water accounts for approximately 60 percent of total body weight (the average for all ages). The total amount of water in the body at any given time is referred to as the total body water (TBW). Water is distributed among various compartments of the body. The largest compartment is the intracellular compartment. This compartment contains the intracellular fluid (ICF), which is all the fluid found inside body cells. Approximately

70 percent of all body water is found within this compartment. The extracellular compartment contains the remaining 30 percent of all body water. It contains the extracellular fluid (ECF), all the fluid found outside the body cells. There are two divisions within the extracellular compartment. The first contains the intravascular fluid (fluid found outside cells and within the circulatory system). It is essentially the same as the blood plasma and accounts for about 5 percent of body water. The remaining compartment contains the interstitial fluid (fluid found outside the cell membranes, yet not within the circulatory system), making up about 25 percent of body water.

Sodium (Na^+). Sodium is the most prevalent cation in the extracellular fluid. It plays a major role in regulating the distribution of water because water is attracted to and moves with sodium.

Potassium (K^+). Potassium is the most prevalent cation in the intracellular fluid. It is also important in the transmission of electrical impulses

Calcium (Ca^{++}). Calcium has many physiologic functions. It plays a major role in muscle contraction as well as nervous impulse transmission.

Magnesium (Mg^{++}). Magnesium is necessary for several biochemical processes that occur in the body and is closely associated with phosphate in many processes.

Chloride (Cl^-). Chloride is an important anion. Its negative charge balances the positive charge associated with the cations. It also plays a major role in fluid balance and renal function. Chloride has a close association with sodium.

Bicarbonate. Bicarbonate is the principal buffer of the body. This means that it neutralizes the highly acidic hydrogen ion (H^+) and other organic acids.

Phosphate. Phosphate is important in body energy stores. It is closely associated with magnesium in renal function. It also acts as a buffer, primarily in the intracellular space, in much the same manner as bicarbonate.

13. **Explain fluid and electrolyte homeostasis and the effects of fluid and electrolyte imbalances.** pp. 41–42

When solutions on opposite sides of a semipermeable membrane are equal in concentration, the relationship is said to be isotonic. When the concentration of a given solute (dissolved substance) is greater on one side of the membrane than on the other, it is said to be hypertonic. When the concentration is less on one side of the cell membrane, as compared to the other, it is referred to as hypotonic. This difference in concentration is known as the osmotic gradient.

The natural tendency of the body is to keep the balance of electrolytes and water equal on both sides of the cell membrane. This is an example of homeostasis, the body's normal tendency to maintain its internal environment in a steady state of balance. If one side of a cell membrane has an increased quantity of a given electrolyte (is hypertonic), there will be a shift of the electrolyte from that side and a shift of water from the other side to restore a balance in concentration.

14. **Explain the movement of water between fluid compartments in the body.** pp. 42–43

The mechanisms by which water and solutes move across cell membranes ensure that the osmolality of body water (the concentration of particles within the water) inside and outside the cells is normally in equilibrium. Sodium, the most abundant ion in the extracellular fluid, is responsible for the osmotic balance of the extracellular space. Potassium plays the same role in the intracellular space.

Within the extracellular compartment, movement of water between the plasma in the intravascular space and the interstitial space is primarily a function of forces at play in the capillary beds. Osmotic pressure is the pressure exerted by the concentration of solutes on one side of a semipermeable membrane, such as a cell membrane or the thin wall of a capillary. Osmotic pressure can be thought of as a "pull" rather than a "push," because a hypertonic concentration of solutes tends to pull water from the other side of the membrane until the osmotic pressure on both sides is equal.

Another force inside the capillaries is hydrostatic pressure, which is the blood pressure, or force against the vessel walls, created by contractions of the heart. Hydrostatic pressure does tend to force some water out of the plasma and across the capillary wall into the interstitial space, a process that is

©2013 Pearson Education, Inc.
Paramedic Care: Principles & Practice, Vol. 2, 4th Ed.

called filtration. Hydrostatic pressure (a force that favors filtration, pushing water out of the capillary) and oncotic force (a force opposing filtration, pulling water into the capillary) together are responsible for net filtration, which is described as the difference between the forces favoring filtration and the forces opposing filtration (Starling's hypothesis).

Edema is the accumulation of water in the interstitial space. It occurs when there is a disruption in the forces and mechanisms that normally keep net filtration at zero or a disruption in the forces that would normally remove water from the interstitial space.

15. Describe the composition and function of blood, including both plasma and formed elements. p. 44

Plasma is made up of approximately 92 percent water, 6 to 7 percent proteins, and a small portion consisting of electrolytes, lipids, enzymes, clotting factors, glucose, and other dissolved substances.

Erythrocytes contain hemoglobin and are responsible for transporting oxygen to the body's peripheral cells. The leukocytes are responsible for immunity and fighting infection. The thrombocytes play a major role in blood clotting.

16. Predict the physiologic effects of infusing various types of intravenous fluids. pp. 45–46

A colloid solution contains proteins, or other high-molecular-weight molecules, that tend to remain in the intravascular space for an extended period of time. In addition, colloids have oncotic force (colloid osmotic pressure), which means they tend to attract water into the intravascular space from the interstitial space and the intracellular space. Thus, a small amount of a colloid can be administered to a patient with a greater-than-expected increase in intravascular volume. Colloids include: plasma protein fraction (Plasmanate), salt-poor albumin, dextran, and hetastarch (Hespan).

Crystalloids are the primary compounds used in prehospital intravenous fluid therapy. Isotonic solutions have electrolyte composition similar to the blood plasma. When placed into a normally hydrated patient, they will not cause a significant fluid or electrolyte shift. Examples include normal saline and lactated Ringer's. Hypertonic solutions have a higher solute concentration than the cells. These fluids will tend to cause a fluid shift out of the interstitial space and intracellular compartment into the intravascular space when administered to a normally hydrated patient. Later, there will be a diffusion of solute in the opposite direction. An example is 7.5 sodium chloride solution. Hypotonic solutions have a lower solute concentration than the cells. When administered to a normally hydrated patient, they will cause a movement of fluid from the intravascular space into the interstitial space and intracellular compartment. Later, solutes will move in an opposite direction. An example is 5 percent dextrose in water (D_5W).

17. **Explain the processes of cellular respiration and energy production to include:**

    a. **glycolysis**

pp. 52–53

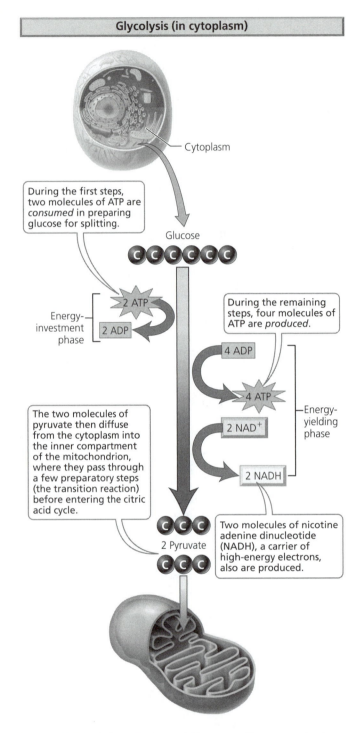

Goodenough, Judith and Betty A. McGuire, *Biology of Humans: Concepts, Applications, and Issues, 3rd Edition,* © 2010. Reprinted and electronically reproduced by permission of Pearson Education, Inc., Upper Saddle River, NJ.

Transition Reaction (in mitochondrion)

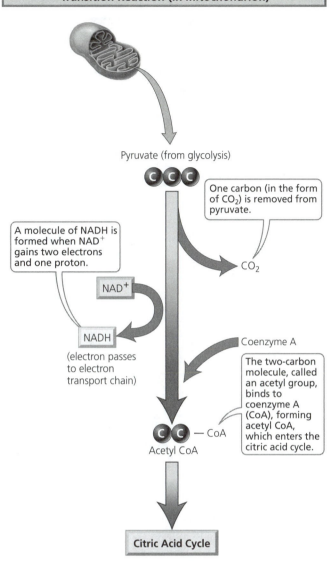

Pyruvate (from glycolysis)

One carbon (in the form of CO_2) is removed from pyruvate.

A molecule of NADH is formed when NAD^+ gains two electrons and one proton.

NAD^+

CO_2

NADH

(electron passes to electron transport chain)

Coenzyme A

The two-carbon molecule, called an acetyl group, binds to coenzyme A (CoA), forming acetyl CoA, which enters the citric acid cycle.

— CoA

Acetyl CoA

Citric Acid Cycle

Goodenough, Judith and Betty A. McGuire, *Biology of Humans: Concepts, Applications, and Issues, 3rd Edition,* © 2010. Reprinted and electronically reproduced by permission of Pearson Education, Inc., Upper Saddle River, NJ.

Citric Acid Cycle (in mitochondrion)

Acetyl CoA, the two-carbon compound formed during the transition reaction, enters the citric acid cycle.

The citric acid cycle also yields several molecules of FADH$_2$ and NADH, carriers of high-energy electrons that enter the electron transport chain.

Acetyl CoA

Oxaloacetate

NADH

NAD$^+$

Malate

FADH$_2$

FAD

Succinate

ATP   ADP + Pi

Citric Acid Cycle

CoA

Citrate

CO$_2$ leaves cycle

NAD$^+$

NADH

α-Ketoglutarate

CO$_2$ leaves cycle

NAD$^+$

NADH

The citric acid cycle yields one ATP from each acetyl CoA that enters the cycle, for a net gain of two ATP.

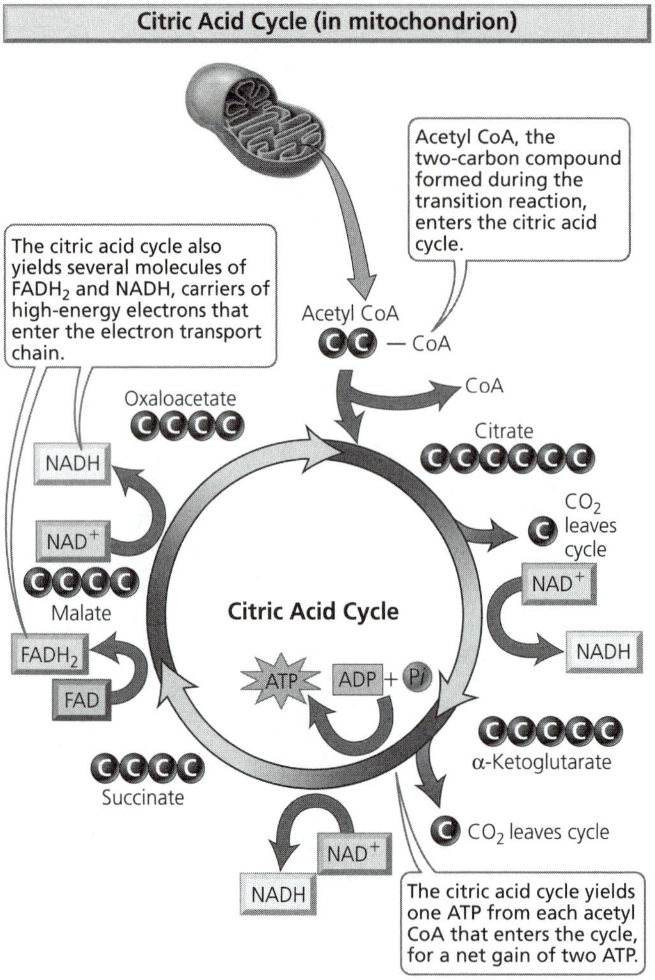

Goodenough, Judith and Betty A. McGuire, *Biology of Humans: Concepts, Applications, and Issues, 3rd Edition,* © 2010. Reprinted and electronically reproduced by permission of Pearson Education, Inc., Upper Saddle River, NJ.

©2013 Pearson Education, Inc.
Paramedic Care: Principles & Practice, Vol. 2, 4th Ed.

Electron Transport Chain (inner membrane of mitochondrion)

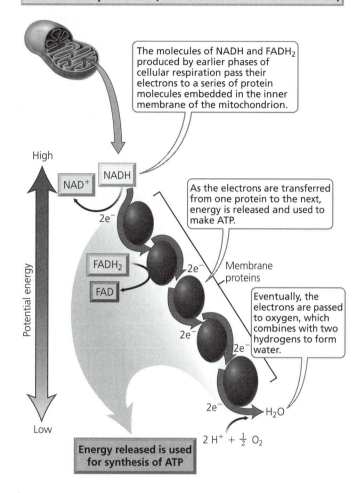

The molecules of NADH and FADH$_2$ produced by earlier phases of cellular respiration pass their electrons to a series of protein molecules embedded in the inner membrane of the mitochondrion.

High

NAD$^+$ NADH

As the electrons are transferred from one protein to the next, energy is released and used to make ATP.

2e$^-$

FADH$_2$ 2e$^-$ Membrane proteins

FAD

Eventually, the electrons are passed to oxygen, which combines with two hydrogens to form water.

2e$^-$

2e$^-$

Potential energy

2e$^-$ H$_2$O

Low $2\,H^+ + \frac{1}{2}\,O_2$

Energy released is used for synthesis of ATP

Goodenough, Judith and Betty A. McGuire, *Biology of Humans: Concepts, Applications, and Issues, 3rd Edition,* © 2010. Reprinted and electronically reproduced by permission of Pearson Education, Inc., Upper Saddle River, NJ.

d. fermentation

pp. 53–55

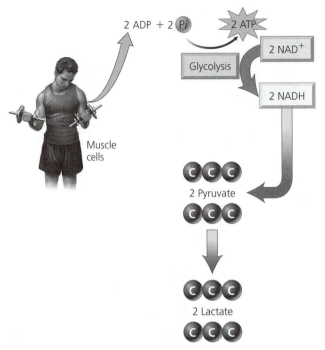

Goodenough, Judith and Betty A. McGuire, *Biology of Humans: Concepts, Applications, and Issues,*
3rd Edition, © 2010. Reprinted and electronically reproduced by permission of Pearson Education, Inc.,
Upper Saddle River, NJ.

18. Describe cellular responses to stress.   pp. 54–58

There are several possible cellular responses to an increase in stress. Some cellular responses can come in the form of normal growth (hyperplasia and hypertrophy), while others involve abnormal changes in size or function (atrophy and metaplasia).

An increase in the number of cells in a tissue or organ is termed hyperplasia. This usually results in the tissue or organ in question increasing in size.

An increase in the size of cells in a tissue or organ is referred to as hypertrophy. Hypertrophy is not due to the cell's swelling. Instead, it is due to the creation of more structural components within the cell.

A decrease in the size of a cell is termed atrophy. Atrophy can result from several factors, including a decreased workload, decreased blood supply, loss of nervous control, inadequate nutritional intake, lack of endocrine stimulation, and aging.

In certain situations, a cell can change from one adult cell type to another adult cell type. This process is called metaplasia and is reversible. Metaplasia is an adaptive response that serves to protect the organism from stress.

When cells are stressed to the point that they can no longer adapt, or when they are exposed to toxic agents, cell injury can result. If cell injury is persistent or severe, cell death may ultimately occur.

The most common type of cellular injury is that due to ischemia and hypoxia. Ischemia results from diminished blood flow, while hypoxia is due to decreased availability of oxygen.

Even when the blood supply and oxygen are restored to cells previously inadequately perfused, these cells still may die. Generally, cells that are reversibly injured may survive, while those that are irreversibly injured will not. However, some cells that are reversibly injured will die even after blood flow resumes—either by necrosis or by apoptosis.

Various chemicals, including drugs, can cause injury to a cell. This occurs through two mechanisms: direct action on cells or through the creation of chemical precursors that are converted to a cytotoxic metabolite.

Apoptosis occurs when a cellular program is activated that causes the release of enzymes that destroy the genetic material within the nucleus of the cell and selected proteins in the cytoplasm.

Abnormal or disordered growth in a cell is referred to as dysplasia. Dysplasia is more common in cells that reproduce rapidly, such as epithelial cells, and is often a precursor to the development of cancer.

Content Self-Evaluation

MULTIPLE CHOICE

_____ 1. The basic unit of all living organism is the
    A. atom.
    B. proton.
    C. electron.
    D. cell.
    E. neutron.

_____ 2. All of the following are functions of the plasma membrane EXCEPT
    A. cell adhesion.
    B. energy production.
    C. movement in and out of the cell.
    D. cell-cell recognition.
    E. cellular structural integrity.

_____ 3. The movement of substances across a membrane from an area of higher concentration on one side to an area of lower concentration on the other side until the concentration is equal is called
    A. osmosis.
    B. facilitated diffusion.
    C. endocytosis.
    D. active transport.
    E. simple diffusion.

_____ 4. The movement of water molecules from an area of high water concentration to an area of low water concentration is called
    A. osmosis.
    B. facilitated diffusion.
    C. endocytosis.
    D. active transport.
    E. simple diffusion.

_____ 5. What percentage of total body weight is made up of total body water?
    A. 30 percent
    B. 40 percent
    C. 50 percent
    D. 60 percent
    E. 70 percent

_____ 6. All of the following are frequent cations EXCEPT
    A. sodium.
    B. calcium.
    C. phosphate.
    D. magnesium.
    E. potassium.

_____ 7. The accumulation of water in the interstitial space is called edema.
    A. True
    B. False

_____ 8. White blood cells include all of the following EXCEPT
    A. eosinophils.
    B. monocytes.
    C. thrombocytes.
    D. lymphocytes.
    E. basophils.

_____ 9. All of the following are colloid solutions EXCEPT
    A. Plasmanate.
    B. lactated Ringer's.
    C. dextran.
    D. Hespan.
    E. salt-poor albumin.

_____ 10. _____ are the "powerhouses" of the cells in that they provide the energy needed for all of a cell's biochemical processes.
A. Golgi apparatus
B. Lysosomes
C. Peroxisomes
D. Ribosomes
E. Mitochondria

_____ 11. The series of reactions that yields two molecules of ATP and several molecules of NADH and FADH$_2$ and releases carbon dioxide as waste occurs during
A. glycolysis.
B. transition reaction.
C. the citric acid cycle.
D. electron transport.
E. fermentation.

_____ 12. An increase in the number of cells in a tissue or organ is termed
A. hypertrophy.
B. hyperplasia.
C. atrophy.
D. metaplasia.
E. atrophy.

_____ 13. If there is damage to the plasma membranes of the cell, enzymes released from the lysosomes will digest the contents of the cell, resulting in cellular
A. atrophy.
B. necrosis.
C. oxidation.
D. hypertrophy.
E. apoptosis.

_____ 14. Ischemia results from decreased availability of oxygen, while hypoxia is due to diminished blood flow.
A. True
B. False

_____ 15. Abnormal or disordered growth in a cell that is a precursor to the development of cancer is known as
A. metaplasia.
B. hyperplasia.
C. dysplasia.
D. atrophy.
E. hypertrophy.

©2013 Pearson Education, Inc.
Paramedic Care: Principles & Practice, Vol. 2, 4th Ed.

Special Project

Cell Structures

Label the structures in the following eukaryotic cell diagram.

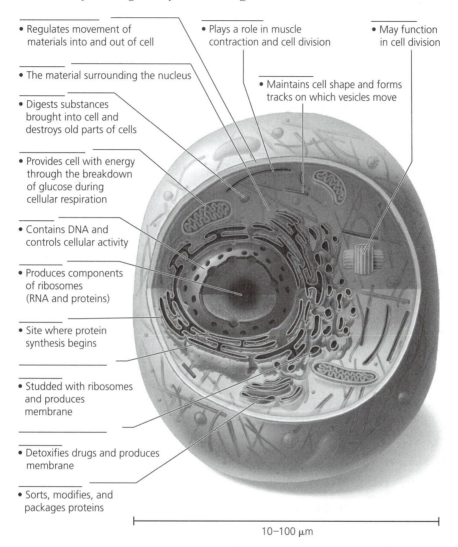

- _____ _____
  - Regulates movement of materials into and out of cell

- _____
  - The material surrounding the nucleus

- _____
  - Digests substances brought into cell and destroys old parts of cells

- _____
  - Provides cell with energy through the breakdown of glucose during cellular respiration

- _____
  - Contains DNA and controls cellular activity

- _____
  - Produces components of ribosomes (RNA and proteins)

- _____
  - Site where protein synthesis begins

- _____
  - Studded with ribosomes and produces membrane

- _____
  - Detoxifies drugs and produces membrane

- _____
  - Sorts, modifies, and packages proteins

- _____
  - Plays a role in muscle contraction and cell division

- _____
  - Maintains cell shape and forms tracks on which vesicles move

- _____
  - May function in cell division

10–100 μm

Part 4: Disease at the Tissue Level, p. 59

Review of Chapter Objectives

After reading this part of the chapter, you should be able to:

19. Describe the embryonic origins of body tissues.   **pp. 59–60**

All the tissues of the body are derived from three distinct cell lines seen during early embryonic development. About two weeks after conception, the cells of the embryo start to differentiate into three germ layers consisting of primitive cell types that differentiate into the various tissues and organs of the body.

The endoderm is the innermost germ cell layer and gives rise to epithelial tissue, most of which is glandular epithelium. Cells from the endoderm eventually form the entire epithelial lining of the digestive tract with the exception of a portion of the mouth and a portion of the rectum. In addition to the digestive tract, the endoderm gives rise to the epithelial cells that line all the exocrine glands including: the liver and associated ducts; pancreas; epithelium of the auditory tube and tympanic cavity; trachea, bronchi, and alveoli (except the nasal cavity); urinary bladder and part of the urethra; and lining of follicles in the thyroid and thymus glands.

The middle germ layer, or mesoderm, gives rise to numerous body tissues. These include: skeletal, cardiac, and smooth muscle; kidney tissue; fibrous tissue; bone and cartilage; fat (adipose) tissue; blood and lymph vessels; and blood cells.

The ectoderm is the outermost germ layer and gives rise to all the tissues that cover the body surfaces as well as the nervous system. There are three parts of the ectoderm, each resulting in different tissues. External ectoderm includes: skin (along with glands, hair, nails); epithelium of the mouth and nasal cavity; and lens and cornea of the eye. Neural crest includes: melanocytes (cells that produce melanin, or pigment); peripheral nervous system; adrenal medulla; meninges; facial cartilage; and dentin (in teeth). Neural tube includes: brain; spinal cord and motor neurons; retina; and posterior pituitary.

The germ layers ultimately differentiate into four primary tissue types: epithelial tissues, connective tissues, muscles tissues, and nervous tissues.

20. **Discuss the basic structure and function of epithelial, connective, muscle, and nervous tissues.**   pp. 60–69

Epithelial tissue. Epithelial tissues cover the body surfaces. In addition, they line all passageways that communicate with the outside. Distribution of the epithelial tissues includes the interior of body cavities, the lining of organs and blood vessels, the outer layers of skin, and others.

Connective tissue. Connective tissues provide a framework on which epithelial tissue rests and within which nerve tissue and muscle tissue are embedded. Blood vessels and nerves travel through connective tissue. Connective tissue not only functions as a mechanical support for other tissues but also provides an avenue for communication and transport among other tissues. Connective tissues play a major role in protecting the body through immunity and inflammation.

Muscle tissue. Muscle tissues are responsible for the movement of the organism and for movement of substances through the organism.

Nerve tissue. Nerve tissues coordinate the activities of the body. They are capable of conducting electrical impulses from one region of the body to another. Most nerve tissue is found within the brain and the spinal cord.

21. **Describe the process of neoplasia, including factors associated with cancer.**   pp. 65–66

Neoplasia is an abnormal type of tissue growth where the cells grow and multiply in an uncontrolled fashion. In neoplasia, the factors that normally control cell and tissue growth are lost, resulting in a continuing increase in the number of dividing cells. This mass of uncontrolled cell growth is referred to as a tumor.

Neoplasia, by definition, means new growth. The tumors may be benign or malignant. Benign and malignant tumors have different characteristics. Benign neoplastic lesions are slow growing, usually encased by cells that are adherent, do not invade local tissue, do not spread to other body areas, and do not recur once removed. Cancerous tumors have the opposite characteristics. They grow fast and are not encapsulated, thus making removal more difficult. Malignant cells do not adhere together well, thus allowing cancerous cells to shed to other areas of the body—often through the bloodstream in a process called metastasis.

©2013 Pearson Education, Inc.
Paramedic Care: Principles & Practice, Vol. 2, 4th Ed.

Content Self-Evaluation

MULTIPLE CHOICE

_____ 1. A group of cells that serve a common purpose is called a tissue.
   A. True
   B. False

_____ 2. Which of the following is NOT developed from the mesoderm?
   A. Bone and cartilage   D. Skeletal muscle
   B. Blood and lymph vessels   E. Adipose tissue
   C. Lining of digestive tract

_____ 3. The tissue type that covers body surfaces is
   A. epithelial tissue.   D. connective tissue.
   B. embryotic tissue.   E. muscle tissue.
   C. nerve tissue.

_____ 4. The tissue type that provides a framework for other tissues is
   A. epithelial tissue.   D. connective tissue.
   B. embryotic tissue.   E. muscle tissue.
   C. nerve tissue.

_____ 5. The tissue type responsible for the movement of the organism and for movement of substances through the organism is
   A. epithelial tissue.   D. connective tissue.
   B. embryotic tissue.   E. muscle tissue.
   C. nerve tissue.

_____ 6. The tissue type that coordinates the activities of the body is
   A. epithelial tissue.   D. connective tissue.
   B. embryotic tissue.   E. muscle tissue.
   C. nerve tissue.

_____ 7. Which of the following is NOT a characteristic of epithelial tissue?
   A. Separated from underlying tissue by basement membrane
   B. Polarized epithelial cells
   C. Several blood vessels
   D. Small intercellular spaces
   E. Covers with an uninterrupted layer of cells

_____ 8. Which of the following is NOT a type of epithelial tissue?
   A. Stratified squamous   D. Stratified columnar
   B. Simple cylindrical   E. Stratified squamous
   C. Simple cuboidal

_____ 9. Collagen fibers are randomly coiled and thus capable of stretching.
   A. True
   B. False

_____ 10. Which of the following are small mobile cells that are found in the connective tissues, often near blood vessels that release chemicals as part of the body's defense system?
   A. Fibroblasts   D. Osteocytes
   B. Macrophages   E. Mast cells
   C. Adipocytes

_____ 11. Dense connective tissue is found in all of the following EXCEPT
   A. bone.   D. blood.
   B. cartilage.   E. ligaments.
   C. tendons.

_____ 12. Skeletal muscle contains striations (alternating dark and light bands) that give them a characteristic appearance under the microscope.
   A. True
   B. False

_____ 13. _____ is an abnormal type of tissue growth where the cells grow and multiply in an uncontrolled fashion.
   A. Apoptosis   D. Dysplasia
   B. Hyperplasia   E. Metaplasia
   C. Neoplasia

_____ 14. Malignant cells do not adhere together well, thus allowing cancerous cells to shed to other areas of the body in a process called
   A. mitosis.   D. metastasis.
   B. endocytosis.   E. exocytosis.
   C. phagocytosis.

_____ 15. The order in which carcinogenesis occurs is
   A. initiation, promotion, progression.   D. promotion, progression, initiation.
   B. promotion, initiation, progression.   E. progression, initiation, promotion.
   C. initiation, progression, promotion.

Special Project

MATCHING

Match the following tissue types with examples of locations where they can be found.

   A. simple squamous epithelial

   B. striated squamous epithelial

   C. simple cuboidal epithelial

   D. striated cuboidal epithelial

   E. simple columnar epithelial

   F. striated columnar epithelial

   G. loose areolar connective

   H. loose adipose connective

   I. dense connective

   J. cartilage connective

   K. bone connective

   J. blood connective

   M. skeletal muscle

   N. cardiac muscle

   O. smooth muscle

   P. nervous

   1. Outer layer of skin

   2. Linings of mouth, esophagus, vagina

3. Rings in respiratory air tubules

4. Muscles attached to bones

5. Most of digestive tract; bronchi

6. Skeleton

7. Excretory ducts of some glands; uterus

8. Under skin, around kidneys and heart

9. Ducts of sweat glands, mammary glands, salivary glands

10. Tendons, ligaments

11. Linings of heart and blood vessels; air sacs of lungs

12. Urethra; junction of esophagus and stomach

13. Kidney tubules; secretary portions of glands and ducts

14. Nose (tip); external ear

15. Within blood vessels

16. Wall of heart

17. Walls of digestive system, blood vessels, and tubules of urinary system

18. Brain, spinal cord, and peripheral nerves

19. Between muscles; surround glands

20. Wrapping small blood vessels and nerves

Part 5: Disease at the Organ Level, p. 69

Review of Chapter Objectives

After reading this part of the chapter, you should be able to:

22. **Describe the risk factors and basic nature of the following types of disorders:**

   a. **immunologic diseases, including rheumatic fever, allergies, and asthma** pp. 70–71
   Rheumatic fever is an inflammatory reaction to an infection but is not an infection itself. There seems to be a hereditary factor, but inadequate nutrition and crowded living conditions are contributing factors.

   Allergies often have a family history factor (and some allergies can be passed from the mother to the fetus during pregnancy). However, allergic reactions are triggered by exposure to allergens and can usually be controlled by avoiding or reducing the presence of allergens as well as with medication.

   Asthma sufferers may inherit the propensity for airway narrowing in response to various stimuli, but other triggering factors may be identified and, perhaps, controlled, including stress, overexertion, exposure to cold air, and stimuli such as pollens, dust mites, cockroach detritus, and smoke.

   b. **common cancers** p. 71
   Widely varying family history and environmental factors are included among the risk factors for cancer. Some kinds of cancer, such as breast and colorectal cancer, tend to cluster in families and seem to have a combination of genetic and environmental causes. Others, such as lung cancer, are more strongly identified with environmental causes.

For breast cancer, the greatest risk factor is female gender. The second highest risk factor is age. Lifestyle factors such as lack of exercise and obesity may contribute slightly to the incidence of breast cancer, but this has not been proven.

As with breast cancer, colorectal cancer risk factors include age (with the incidence rising after age 40 and peaking between 60 and 75) and family history (incidence in a first-degree relative increases the risk by two or three times). There are gender factors, with rectal cancer being more common in men and colon cancer more common in women. Diet may also be a risk factor, although recent studies have failed to confirm a link between a high-fat, low-fiber diet and colorectal cancer. (However, a high-fat, low-fiber diet has been positively linked to heart disease and other health problems.)

The causes of lung cancer are overwhelmingly environmental. Smoking has been identified as the main cause of 90 percent of lung cancers in men and 70 percent of lung cancers in women. Lung cancer can also be caused by inhaling substances such as asbestos, arsenic, and nickel, usually in the workplace.

c. type I and type II diabetes mellitus   p. 71

There are two major types of diabetes: type I and type II. Type I diabetes usually occurs before age 40, sometimes in childhood. Although it is less prevalent than type II diabetes, it is more severe.

In the type I diabetic, the pancreas produces no or almost no insulin, which is required for the cellular utilization of glucose, the body's chief source of energy. Type I diabetics must take insulin daily. There is some association of type I diabetes with family history, and medical researchers have pinpointed some possible genetic factors. Other causative factors may include autoimmunity disorders and viral infections that invade the pancreas and destroy the insulin-producing cells.

Type II diabetes usually occurs after age 40 and the incidence increases with age. It clusters much more strongly in families than does type I diabetes. In contrast to type I diabetes, in which there is a total lack of insulin, type II diabetes is associated with a decreased insulin receptor response or a decrease in insulin production. Diet and exercise may also be factors, since the majority of type II diabetics are obese. Type II diabetes can often be controlled with diet and exercise or with oral medications.

d. hematologic disorders, including disorders of coagulation and hemochromatosis   p. 71

Hemophilia is a bleeding disorder that is caused by a genetic clotting factor deficiency. It can be mild, but if severe it can cause not only serious bruising but also bleeding into the joints, which can lead to crippling deformities. The heredity is sex-linked, inherited through the mother, and affects male children almost exclusively. There is no cure, but administration of concentrated clotting factors can improve the condition.

Hemochromatosis is another genetic disorder, but this time caused by a histocompatibility complex dysfunction. It is marked by an excessive absorption and accumulation of iron in the body, causing weight loss, joint pain, abdominal pain, palpitations, and testicular atrophy in males. It is treated by removing blood from the body at intervals.

Not all blood disorders are genetic. Environmental factors, for example, can cause anemia (reduction in circulating red blood cells). In addition, some antihypertensive medications and other drugs may cause a drug-induced hemolytic (erythrocyte-destroying) anemia.

e. cardiovascular disease   pp. 71–72

Disorders such as prolongation of the QT interval (a delay between depolarization and repolarization of the ventricles as revealed in an electrocardiogram) and mitral-valve prolapse (an upward ballooning of the valve between the left ventricle and atrium that allows blood to regurgitate back into the atrium when the ventricle contracts) tend to cluster in families.

The American Heart Association lists heredity as a major risk factor for cardiovascular disease. Those with parents who have coronary artery disease (deposits on the walls of the coronary arteries that reduce blood flow to the heart muscle) have an approximately fivefold risk of developing the disease. This is why it is important to ask about family history of congenital heart disease (CHD), hypertension, and stroke when assessing patients with possible cardiovascular disease. Environmental factors, such as a diet high in saturated fats and cholesterol and lack of exercise, also play a large role in cardiovascular disease.

Hypertension (high blood pressure) is a major risk factor not only for cardiac disease but also for stroke and kidney disease. Studies of family history show that approximately 20 to 40 percent of

©2013 Pearson Education, Inc.
Paramedic Care: Principles & Practice, Vol. 2, 4th Ed.

the causation of hypertension is genetic. The remaining causative factors, then, are environmental, and may include high sodium ingestion, lack of physical activity, stress, and obesity.

Cardiomyopathy (disease affecting the heart muscle) is thought to occur secondarily to other causes such as infectious disease, toxin exposure, connective tissue disease, or nutritional deficiencies, which may be partially or totally environmental.

f. renal disorders p. 72

Renal (kidney) failure is caused by a variety of factors (primarily hypertension) that may eventually require a patient to receive dialysis treatment several times a week. Complications of dialysis include problems with vascular access devices (shunts, fistulas), localized infection and sepsis, and electrolyte abnormalities (hyperkalemia), which can result in cardiac arrest.

g. rheumatic disorders p. 72

Gout is a condition that may have both genetic and environmental causes. It is characterized by severe arthritic pain caused by deposit of crystals in the joints, most commonly the great toe. The crystals form as the result of an abnormally high level of uric acid in the blood that may be caused when the kidneys do not excrete enough uric acid or by high production of uric acid. High production of uric acid may be caused by a hereditary metabolic abnormality. Although the underlying cause may be genetic, attacks of gout can be triggered by environmental factors such as trauma, alcohol consumption, ingestion of certain foods, and stress, or other illnesses. Patients with gout also have a tendency to develop kidney stones.

h. gastrointestinal disorders p. 72

Lactose intolerance is usually identified by the inability of the patient to tolerate milk and some other dairy products. The patient lacks lactase, the enzyme that usually breaks down lactose in the digestive tract. This enzyme deficiency may be congenital (inborn) or may develop later on. It is more common in those of Asian, African, Native American, or Mediterranean ancestry than it is among northern and western Europeans.

Crohn's disease is a chronic inflammation of the wall of the digestive tract that usually affects the small intestine, the large intestine, or both. The cause is not known, but medical researchers have focused on immune system dysfunction, infection, and diet as the major probabilities.

In ulcerative colitis, a disease similar to Crohn's disease, the large intestine becomes inflamed and develops ulcers. As with Crohn's disease, the cause is not known, but an overactive immune response is suspected, and heredity seems to play a role.

Peptic ulcers develop when the normal protective structures and mechanisms, such as mucous production, break down and stomach acid and digestive juices. Environmental factors, bacterial infection (by *Helicobacter pylori*), diet, stress, and alcohol consumption are thought to play roles in the development of peptic ulcers. Many medications, particularly nonsteroidal anti-inflammatory medications, are associated with ulcer formation.

Cholecystitis is an inflammation of the gallbladder that usually results from blockage by a gallstone. There may be a genetic predisposition for gallstone formation. Gallstones are more prevalent in women and in some groups such as Native Americans and Mexican Americans. Other risk factors include age, a high-fat diet, and obesity.

Obesity can be defined as being more than 20 percent over the ideal body weight. Obesity has both an environmental and familial risk transmission. Research has shown that children whose parents are obese have a much-increased chance of developing obesity. Environmental factors such as proper nutrition and exercise may not be modeled or taught by obese parents, but there also seems to be a genetic factor to many cases of obesity. Obesity has been linked to, or defined as a cause for, diseases such as hypertension, heart disease, and vascular diseases.

i. neuromuscular disorders p. 72

Huntington's disease (which results in uncontrollable jerking and writhing movements) and muscular dystrophy (which results in progressive muscle weakness) are both known to be caused by genetic defects.

Multiple sclerosis (which affects the nerves of the eye, brain, and spinal cord) seems to have some hereditary factor with clustering among close relatives. Its exact cause is unknown, but it seems to result when the virus-triggered autoimmune response begins to attack the myelin sheath that protects the nerves.

Alzheimer's disease is thought to cause about 50 percent of dementias, or progressive mental deterioration. Its cause is unknown, but it does cluster strongly in families and appears to be either caused or influenced by specific gene abnormalities.

j. psychiatric disorders   pp. 72–73

Schizophrenia affects about 1 percent of the population worldwide and is more prevalent than Alzheimer's disease, diabetes, or multiple sclerosis. The schizophrenic loses contact with reality and suffers from hallucinations, delusions, abnormal thinking, and disrupted social functioning. People who develop schizophrenia are now thought to be "biologically vulnerable" to the disease, but what makes them vulnerable is not fully understood. The cause may be a genetic predisposition or some problem that occurs before, during, or after birth or a viral infection of the brain.

Another common psychiatric disorder is manic-depressive illness, also called bipolar disorder, in which the person experiences alternating periods of depression and mania or excitement. It can be mild or severe enough to interfere with the patient's ability to work or function socially. Manic-depressive illness affects about twice as many people as schizophrenia. It is believed to be hereditary, but the exact gene deficit has not yet been discovered.

23. Describe the physiology of perfusion.   pp. 73–76

All body cells require a constant supply of oxygen and other essential nutrients (primarily glucose), while waste products, such as carbon dioxide, must be constantly removed. It is the circulatory system, in conjunction with the respiratory and gastrointestinal systems, that provides the body's cells with these essential nutrients and removal of wastes. This is accomplished by the passage of blood through the capillaries while oxygen, carbon dioxide, nutrients, and wastes are exchanged by movement across the capillary walls and cell membranes. This constant and necessary passage of blood through the body's tissues is called perfusion.

Perfusion is dependent on a functioning and intact circulatory system. The three components of the circulatory system are: the pump (heart), the fluid (blood), and the container (blood vessels).

Factors affecting the pump include preload (amount of blood delivered to the heart during diastole), cardiac contractile force (strength of the contraction), and afterload (the resistance against which the ventricle must contract). Factors affecting the fluid include viscosity (thickness) and amount of blood. Factors affecting the container include condition and tone of the arteries, veins, and capillaries; peripheral vascular resistance (the pressure against which the heart must pump); and pressure within the system.

24. Explain the etiologies and pathophysiology of hypoperfusion.   pp. 76–77

Inadequate perfusion of body tissues is hypoperfusion, which is commonly called shock. Shock occurs first at a cellular level. If allowed to progress, the tissues, organs, organ systems, and ultimately the entire organism are affected.

Hypoperfusion (shock) is almost always a result of inadequate cardiac output. A number of factors can decrease effective cardiac output, including inadequate pump (inadequate preload, inadequate cardiac contractile strength, inadequate heart rate, and excessive afterload), inadequate fluid (hypovolemia—abnormally low circulating blood volume), or inadequate container (dilated container without change in fluid volume and leaking container).

25. Describe the body's compensatory mechanisms in the face of hypoperfusion.   pp. 77–79

Compensated shock. A decrease in arterial blood pressure by the baroreceptors activates several body systems that attempt to re-establish a normal blood pressure. The sympathetic nervous system stimulates the adrenal gland of the endocrine system to secrete the catecholamines epinephrine and norepinephrine. These chemicals profoundly affect the cardiovascular system, causing an increased heart rate, increased cardiac contractile strength, and arteriolar constriction—all of which serve to elevate the blood pressure. Another compensatory mechanism, the renin-angiotensin system, aids the body in maintaining an adequate blood pressure. Another endocrine response by the pituitary gland results in the secretion of antidiuretic hormone (ADH), which also causes the kidneys to reabsorb water, creating an additive effect to that of aldosterone.

©2013 Pearson Education, Inc.
Paramedic Care: Principles & Practice, Vol. 2, 4th Ed.

The spleen, capable of storing over 300 mL of blood, can expel up to 200 mL of blood into the venous circulation and can contract, consequently increasing blood volume, preload, cardiac output, and blood pressure, in response to a sudden drop in blood pressure. Some passive compensatory responses also occur, with beneficial fluid shifts taking place as a result of simple diffusion. With volume loss, the hydrostatic pressure in capillary beds is reduced, and water from the interstitial spaces diffuses into the capillaries.

Decompensated shock. If the conditions causing shock are too serious, or progress too rapidly, compensatory mechanisms may not be able to restore normal function. In those cases, decompensation is said to occur, and the patient is in a state of decompensated shock, also called progressive shock. During decompensated or progressive shock, medical intervention may still be able to correct the condition.

Irreversible shock. Since all the "responding" systems have a point at which they can no longer sustain their action, the shock state may progress to a condition where correction, either by the body's own compensatory mechanisms or through medical intervention, is no longer possible. Cellular deterioration progresses to tissue deterioration, which progresses to organ failure. Medical intervention may save the patient if initiated early enough, but when enough damage has been done to cells, tissues, and organs, no known treatment can help the patient to recover. Medical therapies may support function for a while, but death becomes inevitable.

26. **Predict the signs, symptoms, and consequences of untreated or inadequately treated shock.**   pp. 76–79

Hypoperfusion is inadequate blood flow to and past the body cells. This means that blood flow is insufficient to provide oxygen and necessary nutrients and to remove carbon dioxide and other metabolic wastes. If permitted to continue, hypoperfusion progresses and leads to failure of compensatory mechanisms, decompensation, irreversible shock, and death. Hypoperfusion (or shock) may be caused by trauma, fluid loss, myocardial infarction, infection, allergic reaction, spinal cord or brain injury, and other causes.

27. **Explain each of the following mechanisms of shock:**

   a. **cardiogenic**   pp. 80–81
   Cardiogenic shock is due to the inability of the heart to pump enough blood to meet the body's needs. It is commonly caused by severe left ventricular failure secondary to a myocardial infarction or congestive heart failure. Cardiac output decreases and workload increases, while coronary artery flow decreases and myocardial oxygen demand increases. These factors begin a vicious cycle that often ends in complete heart failure.

   b. **hypovolemic**   pp. 81–82
   Hypovolemic shock is due to the loss of blood volume through internal or external hemorrhage, dehydration, plasma losses from burns, excessive sweating, or third space losses. As the vascular volume decreases, the body compensates by releasing catecholamines, increasing heart rate and inducing vasoconstriction. This produces the classic signs and symptoms of shock—a rapid, weak pulse; cool, clammy, ashen skin; dyspnea; anxiety; combativeness; and, ultimately, hypotension.

   c. **neurogenic**   p. 82
   Neurogenic shock results from injury to the brain or spinal cord that interrupts the body's control over the vascular system. The vessels lose tone and dilate, increasing the size of the vascular container and producing a relative hypovolemia. The body's normal response is muted because the adrenal glands do not secrete catecholamines and the central nervous system cannot induce vasoconstriction. The injury may also affect the heart and respiratory system.

   d. **anaphylactic**   pp. 82–84
   Anaphylactic shock is an exaggerated and severe allergic reaction to a foreign substance that enters the body. It usually occurs rapidly and may be triggered by many substances. The most severe of anaphylactic reactions are triggered when substances are injected directly into the bloodstream, as with bee and wasp stings and injected medications.

e. **septic** p. 84

Septic shock is caused by an infection that progresses and enters the bloodstream. The toxins produced by the overwhelming infection increase capillary permeability and overcome the compensatory mechanisms, and shock results.

28. **Describe the evaluation and treatment goals for patients with cardiogenic, hypovolemic, neurogenic, anaphylactic, and septic shock.** **pp. 80–84**

Cardiogenic shock. A major difference between cardiogenic and other types of shock is the presence of pulmonary edema (excess fluid in the lungs), which will probably result in a complaint of difficulty breathing. There may be diminished lung sounds as fluid enters the interstitial spaces of the lungs. As fluid levels rise, wheezes, crackles, or rales may be heard. A productive cough may develop, characterized by white- or pink-tinged foamy sputum. Cyanosis (a dusky blue-gray skin color) is typical, resulting from the decreased diffusion of oxygen across the alveolar-capillary interface, decreasing oxygen delivery to cells that are already hypoxic because of decreased blood pressure and perfusion. Other signs of shock include altered mentation (resulting from reduced perfusion of the brain) and oliguria (diminished urination resulting from compensatory mechanisms that stimulate reabsorption of water by the kidneys to enhance circulating volume).

Treatment of cardiogenic shock includes the supportive measures that should be provided for shock of any origin: Ensure an open airway, administer supplemental oxygen if the patient is hypoxic and assist ventilations if necessary (to support oxygenation of myocardial and other body cells), and keep the patient warm (because impaired cellular metabolism is no longer producing enough energy to keep body temperature normal).

Hypovolemic shock. The signs of hypovolemic shock are considered the "classic" signs of shock. The mental status becomes altered, progressing from anxiety to lethargy or combativeness to unresponsiveness. The skin becomes pale, during compensated shock, but then begins to fall. The pulse may be normal in the beginning, and then become rapid, finally slowing and disappearing. As the kidneys continue to reabsorb water, urination decreases. Cardiac arrhythmias may develop in late shock, deteriorating to asystole (absence of heartbeat).

While it is accepted practice to administer crystalloid or colloid solutions to replace fluids lost through vomiting, diarrhea, burns, excessive sweating, or osmotic diuresis, the replacement of fluids in trauma patients is quite controversial. It has been demonstrated that the body provides a natural compensation for low-flow states when the systolic pressure is maintained between 70 and 85 mmHg. In a few studies, elevating the systolic blood pressure to greater than 85 mmHg has been associated with worsened outcomes. The worsened outcomes are attributed to the fact that aggressive fluid resuscitation, before the source of bleeding is repaired, causes progressive dilution of the blood, which decreases the oxygen-carrying capacity of the blood. Thus, many surgeons and EMS medical directors are now recommending administering only enough fluid to maintain a systolic blood pressure between 70 and 85 mmHg—a process called "permissive hypotension."

Neurogenic shock. The vasodilation in neurogenic shock causes warm, red skin, and sweat gland malfunction causes dry skin—in contrast to the cool, pale, sweaty skin associated with hypovolemic shock. Because of the lack of compensatory stimulation from catecholamine release, the patient will have a low blood pressure and a slow pulse even in the early stages—again, in contrast to hypovolemic shock.

Treatment for neurogenic shock or spinal shock is similar to treatment for other types of shock and includes support of the airway, oxygenation, ventilation, maintenance of body temperature, and intravenous access. Spinal shock is characterized by hypotension, reflex bradycardia, and warm, dry skin.

Anaphylactic shock. Because the immune responses involved in anaphylaxis can affect different body systems, the signs and symptoms can vary widely, including: skin (flushing, itching, hives, swelling, and cyanosis); respiratory system (breathing difficulty, sneezing, coughing, wheezing, stridor, laryngeal edema, and laryngospasm); cardiovascular system (vasodilation, increased heart rate and decreased blood pressure); gastrointestinal system (nausea, vomiting, abdominal cramping, and diarrhea); and nervous system (altered mental status, dizziness, headache, seizures, and tearing). The patient may present with an altered mental status that can progress to unresponsiveness, so gather a brief history as soon as possible, including previous allergic reactions and any information about what the patient may have ingested or been exposed to that could have caused the present reaction. Be sure the patient is no longer in contact with the allergen; if a stinger is in the skin, scrape it away with a fingernail or scalpel blade.

Since laryngeal edema is often a problem, protecting the patient's airway will be your first concern. Administer oxygen by nonrebreather mask or, as necessary, by endotracheal intubation. The anaphylactic response causes depletion of circulatory volume by promoting capillary permeability and leaking of fluid into interstitial spaces, so establish an IV of crystalloid solution (normal saline or lactated Ringer's) for volume support. The primary treatment for anaphylaxis is pharmacological. In addition to oxygen, epinephrine is usually administered (if the patient has a history of anaphylaxis, he may be carrying a prescribed spring-loaded epinephrine injector), as are antihistamines (diphenhydramine), corticosteroids (methylprednisolone, hydrocortisone, dexamethasone), and vasopressors (dopamine, norepinephrine, epinephrine). Occasionally an inhaled beta agonist (albuterol) may be required.

Septic shock. The signs and symptoms of septic shock are progressive. In the beginning, cardiac output is increased, but toxins causing vasodilation may prevent an increase in blood pressure. The person may seem to be sick, but not alarmingly so.

By the last stages, toxins have increased permeability of the blood vessels to the point where great amounts of fluid are lost from the vasculature and blood pressure falls drastically. Signs and symptoms can vary widely as the patient progresses from early to late stages of septic shock. Some patients may have a high fever, but others, especially the elderly or the very young, may have no fever or may even be hypothermic. The skin can be flushed, if fever is present, or very pale and cyanotic in the late stages. The most susceptible organ system is the lungs and respiratory system, so the patient may present with breathing difficulty and altered lung sounds. The brain may be infected, resulting in altered mental status. Suspicion of septic shock is usually based on a history of recent infection or illness.

Treatment for septic shock includes the supportive measures that should be provided for shock of any origin: Ensure an open airway, administer supplemental oxygen if the patient is hypoxic and assist ventilations if necessary, and keep the patient warm. In addition, treatment is focused on investigating and treating the underlying infection.

29. Describe the pathophysiology of multiple organ dysfunction syndrome (MODS).   pp. 84–86

Multiple organ dysfunction syndrome (MODS) is a progressive impairment of two or more body organs, usually after an initial insult and apparently successful resuscitation. It is caused by an uncontrolled inflammatory response and occurs most commonly after septic shock. The syndrome is caused by an exaggerated immune response in which hormones are released, causing vasodilation, increased capillary permeability, and increased metabolic demands. The syndrome usually begins within 24 hours of the initial insult and progresses over several weeks.

Content Self-Evaluation

MULTIPLE CHOICE

_____   **1.** Which of the following is a factor that can influence disease risk?
    A. Family history   **D.** Lifestyle
    B. Environment   **E.** All of the above
    C. Gender

_____   **2.** Which of the following is a disease with a genetic predisposition?
    A. Septic shock   **D.** Hansen's disease
    B. Rubella   **E.** All of the above
    C. Cystic fibrosis

_____   **3.** Most disease processes are simply caused by either an environmental or genetic factor, rarely both.
    A. True
    B. False

4. The death rate from disease is reported as its
   A. prevalence.
   B. morbidity.
   C. mortality.
   D. incidence.
   E. none of the above.

5. People with genetic predispositions to certain diseases can frequently take actions that modify the risk factors associated with acquiring the disease.
   A. True
   B. False

6. A history of breast cancer in a first-degree relative (mother, sister, or daughter) increases the risk of breast cancer in a woman by
   A. one to two times.
   B. two to three times.
   C. three to four times.
   D. four to five times.
   E. five to six times.

7. What percent of diabetics have type II diabetes?
   A. 50 percent
   B. 60 percent
   C. 70 percent
   D. 80 percent
   E. 90 percent

8. The risk of acquiring heart disease for a person with a familial history of coronary artery disease is how many times greater than for someone without such a family history?
   A. Two
   B. Three
   C. Four
   D. Five
   E. Eight

9. What is the primary cause of renal failure?
   A. Hypotension
   B. Hypertension
   C. Cardiomyopathy
   D. Renal calculi
   E. *Helicobacter pylori*

10. The term *shock* is synonymous with
    A. hypotension.
    B. hypoperfusion.
    C. hypovolemia.
    D. hyperperfusion.
    E. hypervolemia.

11. Perfusion involves the exchange of which of the following between the bloodstream and body cells?
    A. Carbon dioxide
    B. Oxygen
    C. Nutrients
    D. Waste products
    E. All of the above

12. Stroke volume of the heart is directly related to all of the following EXCEPT
    A. preload.
    B. afterload.
    C. oxygen saturation.
    D. cardiac contractile force.
    E. circulating catecholamines.

13. The stretching of the myocardial wall increases the strength of cardiac contraction in the mechanism known as
    A. peripheral vascular resistance.
    B. the Hering-Breuer response.
    C. the Frank-Starling mechanism.
    D. cardiac preload.
    E. the catecholamine response.

14. The oxygen concentration in air within the alveoli is approximately
    A. 10 percent.
    B. 14 percent.
    C. 17 percent.
    D. 19 percent.
    E. 21 percent.

©2013 Pearson Education, Inc.
Paramedic Care: Principles & Practice, Vol. 2, 4th Ed.

15. Which of the following is NOT one of the conditions for movement and utilization of oxygen described by the Fick principle?
    A. Adequate inspired oxygen
    B. Adequate cardiac stretching
    C. Proper tissue perfusion
    D. Efficient oxygen off-loading
    E. Adequate red blood cells

16. Hypoperfusion may occur with all of the following EXCEPT
    A. inadequate heart rate.
    B. dilated vascular container.
    C. excessive vascular constriction.
    D. reduced blood volume.
    E. excessive afterload.

17. The catecholamines epinephrine and norepinephrine are responsible during the body's response to hypoperfusion for
    A. decreasing heart rate.
    B. decreasing cardiac contractile strength.
    C. arteriolar dilation.
    D. increasing blood pressure.
    E. decreasing blood volume.

18. During shock, the spleen may expel blood back into the circulatory system up to a volume of
    A. 200 mL.
    B. 300 mL.
    C. 400 mL.
    D. 500 mL.
    E. 600 mL.

19. During decompensated shock, which of the following is likely to occur?
    A. Fluid shift from the interstitial spaces
    B. Systemic alkalosis
    C. Cardiac excitation
    D. Drop in blood pressure
    E. All of the above

20. What type of shock is due to plasma loss from burns?
    A. Cardiogenic
    B. Hypovolemic
    C. Neurogenic
    D. Septic
    E. Anaphylactic

21. What type of shock is due to a severe allergic reaction?
    A. Cardiogenic
    B. Hypovolemic
    C. Neurogenic
    D. Septic
    E. Anaphylactic

22. Which type of shock results from infection that enters the bloodstream and is carried throughout the body?
    A. Cardiogenic
    B. Hypovolemic
    C. Neurogenic
    D. Septic
    E. Anaphylactic

23. The reason we are aware of multiple organ dysfunction syndrome (MODS) is that modern medicine is able to help patients survive the initial serious illness or injury.
    A. True
    B. False

24. The first evidence of MODS usually presents within
    A. 12 hours.
    B. 24 hours.
    C. 72 hours.
    D. 7 to 10 days.
    E. 14 to 21 days.

25. Death from MODS usually occurs after
    A. 24 hours.
    B. 48 hours.
    C. 72 hours.
    D. 10 days.
    E. 21 days.

Special Project

MATCHING

Match the type of shock with the characteristic of its presentation.

Type of Shock

A. cardiogenic

B. hypovolemic

C. eurogenic

D. septic

E. anaphylactic

Pathology or Presentation

_____ **1.** Pulmonary edema

_____ **2.** Warm, red skin

_____ **3.** Itching and skin flushing

_____ **4.** History of recent illness

_____ **5.** Hives

_____ **6.** Possible high fever

_____ **7.** Classic signs of shock

_____ **8.** Laryngeal edema

_____ **9.** Dry skin

_____ **10.** History of diarrhea

Part 6: The Body's Defenses Against Disease and Injury, p. 86

Review of Chapter Objectives

After reading this part of the chapter, you should be able to:

30. Describe the basic characteristics of bacteria, viruses, fungi, parasites, and prions that act as human pathogens.   **pp. 86–87**

Bacteria are single-cell organisms that consist of internal cytoplasm surrounded by a rigid cell wall. Bacteria are prokaryotic cells that, unlike the eukaryotic cells of the human body, lack an organized nucleus and other intracellular organelles. Bacteria can reproduce independently, but they need a host to supply food and other support. Inside the body, they achieve this by binding to host cells.

Viruses are much smaller than bacteria and can only be seen with an electron microscope. In addition, they cannot grow without the assistance of another organism. In fact, viruses are referred to as intracellular parasites, since they must invade the cells of the organism they infect. A virus has no organized cellular structure except a protein coat (capsid) surrounding the internal genetic material, deoxyribonucleic acid (DNA) or ribonucleic acid (RNA). With no organized cellular structure or cellular organelles, viruses are incapable of metabolism. Once inside a cell, they take over, using the cellular enzymes to replicate and produce more viruses, which decreases synthesis of macromolecules vital to the host cell.

Fungi, which include yeasts and molds, are more like plants than animals. Fungi rarely cause human disease other than minor skin infections such as athlete's foot and some common vaginal infections.

Parasites range in size from protozoa (single-cell animals not much larger than bacteria) to large intestinal worms. Parasites tend to be more common in developing nations than in the United States. Treatment depends on the organism and the location.

Prions are the most recently recognized classification of infectious agents. Initially thought to be slow-acting viruses, prions differ from viruses in that they are smaller, are made entirely of proteins, and do not have protective capsids.

31. Describe the body's three lines of defense against pathogens. p. 88

There are three chief lines of self-defense against infection and injury. One involves anatomic barriers. The other two—the inflammatory response and the immune response—rely on actions of the leukocytes (white blood cells).

The anatomic defenses are external and nonspecific. They are considered external because they prevent substances from penetrating the skin or the coverings of internal passageways (mucous membranes that line the respiratory, gastrointestinal, and genitourinary tracts). They are nonspecific because they defend against all invaders, such as foreign bodies, chemicals, or microorganisms, without targeting any specific type of invader.

The inflammatory response, or inflammation, begins within seconds of injury or invasion by a pathogen. It is nonspecific, attacking any invader by surrounding it with cells and fluids to isolate, destroy, and eliminate it. Inflammation is mediated by multiple plasma protein systems, especially the complement system, the coagulation system, and the kinin system, and involves a variety of cell types as it attacks the invader.

The immune response develops more slowly (one type of response requires a second exposure after priming by the first exposure to the invader). The immune response is specific, in that it will develop a specialized response for each different invader. It is mediated by just one plasma protein system (immunoglobulin) and attacks the invader mainly with a single cell type (lymphocytes, which are one type of leukocyte, or white blood cell).

32. Explain the function of the immune system. pp. 88–97

Most viruses, bacteria, fungi, and parasites, as well as noninfectious substances such as pollens, foods, venoms, drugs, and others that may enter the body, have proteins on their surface called antigens. The immune system detects these antigens as being foreign, or "non-self," and responds to produce substances called antibodies that combine with antigens to control or destroy them. This is known as the immune response. As part of this process, memory cells "remember" the antigen and will trigger an even faster and more effective response to destroy the same antigen if it enters the body again. Such long-term protection against specific foreign substances is known as immunity.

Natural immunity is inborn, part of the genetic makeup of the individual or of the species in general. Active acquired immunity is generated by the host's (infected person's) immune system after exposure to an antigen. Passive acquired immunity is transferred to a person from an outside source (such as mother to fetus).

On first exposure to an antigen, after a lag-time of five to seven days, the presence of IgM antibodies can be detected in the blood, with a lesser presence of IgG antibodies. This constitutes the primary immune response, also called the initial immune response. If there is a second exposure to the antigen, the body responds much faster, and a far greater quantity of IgG antibodies is produced. The level of IgG antibodies, with their memory for the specific antigen, will remain elevated for many years. This constitutes the secondary immune response, also called the anamnestic (or memory assisting) immune response.

T lymphocytes do not produce antibodies. Instead, they recognize the presence of a foreign antigen and attack it directly. This type of immunity is called cell-mediated immunity. B lymphocytes do not attack antigens directly. Instead, they produce the antibodies (immunoglobulins) that attack antigens. B lymphocytes also develop memory, and confer long-term immunity to specific antigens. This type of immunity is called humoral immunity.

33. Describe the process of inflammation. pp. 97–107

Inflammation, also called the inflammatory response, is the body's response to cellular injury.

Inflammation develops swiftly; is nonspecific (it attacks all unwanted substances in the same way); is temporary, lasting only until the immediate threat is conquered (usually only a few days to two weeks); involves platelets and many types of white blood cells (the granulatory cells called neutrophils, basophils, and eosinophils; and the monocytes that mature into macrophages); and involves several plasma protein systems (complement, coagulation, and kinin).

The functions of inflammation include: destroy and remove unwanted substances; wall off the infected and inflamed area; stimulate the immune response; and promote healing.

34. Explain the pathophysiology of hypersensitivity reactions and deficiencies in immunity and inflammation. pp. 107–111

Hypersensitivity is an exaggerated and harmful immune response. The word *hypersensitivity* is often used as a synonym for *allergy*. However, hypersensitivity is also used as an umbrella term for allergy and two other categories of harmful immune response: allergy (an exaggerated immune response to an environmental antigen, such as pollen or bee venom); autoimmunity (a disturbance in the body's normal tolerance for self-antigens, as in hyperthyroidism or rheumatic fever); and isoimmunity, also called allo-immunity (an immune reaction between members of the same species, commonly of one person against the antigens of another person, as in the reaction of a mother to her infant's Rh negative factor or in transplant rejections).

Hypersensitivity reactions are classified as immediate hypersensitivity reactions or delayed hyper-sensitivity reactions, depending on how long it takes the secondary reaction to appear after re-exposure to an antigen. Usually, when a hypersensitivity reaction takes place, inflammation is triggered that results in destruction of healthy tissues. Four mechanisms, or types, of hypersensitivity that cause this destructive reaction have been identified: IgE-mediated allergen reactions (Type I), tissue-specific reac-tions (Type II), immune-complex-mediated reactions (Type III), and cell-mediated reactions (Type IV).

Congenital, or primary, immune deficiency develops if the development of lymphocytes in the fetus or embryo is impaired or halted. Different immune-deficiency diseases may develop, depending on whether the T cells, the B cells, or both have been affected.

In the DiGeorge syndrome, there is a lack or partial lack of thymus development, resulting in a severe decrease in T cell production and function. Bruton agammaglobulinemia is caused by impaired development of B cell precursors, resulting in B cells that cannot produce IgM or IgD antibodies. In bare lymphocyte syndrome, lymphocytes and macrophages are unable to produce Class I or Class II HLA antigens, which disrupts the ability of cells to recognize self or non-self substances, resulting in severe infections that are usually fatal before age 5. In Wiskott-Aldrich syndrome, IgM antibody production is reduced. Selective IgA deficiency is the most common immune deficiency. IgA is the an-tibody present in mucous membranes. People with IgA deficiency frequently suffer from sinus, lung, and gastrointestinal infections. In chronic mucocutaneous candidiasis, the T lymphocytes are unable to respond against *candida* infections.

Acquired, or secondary, immune deficiencies develop after birth and do not result from genetic factors. They can be caused by or associated with pregnancy, infections, and diseases such as diabetes or cirrhosis. The elderly are more prone to acquired immune deficiencies than the young. Among the factors that can severely affect immune function are nutritional deficiencies, medical treatment, trauma, and stress. Of special interest is the fatal acquired immune disorder AIDS.

35. Describe the impact of age and stress on disease. pp. 106–107

Newborns and the elderly are particularly susceptible to problems of insufficient immune and inflam-matory responses.

©2013 Pearson Education, Inc.
Paramedic Care: Principles & Practice, Vol. 2, 4th Ed.

Neonates generally go through a phase at about five or six months of age when immune system protection received from the mother is depleted and their own immune systems are still immature, making them particularly susceptible to respiratory tract infections. Inflammatory responses are similarly immature in the neonate.

The elderly also have difficulties with both the immune and the inflammatory responses. B cell and especially T cell functions of the immune system decrease markedly after age 60. The elderly are also prone to impaired wound healing. This is thought not to be due to the normal processes of aging but rather to the higher incidence of chronic diseases such as diabetes and cardiovascular disease in the elderly. Also, many elderly persons take prescribed anti-inflammatory steroids for conditions such as arthritis, and these inhibit inflammation. Decreased perfusion contributes to hypoxia in the wound bed, inhibiting inflammation and healing.

36. Describe the stress response.   **pp. 113–117**

The stress response is initiated by a stressor. The input of the stressor into the central nervous system, as mediated by the person's psychological response, leads to production of corticotropin-releasing factor (CRF) from the hypothalamus, which in turn stimulates responses by the sympathetic nervous system and the endocrine system (neuroendocrine regulation), which then affect the immune system.

Sympathetic nervous system stimulation results in the release of catecholamines norepinephrine (noradrenalin) and epinephrine (adrenalin). All the effects of the catecholamines prepare the body to "fight-or-flight" in response to a stressor.

Cortisol is another hormone produced in response to stress. The corticotropin-releasing factor (CRF) that stimulates the sympathetic nervous system, as previously discussed, simultaneously stimulates the anterior pituitary gland to produce adrenocorticotropic hormone (ACTH), which in turn stimulates the adrenal cortex to produce a variety of steroid hormones, primarily cortisol. One of the primary functions of cortisol is the stimulation of gluconeogenesis. It enhances the elevation of blood glucose by other hormones and also inhibits peripheral uptake and oxidation of glucose by the cells. Cortisol also affects protein metabolism, increasing synthesis of proteins in the liver but increasing breakdown of proteins in the muscle, lymphoid tissue, fatty tissues, skin, and bone.

Other hormones are associated with decreased pain sensitivity, increased feelings of well-being, and changes in metabolism (proteins, lipids, and carbohydrates).

Content Self-Evaluation

MULTIPLE CHOICE

_____ 1. Which of the following are single-cell organisms consisting of cytoplasm surrounded by a rigid cell membrane?
   A. Viruses
   B. Bacteria
   C. Fungi
   D. Parasites
   E. Prions

_____ 2. Which of the following are released by bacterial cells during their growth?
   A. Antibiotics
   B. Gram-negative material
   C. Exotoxins
   D. Endotoxins
   E. None of the above

_____ 3. Which of the following are more like plants than animals and rarely cause serious human disease?
   A. Viruses
   B. Bacteria
   C. Fungi
   D. Parasites
   E. Prions

_____ 4. The body's anatomical barrier against infection (the skin and linings of the respiratory and digestive systems) is considered
  A. an external, specific barrier.
  B. an external, nonspecific barrier.
  C. an internal, specific barrier.
  D. an internal, nonspecific barrier.
  E. none of the above.

_____ 5. The body's immune response against infection is considered
  A. an external, specific response.
  B. an external, nonspecific response.
  C. an internal, specific response.
  D. an internal, nonspecific response.
  E. none of the above.

_____ 6. The proteins located on the surface of many substances that enter the body and are used during the immune response to identify foreign organisms are
  A. antigens.
  B. antibodies.
  C. B cells.
  D. T cells.
  E. lymphocytes.

_____ 7. Which of the following types of immunity is genetic?
  A. Primary
  B. Acquired
  C. Natural
  D. Secondary
  E. Extrinsic

_____ 8. Which type of immunity refers to the body's initial response to exposure to an antigen?
  A. Primary
  B. Acquired
  C. Natural
  D. Secondary
  E. Humoral

_____ 9. The type of immunity, resident in the blood, that produces antibodies and remembers a specific antigen is
  A. cell-mediated.
  B. humoral.
  C. natural.
  D. primary.
  E. extrinsic.

_____ 10. Which of the following is NOT an essential characteristic of an antigen required to trigger an immune response?
  A. Sufficient foreignness
  B. Sufficient size
  C. Sufficient complexity
  D. Sufficient quantity
  E. Sufficient lability

_____ 11. The antigens that help the body recognize a substance as "self" or "non-self" are called HLA (histocompatibility locus antigens) antigens.
  A. True
  B. False

_____ 12. Under the ABO classification system, the universal blood donor is identified as having blood type(s):
  A. A.
  B. B.
  C. O.
  D. AB.
  E. B and O.

_____ 13. An antibody attaching to an antigen may result in all of the following EXCEPT
  A. agglutination.
  B. debridement.
  C. neutralization.
  D. enhancement of phagocytosis.
  E. precipitation.

_____ 14. Some antibodies are present in tears, saliva, and breast milk.
  A. True
  B. False

©2013 Pearson Education, Inc.
Paramedic Care: Principles & Practice, Vol. 2, 4th Ed.

_____ 15. Which cells are associated with the cell-mediated response of the immune system?
- **A.** B cells
- **B.** T cells
- **C.** Phagocytes
- **D.** Y cells
- **E.** Both A and B

_____ 16. The infant's antibody levels are lowest at what age?
- **A.** Birth
- **B.** 1 to 2 months
- **C.** 5 to 6 months
- **D.** 6 to 8 months
- **E.** 10 to 12 months

_____ 17. Which of the following is NOT a function of the inflammatory response?
- **A.** To destroy and remove unwanted substances
- **B.** To wall off the infected and inflamed area
- **C.** To stimulate the immune response
- **D.** To promote healing
- **E.** To agglutinate viruses

_____ 18. Degranulation by the mast cells occurs when the cell is stimulated by all of the following EXCEPT
- **A.** physical injury.
- **B.** toxins.
- **C.** allergic reactions.
- **D.** histamines.
- **E.** venoms.

_____ 19. The impaired wound healing experienced by the elderly is thought to be a natural consequence of aging.
- **A.** True
- **B.** False

_____ 20. The common allergic and anaphylactic responses are caused by which immunoglobulin (antibody)?
- **A.** IgM
- **B.** IgG
- **C.** IgA
- **D.** IgE
- **E.** IgD

_____ 21. The common clinical signs of a severe allergic reaction include all of the following EXCEPT
- **A.** skin flushing.
- **B.** dyspnea.
- **C.** nausea.
- **D.** dizziness.
- **E.** bradycardia.

_____ 22. The initial stage of the general adaptation syndrome in response to stress is
- **A.** exhaustion.
- **B.** resistance.
- **C.** withdrawal.
- **D.** alarm.
- **E.** turnover.

Special Project

Complete the diagram below summarizing the immune response process. Write the letter of the label in the appropriate place on the diagram.

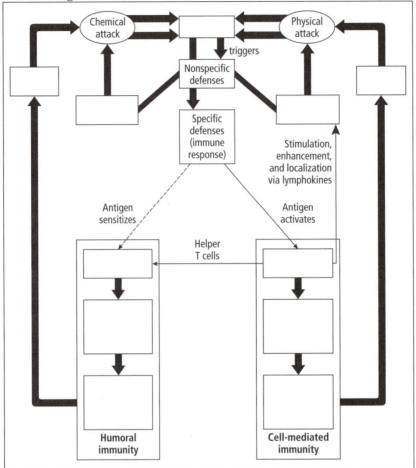

A. Activation of B cells

B. Cytotoxic T cells

C. Maturation of plasma cells and production of antibodies

D. Production of memory T cells and cytotoxic T cells

E. Antigen

F. Complement system

G. NK cells/macrophages

H. Production of memory B cells and plasma cells

I. Activation of T cells

J. Maturation and migration of cytotoxic T cells

K. Circulating antibodies

©2013 Pearson Education, Inc.
Paramedic Care: Principles & Practice, Vol. 2, 4th Ed.

2

Human Life Span Development

Review of Chapter Objectives

After reading this chapter, you should be able to:

1. Define key terms introduced in this chapter.

Knowing and being able to apply the key terms in each chapter is critical to understanding chapter concepts. Write the list of key terms. Then write the definition of each one in your own words. Check your understanding by confirming the definitions in the text glossary. Correct any misunderstandings. Create a study aid by writing each key term on the front of an index card and the definition on the back. Use the cards to quiz yourself or to have someone quiz you.

2. Describe the physiologic characteristics of infants.   **pp. 123–125**

Infancy is the period from birth to one year of age in which the vital signs are pulse rate 100 to 160, respiratory rate 30 to 60, systolic blood pressure 87 to 105, and body temperature of 98 to 100°F. The weight of the infant decreases immediately after birth and then increases, doubling birth weight after 4 to 6 months and tripling it after 9 to 12 months. Immediately after birth, the cardiovascular system changes dramatically from the maternal circulation, with the left ventricle increasing in strength throughout the first year. The infant airway is less stable than the adult's, and the infant is an obligate nasal breather and has delicate lung tissue that is prone to barotrauma. Acquired immunity from the mother somewhat protects the infant from 6 months up to about 1 year. The infant has well-developed reflexes including the startle (Moro), palmar grasp, rooting, and sucking reflexes, which usually disappear after the first few months. The infant's skull is not completely closed, and the openings (the fontanelles) may demonstrate dehydration when sunken. They close by 9 to 18 months.

3. Describe the psychosocial characteristics of infants.   **pp. 125–126**

Psychosocially, the infant develops based on instincts, drives, capacities, and interactions with the environment. Bonding occurs as the infant senses that his needs will be met by caregivers and develops attachments to family. The infant learns as caregivers gradually increase their expectations of the infant and child. In crisis, the infant will often follow a predictable sequence of responses: protest, despair, and withdrawal.

4. Discuss the impact of family processes on the psychosocial development of infants.   **p. 125**

A key component of the infant's environment is the family. The interactions babies have with their families help them to grow and change and help their families do the same. This is called "reciprocal socialization," a model that recognizes the child's active role in his or her own development.

Raising a baby requires a lot of hard work, but studies show that healthy, happy, and self-reliant children are the products of stable homes in which parents give a great deal of time and attention to their children.

5. Describe the physiologic characteristics of toddlers and preschoolers. pp. 126–127

The toddler is a child from 1 to 3 years of age with vital signs normally of a pulse rate of 80 to 110, respirations at 24 to 40, systolic blood pressure at 95 to 105, and temperature of 96.8 to 99.6°F. The preschooler is between 3 and 6 years of age and has vital signs of a pulse rate of 70 to 110, respirations of 22 to 34, a systolic blood pressure between 95 and 110, and a body temperature of 96.8 to 99.6°F. The toddler and preschooler gain about 2 kg in body weight per year. Their cardiovascular systems are better developed, and thermoregulation is more efficient than in infants. The lungs are increasing in surface area, yet rapid respirations will tire the child quickly. Passive immunity is lost, and the toddler and preschooler become more susceptible to minor respiratory and gastrointestinal infections, though they now begin to develop their own immunities.

6. Describe the psychosocial characteristics of toddlers and preschoolers. pp. 127–128

Psychosocially, the toddler and preschooler begin to use words and understand their meaning. By the age of 3 or 4 years they have mastered the basics of language. They begin to understand cause and effect, develop separation anxiety, and engage in playacting and magical thinking. They become progressively more influenced by peers and television. Divorce may have an important impact on their psychosocial development, because they may feel abandoned or responsible.

7. Explain the impact of relationships with others, including parents, on toddlers and preschoolers. p. 128

Interaction with children of similar age is very important to the development of toddler and school-age children. As childhood progresses, peer groups actually become more important. Interaction with peers offers an awareness of others, as well as opportunities for learning skills, comparing oneself to others, and feeling like part of a group.

8. Describe the impact of parenting styles, divorce, television and video games, and modeling on toddlers and preschoolers. p. 128

Authoritarian parents are demanding and desire instant obedience from a child. No consideration is given to the child's view, and no attempt is made to explain why. This parenting style often leads to children with low self-esteem and low competence.

Authoritative parents respond to the needs and wishes of their children. While they believe in parental control, they attempt to explain their reasons to the child. They expect mature behavior and will enforce rules, but they still encourage independence and actualization of potential. These parents believe that both they and children have rights and try to maintain a happy balance between the two. This parenting style usually leads to children who are self-assertive, independent, friendly, and cooperative.

Permissive parents take a tolerant, accepting view of their children's behavior, including aggressive behavior and sexual behavior. They rarely punish or make demands of their children, allowing them to make almost all of their own decisions. This parenting style may lead to impulsive, aggressive children who have low self-reliance, low self-control, low maturity, and lack responsible behavior.

As a result of divorce, a child's physical way of life often changes and the child's psychological life is also touched. The effects on the child's development, however, depend greatly on the child's age, his cognitive and social competencies, the amount of dependency on his parents, how the parents interact with each other and the child, and even the type of child care. Toddlers and preschoolers commonly express feelings of shock, depression, and a fear that their parents no longer love them. They may feel they are being abandoned. They are unable to see the divorce from their parents' perspective, and therefore believe the divorce centers on them. The parents' ability to respond to a child's needs greatly influences the ultimate effects of divorce on the child.

Virtually every family has at least one television in the home, and many have video game players of one kind or another. Most children watch television and/or play video games for several hours each day, many with few, if any, parental restrictions.

©2013 Pearson Education, Inc.
Paramedic Care: Principles & Practice, Vol. 2, 4th Ed.

Television violence increases levels of aggression in toddlers and preschoolers, and it increases passive acceptance of the use of aggression by others. Parental screening of the television programs children watch may be effective in avoiding these outcomes. Some video games also feature violent scenarios that parents may do well to monitor.

Toddlers and preschool-age children begin to recognize sexual differences, and, through modeling, they begin to incorporate gender-specific behaviors they observe in parents, siblings, and peers.

9. Describe the physiologic development of school-age children.   p. 128

The school-aged child is between 6 and 13 years old and has vital signs of a pulse rate of 65 to 110, respirations of 18 to 30, systolic blood pressure of 97 to 112, and a body temperature of 98.6°F. As the vital signs continue to move toward normal adult values, the school-aged child grows at a rate of 6 cm and 3 kg per year. Brain function continues to increase, and primary teeth are replaced by permanent ones.

10. Describe the psychosocial characteristics of school-age children.   pp. 128–129

The school-aged child develops advanced decision-making skills and develops his own self-concept. Factors in this development include self-esteem, moral reasoning and judgment, and self-control.

11. Describe the physiologic characteristics of adolescents.   pp. 129–130

The adolescent is between 13 and 19 years of age and has normal vital signs of a pulse rate of 60 to 90, respirations of 12 to 26, a systolic blood pressure of 112 to 128, and a body temperature of 98.6°F. The adolescent may experience a rapid growth spurt, with maximum growth occurring for the female by age 16 and by age 18 for the male. During this stage, children reach reproductive maturity. In females, the breasts enlarge and menstruation begins.

12. Describe the psychosocial characteristics of adolescents.   p. 130

Adolescence is a time of great psychosocial change. The adolescent strives for autonomy, becomes interested in the opposite sex, and develops an individual identity. The development of logical, analytical, and abstract thinking continues, and the adolescent becomes disappointed when others, especially adults, do not live up to their personal code of ethics.

13. Describe the physiologic and psychosocial characteristics of early adulthood and middle adulthood.   pp. 130–131

The early adult years are between ages 19 and 40. During this stage of life, normal vital signs are a pulse rate of 60 to 100, respirations of 12 to 20, blood pressure of 120/80, and body temperature of 98.6°F. The body reaches peak performance between 19 and 26 years of age, then begins to slow. Spinal disks settle, leading to a loss in body height, and fatty tissues increase, leading to weight gain.

During this time period, most lifelong habits and routines develop and job stress is at its greatest. The family is also stressed by childbirth and the challenges it brings.

14. Describe the physiologic characteristics associated with aging and late adulthood.   pp. 131–134

The middle-aged adult years are between 40 and 60. During this stage, normal vital signs include a pulse rate of 60 to 100, respirations of 12 to 20, a blood pressure of 120/90, and a body temperature of 98.6°F. During middle age, some degradation of vision and hearing occur, and cardiovascular disease and cancer become health risks.

Middle-aged adults become concerned about the social clock and become more task oriented, aiming to accomplish their lifelong goals. They may experience the "empty-nest syndrome," in which the children leave home and parental responsibilities become much reduced. Financial commitments associated with elderly parents and young children may add stress.

The late-aged adult is older than 60 years and has vital signs that are dependent on individual health status. The walls of the blood vessels thicken, increasing peripheral vascular resistance and reducing blood flow to the organs. The heart begins to show signs of disease of the valves, coronary arteries, electrical system, and the heart muscle itself. Blood volume decreases, as does the number of platelets and red blood cells. The respiratory surface area decreases, as does lung elasticity. The chest expands, and the chest wall stiffens. Respiratory workload increases, while efficiency decreases and coughing becomes less effective. The endocrine system works less efficiently, and glucose metabolism and insulin production decrease. The senses continue to deteriorate, including smell, eyesight, and hearing. Reaction time also diminishes.

15. **Describe the psychosocial characteristics and concerns associated with aging and late adulthood.**

Late-aged individuals are affected by concerns regarding housing, self-reliance, and financial burdens. They may be "forced" into retirement while they are still able to perform.

Case Study Review

Reread the case study on page 122 in Paramedic Care: Paramedicine Fundamentals; *then, read the following discussion.*

This case study helps us appreciate the life span differences that paramedics must be prepared to address with any emergency response.

This call requires you and your partner to care for a newborn infant and her mother. These are two very different patients with very different normal vital signs, different abilities to respond to environmental stimuli, and different levels of physiological and psychosocial development. Your assessment and care must be different for each, and so you must understand the physiological differences between the two. A pulse rate of 140 and a respiratory rate of 46 would signal extreme distress in the mother but are considered in the normal range in the newborn. It is also important to understand that an active cry is a good sign of adequate respiration in the newborn, while slow, quiet respiration in the toddler may be a sign of respiratory exhaustion and failure.

While the human body maintains a relatively uniform anatomy and physiology throughout life, we must appreciate the subtle differences associated with the infant, toddler, preschooler, school-aged child, adolescent, and the early, middle-aged, and late-aged adult. Not only do vital signs change with age, but the effectiveness of the cardiovascular, respiratory, gastrointestinal, and endocrine systems do also. Further, psychosocial development affects the way the various age-grouped individuals respond to the environment and to the stresses of life and disease. Understanding life span development will increase your understanding of patients and their responses to disease.

Content Self-Evaluation

MULTIPLE CHOICE

_____ 1. In which age group does normal body temperature become that which is found in adults?
   A. Infant
   B. Toddler
   C. Preschooler
   D. School age
   E. Adolescent

_____ 2. The toddler represents a child between the ages of
   A. birth and 1 year.
   B. 1 and 3 years.
   C. 3 and 5 years.
   D. 6 and 12 years.
   E. 13 and 18 years.

_____ 3. The adolescent represents a child between the ages of
   A. birth and 1 year.
   B. 1 and 3 years.
   C. 3 and 5 years.
   D. 6 and 12 years.
   E. 13 and 18 years.

_____ **4.** Blood pressure generally rises with age.
   A. True
   B. False

_____ **5.** The respiratory rate generally rises with age.
   A. True
   B. False

_____ **6.** During the first week of life, the infant's weight is expected to
   A. increase by 2 kg per week.
   B. decrease by 5 to 10 percent.
   C. double.
   D. triple.
   E. none of the above.

_____ **7.** When compared to the airway at any other stage of life, the infant's airway is
   A. shorter.   **D.** more easily obstructed.
   B. narrower.   **E.** all of the above.
   C. less stable.

_____ **8.** The reflex sometimes referred to as the "startle reflex" is the
   A. Moro reflex.   **D.** sucking reflex.
   B. palmar reflex.   **E.** reflux reflex.
   C. rooting reflex.

_____ **9.** The anterior fontanelle closes between
   A. 1 and 2 months.
   B. 2 and 4 months.
   C. 9 and 18 months.
   D. 1 and 2 years.
   E. none of the above.

_____ **10.** The process of learning used by children in which they build upon what they already know is called
   A. bonding.
   B. secure attachment.
   C. scaffolding.
   D. benchmarking.
   E. modeling.

_____ **11.** The toddler is very susceptible to minor respiratory and gastrointestinal infections.
   A. True
   B. False

_____ **12.** The weight of the toddler's brain is approximately what percentage of the weight of the adult brain?
   A. 60 percent   **D.** 90 percent
   B. 70 percent   **E.** 96 percent
   C. 80 percent

_____ **13.** Children begin to develop magical thinking at about
   A. 1 to 2 years.
   B. 2 to 3 years.
   C. 3 to 4 years.
   D. 4 to 5 years.
   E. 5 to 6 years.

_____ **14.** The school-aged child gains about how much weight per year?
   A. 1 kg   **D.** 4 kg
   B. 2 kg   **E.** 5 kg
   C. 3 kg

15. At what age does the female generally finish growing?
   - **A.** 12
   - **B.** 14
   - **C.** 16
   - **D.** 18
   - **E.** 20

16. In late adolescence, the average male is taller and stronger than the average female.
   - **A.** True
   - **B.** False

17. Peak physical condition occurs among
   - **A.** preschool-age children.
   - **B.** school-age children.
   - **C.** adolescents.
   - **D.** early adults.
   - **E.** middle-aged adults.

18. The leading cause of death among early adults is
   - **A.** accidents.
   - **B.** cardiovascular disease.
   - **C.** cancer.
   - **D.** respiratory disease.
   - **E.** drug overdose.

19. The maximum life span for a human being is about
   - **A.** 76 years.
   - **B.** 84 years.
   - **C.** 96 years.
   - **D.** 100 years.
   - **E.** 120 years.

20. By the age of 80, the vessels of the cardiovascular system decrease their elasticity by about 50 percent.
   - **A.** True
   - **B.** False

21. During late adulthood, which of the following is expected?
   - **A.** Decreased blood volume
   - **B.** Decreased platelet count
   - **C.** Decreased number of red blood cells
   - **D.** Poor iron levels
   - **E.** All of the above

22. Which of the following is NOT expected of the respiratory system during late adulthood?
   - **A.** Enlarged alveoli
   - **B.** Decreased airway diameter
   - **C.** Reduced lung surface area
   - **D.** Stiffening of the chest wall
   - **E.** Increased likelihood of respiratory disease

23. Which of the following is a likely result of tooth loss in the elderly?
   - **A.** An increased swallowing time
   - **B.** Decreased peristalsis
   - **C.** Less effective esophageal sphincter
   - **D.** The swallowing of larger pieces of food
   - **E.** All of the above

24. The individual in late adulthood is likely to be sensitive to loud noises and yet less able to hear indistinct speech or normal conversation in the presence of loud noises.
   - **A.** True
   - **B.** False

©2013 Pearson Education, Inc.
Paramedic Care: Principles & Practice, Vol. 2, 4th Ed.

_____ **25.** Arteriosclerotic heart disease is the major killer after age 40 in all age, gender, and racial groups.
- **A.** True
- **B.** False

MATCHING

Write the letter of the development stage in the space provided next to the characteristic most commonly associated with that age group.

- **A.** infant
- **B.** toddler
- **C.** preschooler
- **D.** school age
- **E.** adolescent
- **F.** early adult
- **G.** middle-aged adult
- **H.** late-aged adult

_____ **26.** Highest level of job stress

_____ **27.** Concerned with "social clock"

_____ **28.** Baby teeth begin to appear

_____ **29.** Sexual maturity

_____ **30.** Permanent teeth

_____ **31.** Hearing loss for pure tones

_____ **32.** Development of self-concept

_____ **33.** Understanding of cause and effect

_____ **34.** Hearing maturity

_____ **35.** Loss of sucking and rooting reflexes

Special Project

Complete the following chart of normal vital signs over the life span. Review the changes that occur in each vital sign as the patient ages.

NORMAL VITAL SIGNS					
Life Stage	**Pulse**	**Respirations**	**Blood Pressure**	**Temperature (Fahrenheit)**	**Temperature (Celsius)**
Infancy (at birth)					
Infancy (at 1 year)					
Toddler (12–36 months)					
Preschool age (3–5 years)					
School age (6–12 years)					
Adolescence (13–18 years)					
Early adulthood (19–40 years)					
Middle adulthood (41–60 years)					
Late adulthood (61+ years)					

©2013 Pearson Education, Inc.
Paramedic Care: Principles & Practice, Vol. 2, 4th Ed.

Emergency Pharmacology

Because Chapter 3 is lengthy, it has been divided into parts to aid your study. Read the assigned text-book pages; then, progress through the objectives and self-evaluation materials as you would with other chapters. When you feel secure in your grasp of the content, proceed to the next section.

Review of Chapter Objectives

After reading this chapter, you should be able to:

1. **Define key terms introduced in this chapter.**

   Knowing and being able to apply the key terms in each chapter is critical to understanding chapter concepts. Write the list of key terms. Then write the definition of each one in your own words. Check your understanding by confirming the definitions in the text glossary. Correct any misunderstandings. Create a study aid by writing each key term on the front of an index card and the definition on the back. Use the cards to quiz yourself or to have someone quiz you.

Part 1: Basic Pharmacology, p. 139

Review of Chapter Objectives

After reading this part of the chapter, you should be able to:

2. **Explain the chemical, generic, brand, and official names of drugs.**   pp. 139–140

   The chemical name of a drug represents its chemical composition and molecular structure. An example is 7-chloro-1,3-dihydro-1-methyl-5-phenyl-2H-1,4-benzodiazepine-2-one.

   The generic name of a drug is suggested by the original manufacturer and confirmed by the United States Adopted Name Council. An example, for which the chemical name is given above, is diazepam.

   The official name of a drug is established by the Federal Drug Administration when it is listed in the *United States Pharmacopeia* (USP). An example is diazepam, USP.

   The brand, trade, or proprietary name of a drug is the name given the drug by a specific manufacturer. This name is a proper name and should be capitalized and may be followed by a trademark insignia. An example is Valium®, a brand name for diazepam.

3. Give examples of drugs from each of the four main sources of drugs. p. 140

The four main sources of drugs are plants, animals, minerals, and synthetics.

Plant extracts such as gums and oils have long been a source of medications. Examples include the purple foxglove, a source of digitalis (a glycoside), and deadly nightshade, a source of atropine (an alkaloid).

Animal extracts are another important source of drugs. For many years, the primary sources of insulin for treating diabetes mellitus were the extracts of bovine (cow) and porcine (pig) pancreas.

Minerals are inorganic sources of drugs such as calcium chloride and magnesium sulfate.

Synthetic drugs are created in the laboratory. They may provide alternative sources of medications for those found in nature, or they may be entirely new medications not found in nature.

4. Identify reliable reference materials for drug information. p. 140

Drug inserts usually accompany prescription drugs and list information as required by the United States Food and Drug Administration.

The *Physician's Desk Reference* (PDR) is a compilation of materials supplied by drug manufacturers (usually the drug insert material). It also contains indexing and some drug photos.

Drug Information is a publication of the Society of Health System Pharmacists. It is an authoritative listing of virtually every drug used in the United States.

The *Monthly Prescribing Reference* is a periodic publication designed to keep physicians informed regarding the prescription of medications and which prescription drugs are used for which diseases.

The *AMA Drug Evaluation* is published by the American Medical Association and is a comprehensive listing of commonly used medications.

5. Describe each of the components of a drug profile. pp. 140–141

Names: The generic, trade, and sometimes the chemical names.

Classification: The broad group to which the drug belongs.

Mechanism of action: The way the drug causes its desired effects (its pharmacodynamics).

Indications: The conditions appropriate for the drug's administration.

Pharmacokinetics: How the drug is absorbed, distributed, and eliminated, including its onset and duration of action.

Side effects/adverse reactions: The drug's untoward or undesired effects.

Routes of administration: How the drug is given.

Contraindications: Conditions that make it inappropriate to administer a drug (including conditions in which administration is likely to cause a harmful outcome).

Dosage: The amount of drug that should be given.

How supplied: The typical concentrations and preparations of the drug.

Special considerations: How the drug may affect pregnant, pediatric, and geriatric patients.

6. Explain how key drug legislation applies to the paramedic's role in administering drugs. pp. 141–142

The Pure Food and Drug Act of 1906 was enacted to improve the quality and labeling of drugs and named the *United States Pharmacopeia* as the country's official source for drug information.

The Harrison Narcotic Act of 1914 restricted the use of addictive drugs by controlling importation, manufacture, sale, and use of opium, cocaine, and their derivatives.

The Federal Food, Drug and Cosmetic Act of 1938 empowered the Food and Drug Administration (FDA) to establish and enforce standards for drugs.

In 1951, the Durham-Humphrey Amendments to the Federal Food, Drug and Cosmetic Act required pharmacists to have written or oral orders (prescriptions) for certain drugs and created a category of over-the-counter drugs.

©2013 Pearson Education, Inc.
Paramedic Care: Principles & Practice, Vol. 2, 4th Ed.

The Comprehensive Drug Abuse Prevention and Control Act of 1970 repealed the Harrison Narcotics Act, established five schedules of controlled substances, and identified levels of control and required recordkeeping for each.

7. Discuss the processes of drug research and bringing a drug to market. pp. 142–143

Initial drug testing begins with the study of both male and female mammals. After testing a drug's toxicity, researchers evaluate its pharmacokinetics—how it is absorbed, distributed, metabolized (biotransformed), and excreted—in animals. These animal studies also help determine the drug's therapeutic index (the ratio of its lethal dose to its effective dose). If the results of animal testing are satisfactory, the FDA designates the drug as an investigational new drug (IND), and researchers can then test it in humans.

Human studies take place in four phases:

Phase 1: The primary purposes of phase 1 testing are to determine the drug's pharmacokinetics, toxicity, and safe dose in humans. These studies are usually carried out on limited populations of healthy human volunteers; some drugs with a high risk of untoward effects will not be tested on healthy individuals.

Phase 2: When phase 1 studies prove that the drug is safe, it is tested on a limited population of patients who have the disease it is intended to treat. The primary purposes of phase 2 studies are to find the therapeutic drug level and watch carefully for toxic and side effects.

Phase 3: The main purposes of phase 3 testing are to refine the usual therapeutic dose and to collect relevant data on side effects. Gathering the significant amounts of data needed for these goals requires a large patient population. Phase 3 studies are usually double-blind. That is, neither the patient nor the researcher knows whether the patient is receiving a placebo or the drug until after the study has been completed. This keeps personal biases from affecting the reporting of results. Some phase 3 studies are controlled studies, which are like placebo studies except that, instead of a placebo, the patient receives a treatment that is known to be effective. Occasionally, a double-blind study will be ended sooner than planned if the early results are convincing. Once phase 3 studies are completed, the manufacturer files a New Drug Application (NDA) with the Food and Drug Administration, which then evaluates the data collected in the investigation's first three phases. At this point the FDA decides whether to conditionally approve manufacturing and marketing the drug in the United States.

Phase 4: Phase 4 testing involves postmarketing analysis during conditional approval. Once a drug is being used in the general population, the FDA requires the drug's maker to monitor its performance. Many drugs have been discontinued after marketing when previously unknown effects became apparent.

8. Explain the paramedic's roles and responsibilities with respect to administering medications. pp. 144–145

There are six basic "rights" of drug administration that indicate the paramedic's essential responsibilities and practices. They are the right medication, the right dose, the right time, the right route, the right patient, and the right documentation.

The right medication. Ensure the medication is what is intended for the patient. Review your standing orders or, if an order is received from medical direction, repeat the order back to the physician so you are both clear on the medication, dose, route, and timing of the administration. Also examine the drug packaging to ensure it is the medication you wish to administer.

The right dose. Carefully calculate the dose (usually weight dependent) for the patient before you draw up the medication and again just before you administer it. Prehospital medications are usually packaged to accommodate a single administration. If the drug package you select has much more or less than you intend to use, recheck the packaging to ensure it is the right drug and right concentration and recheck your calculations to ensure the right dosage.

The right time. Usually prehospital medications are given rather rapidly and not on a schedule. Check the packaging and your protocols for administration rate and ensure you follow the sequencing, time intervals, and drip rates for emergency drugs.

The right route. While most emergency drugs are administered by the IV route, be aware of the alternative routes of drug administration, the drugs administered via those routes, and the circumstances requiring the use of those routes. With each medication administration, ensure you are using the right route.

The right patient. It is imperative to ensure that the patient is properly matched to medication. A patient/drug mismatch is an infrequent problem in prehospital care, but as EMS moves to the out-of-hospital environment, paramedics may be treating some patients on a routine basis. Always ensure that the medication order is for the patient you are attending.

The right documentation. Thoroughly document all aspects of patient care, including what drugs (medication, dose, time, and route) were administered in what dosage.

9. **Discuss special considerations in administering drugs to pregnant, lactating, pediatric, and geriatric patients.** pp. 145–146

Pregnancy alters the mother's physiology and also adds a second party, the developing fetus, to the concerns regarding medication administration. The increased maternal heart rate, cardiac output, and blood volume can affect the onset and actions of many medications. Drugs may also alter fetal development and result in fetal injury, deformity, or death. During the third trimester, some drugs may pass through the placenta and affect the fetus directly.

Several anatomical and physiological differences between pediatric patients and adults result in differences in the ways drugs are absorbed and metabolized. Differences in gastric pH and emptying time and lower digestive enzyme levels in children change the way enteral medications are absorbed. A child's thinner skin causes topical agents to be absorbed more quickly. Lower plasma protein levels in children affect the availability of agents that usually bind to them. Higher water content in the neonate also affects drug absorption and distribution, as does the slower, then faster metabolism of the neonate and child, respectively. Organ maturity also affects drug metabolism and elimination. For children, drug administration is often guided by weight and in some cases guided by height (the Broselow tape).

With advancing age, the body's metabolism, gastric motility, decreased plasma proteins, reduced body fat and muscle mass, and depressed liver function all affect the absorption, metabolism, and elimination of drugs. Older patients are also likely to be on multiple medications for multiple diseases, thereby increasing the likelihood of adverse medication interactions.

10. **Explain key principles of pharmacokinetics.** pp. 146–151

Pharmacokinetics examines the absorption, distribution, biotransformation, and elimination of drugs.

For a drug to perform its action, it must first reach its site of action, a process referred to as absorption. While some drugs affect target tissue directly (such as antacids in the stomach), most must first find their way to the bloodstream. Drugs administered directly into a venous or arterial vessel are quickly transported to the heart, mixed with the blood, and distributed throughout the body. A drug injected into the muscle tissue and, to a somewhat lesser degree, into the subcutaneous tissue, is transported quickly to the bloodstream because of the more than adequate circulation in these tissues. However, shock and hypothermia may slow the process, whereas fever and hyperthermia may speed it. Oral medications must survive the gastric acidity and be somewhat lipid soluble to be transported across the intestinal membrane. The differing acid content of the digestive tract also affects the dissociation of the drug into ions that are more difficult to move into the circulation. And, finally, the drug's concentration affects its uptake by the bloodstream and, ultimately, its distribution. The end result of the absorption process is the concentration of the drug in the bloodstream and its availability for activation of the target tissue, called its bioavailability.

Once a drug enters the bloodstream, it must be carried throughout the body and to its site of action. The term for this process is distribution. Many factors affect the release and uptake of a drug by the body's cells. Some drugs bind to the plasma proteins of the blood and are released over a prolonged period of time. An increase in the blood's pH may increase the rate of release of the drug, or competition from other drugs for binding sites may cause more of a drug to become available. Distribution of some drugs is dependent on their ability to cross the blood-brain or placental barriers. Other drugs are easily deposited in fatty tissue, bones, and teeth.

©2013 Pearson Education, Inc.
Paramedic Care: Principles & Practice, Vol. 2, 4th Ed.

Once in the body, drugs are broken down into metabolites in a process called biotransformation. This process makes the drug more or less active and can make the drug more water soluble and easier to eliminate. Some drugs are totally metabolized, some are partially metabolized, and still others are not metabolized at all. The liver is responsible for most biotransformation, while the lungs, kidneys, and GI tract do some limited biotransformation.

Elimination is the excretion of the drug in urine, expired air, or in feces. Renal excretion is the major mechanism for eliminating drugs from the body. Drugs are eliminated as the blood pressure pushes and filters blood through kidney structures. This effect is enhanced by special cells that "pump" (active transport) some metabolites into the tubules. Kidney reabsorption also plays a part in drug excretion. Protein-soluble molecules and electrolytes are easily absorbed, but the uptake may be affected by the blood's pH.

11. Describe each of the routes of drug administration. p. 151

Enteral routes deliver medications by absorption through the gastrointestinal tract. There are several routes of enteral administration. Oral routes are the most common for drug administration and are well suited for self-administration of medication. Nasogastric or orogastric tube administration uses either type of tube to direct medications into the stomach. Sublingual administration permits the drug to be absorbed by the capillaries under the tongue. Buccal (between the cheek and gum) absorption is similar to sublingual drug administration. Rectal administration is a route used for unconscious, vomiting, seizing, or uncooperative patients.

Routes outside the gastrointestinal tract are referred to as parenteral and typically use needles to inject medications into the circulatory system or tissues. With intravenous drug administration, a drug is injected directly into the veins, leading to rapid distribution of the medication. Endotracheal medication administration uses the endotracheal tube to place the medication into the lung field, where it is quickly absorbed by the bloodstream. Intraosseous administration directs medication into the medullary space of a long bone in the pediatric patient. Umbilical drug administration uses the umbilical artery or vein as an alternative IV site in the neonate. With intramuscular administration, the medication is injected into the muscle tissue, where it is rapidly absorbed by the bloodstream. Subcutaneous administration is just slightly slower than intramuscular administration. Transdermal administration is slightly slower than subcutaneous, and topical administration has the slowest absorption rate of all routes. With administration by inhalation/nebulization, a drug is introduced into the lung field, where it is absorbed. Nasal medications are introduced into the mucous membranes of the nose and are rapidly absorbed. With instillation, a drug is placed (topically) into a wound or the eye. Intradermal medications are delivered between dermal layers.

12. Describe the various forms of drugs. pp. 151–152

Drugs come in many different forms. Solid drug forms include the following:

- Pills are drugs that are shaped spherically for easily swallowing.
- Powders are drugs simply in a powder form.
- Tablets are powders compressed into a disk-like form.
- Suppositories are drugs mixed with a wax-like base that melts at body temperature. They are usually inserted into the rectum or vagina.
- Capsules are gelatin containers filled with the drug powder or tiny pills. When the container dissolves, the drug is released into the gastrointestinal tract.

Liquid forms include the following:

- Solutions are drugs dissolved in a solvent, usually water or oil based.
- Tinctures are medications extracted using alcohol, with some alcohol usually remaining.
- Suspensions are mixtures of a solvent and drug in which the solid portion will precipitate out.
- Emulsions are suspensions with an oily substance in the solvent that remains as globules even when mixed.
- Spirits are solutions of volatile drugs in alcohol.
- Elixirs are drugs mixed with alcohol and water, often with flavorings to improve taste.
- Syrups are solutions of sugar, water, and drugs.

13. **Describe considerations in drug storage.** p. 152

Temperature, humidity, ultraviolet radiation (sunlight), and time affect the potency of many drugs. It is important that they be stored under proper conditions and that they are rotated so they are utilized (or discarded) before their shelf life expires.

14. **Explain key principles of pharmacodynamics.** pp. 152–155

Pharmacodynamics examines how drugs interact with the body to cause their effects.

Drugs may cause their effects by binding on a receptor site, by changing physical properties, by chemically combining with other substances, or by altering a normal metabolic pathway.

Most drugs effect their actions by binding to receptor sites, especially those of the autonomic nervous system. The drug either inhibits or stimulates the cells or tissue. The force of attraction of a drug is referred to as its affinity. Affinity becomes important when different drugs compete for a site. The drug's efficacy is its ability to cause the expected response. Binding to a receptor site causes a change within the cell and induces the drug's effect. However, some drugs may establish a chain-reaction effect whereby other drugs are released and cause the desired effect. The number of receptor sites may change as the drug becomes available and uses them, thereby reducing the drug's continuing effect. Chemicals that bind to the receptor and cause the expected response are termed agonists. Antagonists bind to the site and do not cause the expected response. Some drugs have both properties. Often drugs compete for a receptor site in a process called competitive antagonism, while a situation in which a drug attaches to a receptor, effectively locking out other drugs, is termed noncompetitive antagonism. Permanent binding to a receptor site is irreversible antagonism.

Drugs also may act by modifying the physical properties of a part of the body. For example, the drug mannitol changes the blood's osmolarity and increases urine output.

Some drugs chemically combine with other substances to cause their desired effect. For example, antacids interact with the hydrochloric acid in the stomach to reduce the pH.

Other drugs act by altering normal biological processes and the metabolic pathways. Such drugs are used to treat cancers and viral infections.

15. **Describe common unintended adverse effects of drug administration.** pp. 154–155

Some common unintended adverse responses to drugs include the following:

Allergic reaction. Also known as hypersensitivity; this effect occurs as the drug is antigenic and activates the immune system, causing effects that are normally more profound than seen in the general population.

Idiosyncrasy. A drug effect that is unique to the individual; different than seen or expected in the population in general.

Tolerance. Decreased response to the same amount of drug after repeated administrations.

Cross tolerance. Tolerance for a drug that develops after administration of a different drug. Morphine and other opioid agents are common examples. Tolerance for one agent implies tolerance for others as well.

Tachyphylaxis. Rapidly occurring tolerance to a drug. May occur after a single dose. This typically occurs with sympathetic agonists, specifically decongestant and bronchodilation agents.

Cumulative effect. Increased effectiveness when a drug is given in several doses.

Drug dependence. The patient becomes accustomed to the drug's presence in his body and will suffer from withdrawal symptoms upon its absence. The dependence may be physical or psychological.

Drug interaction. The effects of one drug alter the response to another drug.

Drug antagonism. The effects of one drug block the response to another drug.

Summation. Also known as an additive effect. Two drugs that both have the same effect are given together, analogous to $1 + 1 = 2$.

©2013 Pearson Education, Inc.
Paramedic Care: Principles & Practice, Vol. 2, 4th Ed.

Synergism. Two drugs that both have the same effect are given together and produce a response greater than the sum of their individual responses, analogous to 1 = 1 = 3.

Potentiation. One drug enhances the effect of another. A common example is promethazine (Phenergan) enhancing the effects of morphine.

Interference. The direct biochemical interaction between two drugs; one drug affects the pharmacology of another drug.

16. **Anticipate how various factors, such as age, body mass, and others, can alter drug responses.** p. 155

Factors altering drug response include the patient's age, body mass, gender, pathological state, genetic factors, and psychological factors, as well as environmental considerations and the time of administration. These factors may increase or decrease the drug's ability to generate its desired effect. Responses to drug administration may include unintended responses, or side effects. These are care-provider induced (iatrogenic) and include allergic reactions, idiosyncratic (unique to an individual) reactions, tolerance, cross-tolerance, tachyphylaxis, cumulative effects, dependency, drug interactions, drug antagonisms, summation, synergistic reactions (a result greater than the expected additive result of two drugs administered together), potentiation, and interference. Some of these effects may be predictable and desired and some may be unexpected.

17. **Describe various types of drug interactions.** p. 155

Drugs have the potential to interact, cause, and alter the effects of other drugs taken by a patient. One drug may alter the effects of another by altering the rate of intestinal absorption, by competing for the same plasma protein binding site, by altering the other's metabolism and hence bioavailability, by causing an antagonistic or synergistic action at a receptor site, by altering the excretion rate of another drug through the kidneys, or by altering the electrolyte balance necessary for the other drug's actions.

Case Study Review

Reread the case study on pages 138–139 in Paramedic Care: Paramedicine Fundamentals; *then, read the following discussion.*

Paramedics Jo Henderson and Scott Parker are presented with a classical myocardial infarction patient in Reverend Allen. They treat Reverend Allen with a great spectrum of drugs in an attempt to relieve discomfort and help the heart continue its coordinated and effective pumping action. These drugs include oxygen, aspirin, nitroglycerin (NitroStat), ondansetron (Zofran), morphine sulfate, and a recombinant tissue plasminogen activator like reteplase (Retavase). To administer these drugs safely, Jo and Scott must understand the pharmacological principles behind their safe and appropriate administration.

They administer supplemental oxygen by the inhalation route to increase the percentage of inspired oxygen, thereby increasing the oxygen available to the hemoglobin of the blood and increasing its saturation. The increased oxygen concentration at the capillary level helps it diffuse into the interstitial compartment and then into the body cells. Oxygen is a very safe drug to use; however, both Jo and Scott know that it may cause the chronic obstructive lung disease (emphysema or chronic bronchitis) patient to slow or stop respirations.

They give Reverend Allen oral chewable aspirin, which they know reduces the tendency of platelets to aggregate and blood to clot. It prevents the creation of new thrombi and helps maintain circulation through the restricted coronary arteries. It, like oxygen, is a very safe drug, though it can contribute to or exacerbate ulcer disease (a problem in chronic, not emergency, administration) and may prolong clotting times in the trauma patient.

They place a saline lock to provide a rapid and direct route for drug administration. The saline lock provides a direct route to the venous circulation, then to the heart and lungs, and then to the entire body through the arterial system. They can then use this route to rapidly make their drugs available to the Reverend Allen's bloodstream and body tissue systems.

Nitroglycerin is given sublingually because it is easily absorbed through the capillary beds found there. It dilates the venous system, reducing cardiac preload and oxygen consumption. Nitroglycerin also may reduce coronary vessel spasm in Prinzmetal's angina. Jo and Scott must be very careful to ensure that Reverend Allen's blood pressure is above 100, because a common side effect of nitroglycerin is orthostatic hypotension. Jo and Scott know that nitroglycerin loses its effectiveness quickly once the container is opened or when it is exposed to light. They ensure the pill has a bitter taste and remember that patients often complain of headaches when the drug is potent. Zofran is a serotonin antagonist that is given to reduce the nausea associated with the heart attack.

As Reverend Allen's chest pain continues, the paramedics administer morphine sulfate to further reduce pain and cardiac workload. Morphine is an opium derivative that reduces the ability of neurons to propagate pain impulses to the spinal cord and brain. Morphine also decreases both cardiac preload and afterload, thereby reducing myocardial oxygen demand in the patient suffering a heart attack. However, morphine's major side effects are respiratory depression and hypotension. Jo and Scott must carefully monitor Reverend Allen's respirations and blood pressure. They must also carefully document the administration of this drug, since it is a controlled substance.

Finally, Jo and Scott administer recombinant tissue plasminogen activator, one of the clot-busting, or thrombolytic, drugs, to dissolve the clot in Reverend Allen's coronary arteries and restore myocardial circulation. While this drug can reduce the impact of a coronary occlusion due to a clot, its administration poses the risk of serious internal bleeding and possible stroke. Jo and Scott evaluate a 12-lead ECG to determine the location of the probable infarct and ask Reverend Allen numerous, carefully worded questions to rule out the various internal hemorrhage risks before the drug is administered. They also carefully document the administration of this medication, because its use will continue during Reverend Allen's hospital stay.

While the steps in the care for Reverend Allen are linear and straightforward, they must be applied with a full understanding of pharmacology. Jo and Scott must ensure that they are giving the right drug to the right patient at the right time through the right route and in the right dose and concentration. They must watch for the expected therapeutic actions as well as expected side effects and untoward (unwanted and nonbeneficial) effects. However, by judiciously using medications, Jo and Scott can relieve Reverend Allen's symptoms, stabilize his vital signs, and begin to treat his disease well before he arrives at the emergency department.

Content Self-Evaluation

MULTIPLE CHOICE

_____ 1. The study of drugs and their interactions with the body is
- A. pharmaceutics.
- B. pharmacokinetics.
- C. pharmacodynamics.
- D. pharmacology.
- E. pharmacopedia.

_____ 2. Which of the following types of drug names is 7-chloro-1,3-dihydro-1-methyl-5-phenyl-2H-1,4-benzodiazepine-2-one?
- A. Chemical name
- B. Generic name
- C. Official name
- D. Brand name
- E. Common name

_____ 3. Which of the following types of drug names is diazepam?
- A. Chemical name
- B. Generic name
- C. Official name
- D. Brand name
- E. Common name

_____ 4. Digitalis is an example of a drug derived from
- A. a plant.
- B. an animal.
- C. a mineral.
- D. synthetic production.
- E. a lipid base.

_____ 5. Bovine insulin is an example of a drug derived from:
   A. a plant.
   B. an animal.
   C. a mineral.
   D. synthetic production.
   E. a lipid base.

_____ 6. The drug reference that presents manufacturer-provided drug information and some photos of drugs is the
   A. *EMS Guide to Drugs*.
   B. *Physician's Desk Reference*.
   C. *AMA Drug Evaluations*.
   D. *Monthly Prescribing Reference*.
   E. all of the above.

_____ 7. The broad group to which a drug belongs is its
   A. indication.
   B. pharmacokinetics.
   C. classification.
   D. mechanism of action.
   E. none of the above.

_____ 8. Conditions in which it is inappropriate to give a drug are referred to as its
   A. mechanisms of action.
   B. indications.
   C. contraindications.
   D. side effects.
   E. special considerations.

_____ 9. Which of the following drugs is classified as a Schedule II controlled substance?
   A. Heroin
   B. Morphine
   C. Codeine
   D. Diazepam
   E. B and C

_____ 10. The assay of a drug in a preparation determines its
   A. potency.
   B. amount and purity.
   C. effectiveness.
   D. availability in a biological model.
   E. effectiveness compared to other like drugs.

_____ 11. The bioequivalence of a drug in a preparation refers to its
   A. potency.
   B. amount and purity.
   C. effectiveness.
   D. availability in a biological model.
   E. effectiveness compared to other like drugs.

_____ 12. Which of the following is NOT one of the six rights of medication administration?
   A. Right dose
   B. Right patient
   C. Right documentation
   D. Right time
   E. Right mechanism

_____ 13. Dosages of many emergency drugs are based on patient weight, so unit dose packaging may not contain the right amount for every patient.
   A. True
   B. False

_____ 14. Children are, for the most part, just small adults, so drug dosages just need to be reduced proportionally by weight.
   A. True
   B. False

_____ 15. Drugs in which of the following FDA categories have demonstrated definite risks to the fetus?
   A. R
   B. A
   C. B
   D. C
   E. D

16. Which of the following is NOT true regarding the newborn patient?
    A. The neonate has less gastric acid than an adult.
    B. The neonate has diminished blood plasma levels.
    C. The neonate has immature renal and hepatic systems.
    D. The neonate has less body water than an adult.
    E. The neonate has lower enzyme levels than an adult.

17. Which of the following is NOT true regarding the geriatric patient?
    A. The geriatric patient has decreased gastrointestinal motility.
    B. The geriatric patient has decreased body fat.
    C. The geriatric patient has decreased muscle mass.
    D. The geriatric patient is more likely to be disease free.
    E. The geriatric patient has decreased liver function.

18. Drugs do not confer any new properties on cells or tissues; they only modify or exploit existing functions.
    A. True
    B. False

19. Which of the following is NOT one of the four basic processes of pharmacokinetics?
    A. Absorption
    B. Distribution
    C. Receptor binding
    D. Biotransformation
    E. Elimination

20. Which of the following represents an energy-consuming movement of ions against the concentration gradient?
    A. Diffusion
    B. Active transport
    C. Osmosis
    D. Filtration
    E. Facilitated transport

21. Which of the following represents movement of molecules across a membrane from an area of higher pressure to an area of lower pressure?
    A. Diffusion
    B. Active transport
    C. Osmosis
    D. Filtration
    E. Facilitated transport

22. The measure of the amount of a drug that is still active after it reaches the target organ is its
    A. bioavailability.
    B. biotransformativity.
    C. metabolism.
    D. pro-drug effect.
    E. active distribution.

23. Which of the following is NOT a significant medium for elimination of drugs from the body?
    A. Urine
    B. Respiratory air
    C. Feces
    D. Sweat
    E. All are significant

24. Which of the following is NOT an enteral route of drug administration?
    A. Oral
    B. Umbilical
    C. Buccal
    D. Sublingual
    E. Rectal

25. Which of the following is the preferred route for medication administration in most emergencies?
    A. Intramuscular
    B. Inhalation
    C. Endotracheal
    D. Intravenous
    E. Subcutaneous

26. Drugs that are mixed with a wax-like base are
    A. pills.
    B. suppositories.
    C. tablets.
    D. capsules.
    E. suspensions.

_____ 27. Drugs that are powders compressed into disks are
     A. pills.   D. capsules.
     B. suppositories.   E. suspensions.
     C. tablets.

_____ 28. Preparations in which the solid does not dissolve in the solvent are
     A. solutions.   D. spirits.
     B. tinctures.   E. elixirs.
     C. suspensions.

_____ 29. Preparations made with alcohol and water solvent, often with flavorings, are
     A. solutions.   D. spirits.
     B. tinctures.   E. elixirs.
     C. suspensions.

_____ 30. Pharmacodynamics are best described as
     A. interactions between drugs.
     B. the processes by which drugs are eliminated from the body.
     C. the effects of a drug on the body.
     D. the processes by which drugs bind to receptor sites.
     E. the processes by which a drug is administered.

_____ 31. The location where a drug combines with a protein, resulting in a biochemical effect, is a
     A. second messenger.   D. agonist.
     B. antagonist.   E. protein block.
     C. receptor.

_____ 32. A drug's ability to cause its expected response is referred to as its
     A. affinity.   D. antagonism.
     B. efficacy.   E. equilibrium.
     C. agonism.

_____ 33. A chemical that binds to a receptor site but does not cause the expected effect is a(n)
     A. partial-antagonist.   D. antagonist.
     B. competitive antagonist.   E. noncompetitive antagonist.
     C. agonist.

_____ 34. A chemical that binds to a receptor site, causes the expected effect, and prevents other drugs from activating the receptor site is a(n)
     A. partial antagonist.   D. antagonist.
     B. competitive antagonist.   E. noncompetitive antagonist.
     C. agonist.

_____ 35. The drug nalbuphine (Nubain) is an example of a(n)
     A. agonist-antagonist.   D. antagonist.
     B. competitive antagonist.   E. noncompetitive antagonist.
     C. agonist.

_____ 36. The drug morphine sulfate is an example of a(n)
     A. agonist-antagonist.   D. antagonist.
     B. competitive antagonist.   E. noncompetitive antagonist.
     C. agonist.

_____ 37. A drug reaction that is unique to an individual is referred to as
     A. idiosyncrasy.   D. synergism.
     B. tachyphylaxis.   E. potentiation.
     C. antagonism.

38. A drug reaction that is greater than expected from the administration of two drugs that have the same effect at the same time is referred to as

A. idiosyncrasy.

B. tachyphylaxis.

C. antagonism.

D. synergism.

E. potentiation.

39. The time span between when a drug drops below its minimum effective concentration and its complete elimination from the body is its

A. onset of action.

B. duration of action.

C. therapeutic index.

D. biological half-life.

E. termination of action.

40. The ratio between a drug's lethal dose and its effective dose is its:

A. onset of action.

B. duration of action.

C. therapeutic index.

D. biological half-life.

E. termination of action.

Special Project

Crossword Puzzle

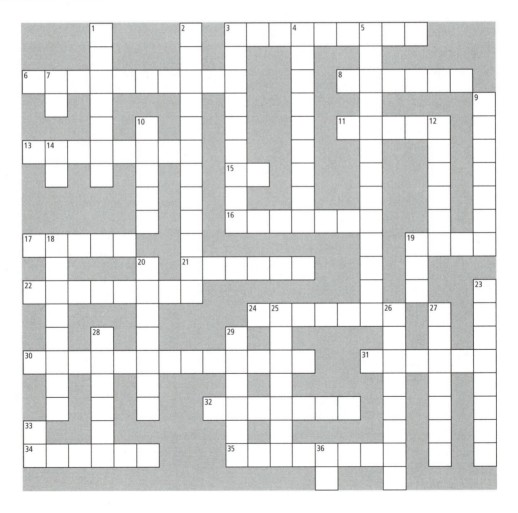

Across

3. Type of drug created in the laboratory

6. Movement of molecules across a membrane down a pressure gradient

8. _____ transport: mechanism to move a substance that requires energy

11. A sugar, water, and drug solution

13. Test that determines a drug's bioequivalency

15. Drug administration to the medullary spaces of bones (abbr.)

16. Generic term for the inorganic source of a drug

17. Route of drug administration via the nose

19. Route of drug administration via the mouth

21. Solution of a volatile drug in alcohol

22. A drug's ability to cause the expected response

24. An agent that binds to a receptor site to cause its intended response

30. Chemically equal to and having the same therapeutic effect as another drug

31. Generic term for the source of drugs extracted from living creatures

32. Drug drawn from a compound by withdrawing a carrier

34. A powder compressed into a disk-like form

35. A protein molecule on the cell wall to which a drug attaches, resulting in a biochemical effect

Down

1. Route of medication delivery via the gastrointestinal tract

2. Drug effect that is unique to an individual

3. Two drugs together producing a response greater than the expected sum of responses

4. Decreased response to the same amount of drug after repeated doses

5. Rapidly occurring tolerance to a drug

7. Route of drug administration that is slower than intravenous injection because the drug passes into the capillaries (abbr.)

9. Route of drug administration via the surface of the skin

10. Test to determine the amount and purity of a chemical in a preparation

12. Fine granular form of a drug

14. Preferred route of drug administration in most emergencies (abbr.)

18. Force of attraction between a drug and a receptor

19. Type of drugs available to the public without a prescription (abbr.)

20. Gelatin container filled with powder or small spheres of drug

23. Suspension of an oily substance in a solvent

25. Name for a drug, suggested by the manufacturer and confirmed by the United States Adopted Name Council

26. Form of a drug prepared by an alcohol extraction process

27. Movement of a solvent, through a semipermeable membrane, from an area of lower to one of higher solute concentration

28. Route of drug administration via the terminal end of the enteral route

29. Drug that is a combination of alcohol and water solvent, commonly mixed with flavorings

33. Endotracheal route of drug administration (abbr.)

36. Oral route of drug administration (abbr.)

Part 2: Drug Classifications, p. 156

Review of Chapter Objectives

After reading this part of the chapter, you should be able to:

18. **Describe the characteristics of common types of drugs used to affect the central nervous system.** pp. 156–172

The central nervous system consists of the brain and spinal column and all neurons that both originate and terminate within these structures. Since this system is responsible for conscious thought and affects many bodily functions, it is the target for many drugs used in medical care. These agents include analgesics, anesthetics, antianxiety and sedative-hypnotic drugs, antiseizure and antiepileptic drugs, CNS stimulants, and psychotherapeutic drugs.

Analgesics are used to reduce the sensation of pain. These drugs include the opioid and nonopioid analgesics, adjunctive medications (to enhance the effects of the analgesics), and opioid agonists-antagonists. Agents that block the actions of analgesics, opioid antagonists and in some cases analgesic antagonists, are used in cases of overdose or to reverse or negate the undesired effects of analgesics.

Anesthetics are used to decrease the sensation of both touch and pain. Anesthetics may be given locally or systemically and in lower doses may produce a decreased sensation of pain while the patient may remain conscious. At higher doses, anesthetics generally induce unconsciousness.

Antianxiety and sedative-hypnotic drugs are used to reduce anxiety, induce amnesia, assist sleeping, and may be used as a part of a balanced approach to anesthesia. These drugs include the benzodiazepines, barbiturates, and alcohol. They decrease (depress) the central nervous system's response to stimuli.

Antiseizure and antiepileptic agents are used to prevent seizure activity and are often associated with undesirable side effects. Antiseizure agents generally act on the sodium and calcium channels in the neural membrane and include phenytoin, carbamazepine, valproic acid, and ethosuximide.

CNS stimulants are used to treat fatigue, drowsiness, narcolepsy, obesity, and attention deficit disorders. They cause their actions by either increasing the release and effectiveness of excitatory neurotransmitters or decreasing the release or effectiveness of inhibitory neurotransmitters. These agents include amphetamines, methylamphetamines, and methylxanthines.

Psychotherapeutic medications treat mental dysfunction, including schizophrenia, depression, and bipolar disorder. Schizophrenia is treated with neuroleptic (affecting the nerves) and antipsychotic drugs (phenothiazines and butyrophenones), which block numerous peripheral neuroreceptor sites. Antidepressants increase the availability, release, or effectiveness of norepinephrine and serotonin and are used to treat depression. These medications include the tricyclic antidepressants (TCAs), the selective serotonin reuptake inhibitors (SSRIs), and monoamine oxidase inhibitors (MAOIs). Bipolar disorder (manic depression) is manifested by dramatic mood swings and is treated with lithium.

Parkinson's disease is another central nervous system disorder caused by the destruction of dopamine-releasing neurons in the portion of the brain controlling fine motor movements. This disease is treated by stimulating the dopamine release (Sinemet) or with anticholinergic agents (benztropine).

19. **Describe the characteristics of common types of drugs used to affect the autonomic nervous system.** pp. 172–186

The autonomic nervous system is located within the peripheral nervous system and consists of the sympathetic (fight-or-flight) and parasympathetic (feed-and-breed) systems. These systems are antagonistic and provide control over body functions. The autonomic nervous system controls virtually every organ and body structure not under conscious control and is responsible for maintaining the internal human environment. The nerves of the two systems do not actually touch other nerves or target organs. Messages are carried through the small space between them (synapse) via chemical messengers (neurotransmitters). Acetylcholine is the neurotransmitter at the target organs of the parasympathetic nervous system, while norepinephrine is the neurotransmitter at the target organs for the sympathetic nervous system.

Stimulation of the parasympathetic nervous system causes pupillary constriction, digestive gland secretion, decreased cardiac rate and strength of contraction, bronchoconstriction, and increased digestive activity. Cholinergic (affecting the acetylcholine receptors) drugs stimulate the parasympathetic nervous system and produce salivation, lacrimation, urination, defecation, gastric motility, and emesis (signs suggested by the acronym SLUDGE). They cause their actions directly by acting on the receptor sites (bethanechol and pilocarpine) or indirectly by inhibiting the degradation of acetylcholine (neostigmine and physostigmine). Anticholinergic (parasympatholytic) drugs oppose the actions of acetylcholine and the parasympathetic nervous system. Atropine is the prototype anticholinergic drug, while scopolamine is used to treat motion sickness and ipratropium bromide (Atrovent) is inhaled to treat bronchoconstriction caused by asthma.

Ganglionic blocking agents compete for the acetylcholine receptors at the ganglia and can effectively turn off the parasympathetic nervous system. Neuromuscular blocking agents produce a state of paralysis without inducing unconsciousness. Ganglionic stimulating agents (nicotine) stimulate the ganglia of both the parasympathetic and sympathetic nervous systems yet have no therapeutic purpose.

Stimulation of the sympathetic nervous system causes an increased heart rate and strength of contraction, bronchodilation, increased blood flow to the muscles, decreased blood flow to the skin and abdominal organs, release of glucose stores from the liver, increased energy production, decreased digestive activity, and the release of epinephrine and norepinephrine. Sympathetic receptors include four adrenergic receptors ($alpha_1$, $alpha_2$, $beta_1$, and $beta_2$) and dopaminergic receptors. $Alpha_1$ stimulation causes peripheral vasoconstriction, mild bronchoconstriction, and increased metabolism. $Alpha_2$ stimulation prevents the over-release of norepinephrine at the synapse. $Beta1$ stimulation exclusively affects the heart and causes increased heart rate, cardiac contractile force, automaticity, and conduction. $Beta_2$ stimulation causes bronchodilation and selective vasodilation. Dopaminergic stimulation causes increased circulation to the kidneys, heart, and brain. Sympathomimetic (adrenergic) drugs stimulate the effects of the sympathetic nervous system, while sympatholytic drugs block the actions of the sympathetic nervous system. $Alpha_1$ drugs increase peripheral vascular resistance, preload, and blood pressure. $Alpha_1$ agonists are used to control blood pressure or to control injury due to the infiltration of an $alpha_1$ drug. $Beta_1$ drugs stimulate the heart and are primarily used in cardiac arrest or cardiogenic shock. $Beta_1$ antagonists are used to control blood pressure, suppress tachycardia, and reduce cardiac workload in angina. $Beta_2$ agonists are used to treat asthma.

20. **Describe the characteristics of drugs used to affect the cardiovascular system.** pp. 186–201

The cardiovascular system consists of the heart, blood vessels, and the blood. The heart is a four-chambered muscular organ that pumps most of the blood around the body. It is controlled by an intrinsic electrical system that coordinates cardiac muscular response and pumping action. The myocardium is unique in that it has the ability to generate an electrical impulse (automaticity) and conduct an impulse to surrounding tissue (conductivity). The heart muscle contracts and relaxes (depolarizes and repolarizes) as sodium, calcium, and potassium ions flow into and out of the cell.

Antidysrhythmic drugs are used to prevent or treat abnormal variations in the cardiac electrical cycle. Sodium channel blockers slow the influx of sodium back into the cell and, in effect, slow conduction through the atria and ventricles. Class IA sodium channel blockers (quinidine, procainamide, and disopyramide) slow repolarization, while class IB drugs (lidocaine, phenytoin, tocainide, mexiletine) speed repolarization and reduce automaticity in the ventricles. Class IC drugs (flecainide, propafenone) decrease conduction velocity through the atria, ventricles, bundle of His, and the Purkinje network and delay ventricular repolarization.

Beta blockers (propranolol, acebutolol, esmolol) are antagonistic to the beta$_1$ actions of the sympathetic nervous system. Since the beta receptors are attached to the calcium channels of the heart, these agents act in a manner very similar to the calcium channel blockers. Potassium channel blockers (bretylium, amiodarone) block the efflux of calcium; these agents prolong repolarization and the effective refractory period (the period before the myocardium can contract again). Calcium channel blockers (verapamil, diltiazem) decrease conductivity through the AV node and slow conduction of atrial flutter or fibrillation to the ventricles. Other antidysrhythmics include adenosine (a fast- and short-acting potassium and calcium blocker), digoxin (decreases SA node firing rate and conduction velocity through the AV node), and magnesium (effective in treating a polymorphic ventricular tachycardia—torsade de pointes).

Antihypertensive drugs manipulate peripheral vascular resistance, heart rate, or stroke volume to reduce blood pressure. Diuretics reduce the amount of circulating blood (and hence the cardiac preload and stroke volume) by increasing the urine output of the kidneys. They include loop diuretics (furosemide), thiazides (HydroDIURIL), potassium-sparing diuretics (spironolactone), and the osmotic diuretics (mannitol). Beta-adrenergic antagonists (metoprolol) act by reducing the heart's rate and contractility as well as by reducing the release of hormones (renin) from the kidneys that ultimately cause vasoconstriction (through the renin-angiotensin-aldosterone system). Centrally acting adrenergic inhibitors (clonidine) stimulate alpha$_2$ receptors and inhibit the release of norepinephrine. Alpha$_1$ antagonists (prazosin, terazosin) competitively block the alpha$_1$ receptors, mediating sympathetic increases in peripheral vascular resistance.

Finally, some drugs (labetalol, carvedilol) have combined alpha and beta antagonistic effects. Angiotensin converting enzyme (ACE) inhibitors (captopril, enalapril, lisinopril, enalaprilat) block the production of angiotensin II, a very potent vasoconstictor, through the renin-angiotensin-aldosterone system. Angiotensin II receptor antagonists act on the renin-angiotensin-aldosterone system by blocking the actions of angiotensin II at its receptor site. Calcium channel blockers (nifedipine) are also effective at controlling hypertension by selectively acting on the smooth muscles of the arterioles and reducing peripheral vascular resistance without reducing cardiac preload. Direct vasodilators (hydralazine, minoxidil, sodium nitroprusside) selectively dilate arterioles and decrease peripheral vascular resistance. Hypertension may also be controlled by agents that block the autonomic nervous system (trimethaphan) or with cardiac glycosides (digoxin, digitoxin) that affect the ion pumps of the myocardium and increase cardiac contraction strength but reduce heart rate.

Angina is treated with calcium channel blockers (verapamil, diltiazem, nifedipine) because they reduce cardiac workload and slow the heart rate. Organic nitrates (nitroglycerin, isosorbide, amyl nitrite) relax vascular smooth muscle, decreasing cardiac preload and workload, and, in Prinzmetal's angina, may increase coronary blood flow.

Three agents are used to prevent and break up blood clots that obstruct either the heart chambers or the blood vessels. Antiplatelet drugs (aspirin, dipyridamole, abciximab, ticlopidine) decrease the formation of platelet plugs during the clotting process. Anticoagulants (heparin, warfarin) interrupt the clotting cascade. Fibrinolytics (streptokinase, alteplase, reteplase, anistreplase) dissolve the fibrin mesh of clots and thereby help break apart clots after they form.

Antihyperlipidemic agents (lovastatin, simvastatin, cholestyramine) are used to reduce the level of low-density lipoproteins, a causative factor for coronary artery disease.

21. **Describe the characteristics of drugs used to affect the respiratory system.** pp. 201–205

The respiratory system is basically a pathway through which air travels in from the exterior to the air-exchange sacs, the alveoli, and then out again. Indications for pharmacological intervention include asthma, rhinitis, and cough.

Asthma is a pathological condition caused by an allergy to pet dander, dust, or mold that causes respiratory restriction or obstruction. The allergic response releases histamine, leukotrienes, and prostaglandins, producing immediate bronchoconstriction and then inflammation. Treatment includes beta$_2$ agonists (albuterol) to reduce bronchoconstriction and epinephrine for severe reactions not responding to beta$_2$ agonists. Anticholinergic agents (ipratropium) act along different pathways to the beta$_2$ agonists

©2013 Pearson Education, Inc.
Paramedic Care: Principles & Practice, Vol. 2, 4th Ed.

and may provide an additive effect in limiting bronchoconstriction. Glucocorticoids (beclomethasone, methylprednisolone, cromolyn) have anti-inflammatory properties that reduce the amount of mucus and the edema in the airway and alveolar walls. Lastly, leukotriene antagonists (zileuton) block the formation of, or the receptors for (zafirlukast), leukotriene. Leukotrienes are mediators released from mast cells that contribute powerfully to both bronchoconstriction and inflammation.

Rhinitis is the inflammation of the mucosa of the nasal cavity and may cause nasal congestion, itching, sneezing, and rhinorrhea (runny nose). Nasal decongestants (phenylephrine, pseudoephedrine, phenylpropanolamine) are alpha₁ agonists that reduce vasodilation and are given in mist or oral form. Antihistamines (alkylamines, ethanolamines, clemastine, phenothiazines, loratadine, cetirizine, fexofenadine) are used for more serious allergic reactions and block the action of histamine and thereby relieve bronchoconstriction, capillary permeability, and vasodilation. Cough suppressants (antitussive agents, both opioid and nonopioid) dull the cough reflex and are designed to treat unproductive coughing due to an irritated oropharynx. Expectorants are intended to increase the productivity of the cough, while mucolytics make the mucus more watery and possibly more effective.

22. Describe the characteristics of drugs used to affect the gastrointestinal system. pp. 205–208

Drugs used to treat the gastrointestinal system are primarily for gastric ulcers, constipation, diarrhea, emesis, and to aid digestion. Peptic ulcer disease occurs as the balance between the protective coating of the stomach and its acidity is no longer maintained. The acid may then eat away at the intestinal lining and tissues underneath. The injury may result in internal hemorrhage. Peptic ulcer disease is treated with antibiotics (bismuth, metronidazole, amoxicillin, tetracycline) to treat the underlying cause and drugs (cimetidine, ranitidine, famotidine, nizatidine, omeprazole, lansoprazole, antacids, pirenzepine) that block or decrease the secretion of acid. Constipation is treated with bulk-forming (methylcellulose, psyllium), surfactant (docusate sodium), stimulant (phenolphthalein, bisacodyl) or osmotic (magnesium hydroxide) laxatives. Diarrhea is often caused by an underlying disease and is usually self-correcting. In severe cases, it is treated with antibiotics. Input from the inner ear, nose, and eyes or a response to anxiety or fear triggers the vomiting reflex (emesis), which can be useful for certain poisonings and overdoses. Antiemetics that reduce the vomiting reflex include serotonin antagonists (Ondansetron), dopamine antagonists (phenothiazines, butyrophenones, metoclopramide), anticholinergic and cannabinoids (dronabinol, nabilone). Finally, drugs used to aid ingestion are enzymes (pancreatin, pancrelipase) similar to endogenous enzymes found in the intestinal tract.

23. Describe the characteristics of drugs used to affect the endocrine system. pp. 208–212

The endocrine system provides the body with hormones essential to maintaining homeostasis and controlling overall body activity. It consists of the following glands: pituitary, pineal, thyroid, thymus, parathyroid, adrenal, pancreas, ovaries, and testes. These organs produce hormones that then circulate throughout the body and affect target organs. Drugs can affect the anterior and posterior pituitary, parathyroid and thyroid, adrenal, pancreas, and reproductive glands or simulate the hormones they produce.

The pituitary gland is made up of the anterior and posterior lobes and resides deep within the skull. The anterior pituitary gland releases hormones related to growth. Dwarfism results from a deficiency in growth hormone and is treated with somatrem and somatropin. Gigantism and acromegaly usually result from a tumor and are treated by surgical removal of the tumor or with the drug octreotide, which inhibits the release of the growth hormone. The posterior pituitary produces oxytocin and antidiuretic hormone (ADH). Oxytocin induces uterine contractions and precipitates delivery, while antidiuretic hormone increases water reabsorption in the kidneys and thereby regulates electrolyte balance, blood volume, and blood pressure. Diabetes insipidus is caused by inadequate circulating ADH and is treated with vasopressin, desmopressin, and lypressin.

The parathyroid gland regulates the levels of calcium and vitamin D. Chronic low calcium and vitamin D levels are treated with supplements, while high levels (usually due to tumors) are treated with surgical removal of all or part of the parathyroid gland.

The thyroid gland hormones play vital roles in growth, maturation, and metabolism. Childhood-onset hyperthyroidism results in dwarfism and mental retardation, while adult-onset hyperthyroidism manifests with a decreased metabolism, weight gain, fatigue, and bradycardia. Hypothyroidism is treated with levothyroxine, a synthetic analogue of thyroxine, the major thyroid hormone. Goiters occur as a result of inadequate iodine in the diet and are treated with iodine supplements. Thyroid tumors often cause hyperthyroidism and are treated with surgery, radiation therapy, or the drug propylthiouracil or a combination of therapies.

The adrenal cortex secretes glucocorticoids that increase the glucose in the bloodstream, mineralocorticoids that regulate the salt/water balance, and androgens that regulate sexual development and maturity. Cushing's disease results in increased glucocorticoid secretion and hyperglycemia, obesity, hypertension, and electrolyte imbalances. It is usually treated surgically, with pharmacological intervention aimed at the symptoms; drugs used for this include antihypertensive agents (spironolactone), ACE inhibitors (captopril), and drugs that inhibit corticoid synthesis. Addison's disease is characterized by hyposecretion of corticoids and presents with hypoglycemia, emaciation, hypotension, hyperkalemia, and hyponatremia. It is treated with cortisone, hydrocortisone, and fludrocortisone.

The pancreas produces two hormones important to glucose metabolism. They are insulin and glucagon. Insulin is essential for the transport of glucose, potassium, and amino acids into the cells. It stimulates cell growth and division and converts glucose into glycogen in the liver and skeletal muscles. Glucagon increases blood glucose levels by promoting the synthesis of glucose from glycerol and amino acids and from breaking down glycogen into glucose. Diabetes is an inappropriate carbohydrate metabolism due to an inadequate release of insulin (type I, juvenile onset) or a decreased responsiveness to insulin (type II, adult onset). Oral hypoglycemic agents stimulate insulin release from the pancreas and are administered to the type II diabetic. They are from four classes: sulfonylureas (tolbutamide, chlorpropamide, glipizide, glyburide), biguanides (metformin), alpha-glucosidase inhibitors (acarbose, miglitol), and thiazolidinediones (troglitazone). Pork, beef, or human insulin is injected subcutaneously daily for the type I diabetic. Hyperglycemic agents (glucagon and diazoxide) act to increase blood glucose levels while 50 percent dextrose in water ($D_{50}W$) is an intravenous sugar solution intended to supply carbohydrates to the hypoglycemic patient.

The genitalia release hormones that regulate human sexuality and reproduction. In the female, the ovaries, ovarian follicles, and, during pregnancy, the placenta, release these hormones. Drug therapy can supplement these hormones, provide contraception, stimulate or relax the pregnant uterus, or assist in fertility. Estrogen is administered postmenopause to reduce the risk of osteoporosis and coronary artery disease. It is also administered in delayed puberty. Progestins counteract the untoward effects of estrogen and are used to treat amenorrhea, endometriosis, and dysfunctional uterine hemorrhage. Estrogen and progestin (or progestin alone) are commonly used as contraceptives. Their side effects include a predisposition to thromboembolisms, hypertension, and uterine bleeding. Oxytocic agents (oxytocin) induce uterine contractions to induce or speed up labor, while tocolytics (terbutaline, ritodrine) relax the smooth muscle of the uterus and delay labor. Female infertility is treated with agents (clomiphene, urofollitropin, menotropin) that promote maturation of ovarian follicles. In the male, testosterone replacement therapy (testosterone enanthate, methyltestosterone, fluoxymesterone) is provided for deficiency or delayed puberty. An enlarged prostate is cared for with surgery or drug (finasteride) therapy.

Recent drugs, such as sildenafil (Viagra), vardenafil (Levitra) and tadalafil (Cialis), are used for erectile dysfunction and act by relaxing vascular smooth muscle. However, in combination with nitrates, these drugs may lead to decreased cardiac preload and profound hypotension.

24. **Describe the characteristics of drugs used to affect the following systems and structures:**

   a. **the eyes** p. 208

   Ophthalmic drugs are used to treat conditions involving the eyes, primarily glaucoma and trauma. In addition, some ophthalmic agents are used in diagnosing and examining the eyes.

   b. **the ears** p. 208

   Most drugs used to treat conditions involving the ear are aimed at eliminating underlying bacterial or fungal infections or at breaking up impacted earwax.

   c. **the female reproductive system** pp. 212–213

   The main groups of drugs affecting the female reproductive system are estrogens, progestins, oral contraceptives, drugs affecting uterine contraction, and those used to treat infertility.

   d. **the male reproductive system** p. 213

   Drugs that affect the male reproductive system include those that treat testosterone deficiency and benign prostatic hyperplasia.

©2013 Pearson Education, Inc.
Paramedic Care: Principles & Practice, Vol. 2, 4th Ed.

e. **the skin** **p. 216**

Dermatologic drugs are used to cleanse, protect, and treat skin irritations.

25. **Describe the characteristics of drugs used to treat the following disorders:**

a. **cancer** **pp. 213–215**

Because cancer is the abnormal growth of normal cells, drugs that kill cancerous cells therefore also kill noncancerous cells. Chemotherapy is thus largely a balancing act aimed at maximizing the kill rate of cancer cells while minimizing the death of normal tissue. The one characteristic that most cancer cells share is rapid cell division and replication. Consequently, most antineoplastic agents have their greatest effect on cancer cells during mitosis and on young, small cancers that are undergoing rapid growth.

The agents used to kill cancer cells are grouped according to their mechanism of action. Antimetabolite drugs mimic some of the enzymes and proteins needed for DNA replication but do not have the same effects; therefore, they prevent cells from reproducing. Their prototype is fluorouracil (Adrucil). Alkylating agents that interfere with DNA splitting include cyclophosphamide (Cytoxan) and mechlorethamine (Mustargen). Mitotic inhibitors also interfere with cell division; they include vinblastine (Velban) and vincristine (Oncovin).

b. **infection and inflammation** **pp. 215–216**

Infectious diseases are typically caused by bacteria, viruses, or fungi and are treated by antimicrobial drugs including antibiotics and antifungal, antiviral, and antiparasitic agents. Symptoms of microbial infection are treated with nonsteroidal anti-inflammatory drugs (NSAIDs), and some diseases are treated prophylactically with serums and vaccines.

Antibiotics either kill the offending bacteria or decrease their ability to grow and reproduce. Penicillin, cephalosporin, and vancomycin act by inhibiting cell wall synthesis and causing the walls to rupture. Macrolide, aminoglycoside, and tetracycline antibiotics prevent cells from replicating.

Antifungal agents inhibit fungal growth (ketoconazole), while antiviral drugs act through various mechanisms (indinavir, acyclovir, zidovudine). Antiparasitic agents are used to treat malaria (chloro-quine, mefloquine, quinine), amebiasis (paromomycin, metronidazole), and helminthiasis (mebendazole, niclosamide).

Other antimicrobials are used to treat diseases such as tuberculosis (isoniazid, refampin) and leprosy (dapsone, clofazimine).

Nonsteroidal anti-inflammatory drugs (ketorolac, piroxicam, naproxen) limit the fever (antipyretics) and pain (analgesics) associated with headache, arthritis, dysmenorrhea, and orthopedic injuries.

c. **poisonings and overdoses** **pp. 219–221**

The treatment for poisoning and overdose depends greatly on the substance involved. In general, therapy aims at eliminating the substance by emptying the gastric contents, by increasing gastric motility in order to decrease the time available for absorption, by alkalinizing the urine with sodium bicarbonate (for tricyclic antidepressant and salicylate overdose), or by filtering the substance from the blood with dialysis. Activated charcoal may be used as a gastric absorbent.

Actual antidotes are few; however, some medications are effective in treating certain overdoses or poisonings. General mechanisms for antidote action include receptor site antagonism, blocking enzyme actions involved with metabolism of the substance, and chelation (binding the substance with a stable compound such as iron so that it becomes inactive).

26. **Describe the characteristics of drugs used to supplement the diet.** **pp. 216–219**

Vitamins are organic compounds necessary for many different physiologic processes including metabolism, growth, development, and tissue repair. The body absorbs most vitamins through the gastrointestinal tract following dietary ingestion. Vitamins must be obtained from the diet, as the body cannot manufacture them.

Water comprises approximately 60 percent of a person's total body weight. The specific composition and amounts of this fluid are vital to a patient's well-being.

The specific amounts of electrolytes such as calcium, potassium, sodium, and chlorine are similarly important.

Content Self-Evaluation

MULTIPLE CHOICE

_____ 1. Drugs can be classified by
A. the body system they affect.
B. the mechanism of their action.
C. their indications.
D. their source.
E. all of the above.

_____ 2. The drug that demonstrates the common properties of a class of drugs is called a
A. root drug.
B. prototype drug.
C. characteristic drug.
D. primary drug.
E. none of the above.

_____ 3. Which of the following is NOT a division of the nervous system?
A. Central nervous system
B. Peripheral nervous system
C. Autonomic nervous system
D. Sympathetic nervous system
E. Antagonistic nervous system

_____ 4. Which nervous system controls motor functions?
A. Somatic
B. Autonomic
C. Sympathetic
D. Parasympathetic
E. Antagonistic

_____ 5. Which nervous system is responsible for the "feed-or-breed" response?
A. Somatic
B. Autonomic
C. Sympathetic
D. Parasympathetic
E. Antagonistic

_____ 6. A drug that relieves pain only is termed a(n)
A. anesthetic.
B. endorphin.
C. analgesic.
D. opioid.
E. antimanic.

_____ 7. The prototype opioid drug is
A. heroin.
B. morphine.
C. aspirin.
D. ibuprofen.
E. acetaminophen.

_____ 8. Naloxone (Narcan) is the principal
A. nonopioid analgesic.
B. opioid agonist.
C. opioid antagonist.
D. prehospital anesthetic.
E. opioid agonist-antagonist.

_____ 9. Anesthetics, as a group, tend to cause which of the following?
A. Reconfigured sensation
B. Respiratory stimulation
C. Central nervous system depression
D. Cardiovascular stimulation
E. Endorphin stimulation

_____ 10. When using neuromuscular blocking agents, it is common to use antianxiety, amnesic, and analgesic agents as well.
A. True
B. False

_____ 11. Which of the following is the only anesthetic gas given in the prehospital setting?
A. Ether
B. Halothane
C. Enflurane
D. Nitrous oxide
E. Sodium pentothal

_____ 12. Hypnotic is a term that describes a drug that
- A. decreases anxiety.
- B. instigates sleep.
- C. reduces sensation.
- D. decreases pain sensation.
- E. is an opioid antagonist.

_____ 13. The antagonist for the benzodiazepines is
- A. naloxone.
- B. flumazenil.
- C. thiopental.
- D. diazepam.
- E. midazolam.

_____ 14. Amphetamines cause which of the following?
- A. Release of epinephrine
- B. Release of dopamine
- C. Decreased wakefulness
- D. Increased appetite
- E. Weight gain

_____ 15. Caffeine is classified as a(n)
- A. methylxanthine.
- B. methylphenidate.
- C. amphetamine.
- D. opioid.
- E. endorphin.

_____ 16. The drug class used to care for patients with mental dysfunctions is
- A. neuroleptic.
- B. psychotherapeutic.
- C. extrapyramidal.
- D. schizophrenic.
- E. antimanic.

_____ 17. It appears that dopamine, norepinephrine, and serotonin play a role in psychotic pathologies.
- A. True
- B. False

_____ 18. As a result of the extrapyramidal effects of antipsychotic drugs, these drugs are termed
- A. Parkinsonian agents.
- B. extrapyramidogenics.
- C. neuroleptics.
- D. dopamine agonists.
- E. neurotransmitters.

_____ 19. The drug of choice for treating the extrapyramidal symptoms associated with antipsychotic drugs is
- A. diazepam.
- B. furosemide.
- C. chlorpromazine.
- D. diphenhydramine.
- E. epinephrine.

_____ 20. Which of the following is NOT a sign or symptom of depression?
- A. Weight loss
- B. Weight gain
- C. Sleep disturbances
- D. Excessive energy
- E. Inability to concentrate

_____ 21. Expected side effects of tricyclic antidepressants include all of the following EXCEPT
- A. blurred vision.
- B. dry mouth.
- C. urinary retention.
- D. bradycardia.
- E. orthostatic hypotension.

_____ 22. Tricyclic antidepressants (TCAs) raise the seizure threshold and are effective antiseizure medications.
- A. True
- B. False

_____ 23. The drug of choice for the management of bipolar disorder is
- A. valium.
- B. lithium.
- C. imipramine.
- D. phenelzine.
- E. morphine sulfate.

_____ **24.** Parkinson's disease may present with which characteristic signs and symptoms?
- **A.** Elation
- **B.** Unsteady gait
- **C.** Postural rigidity
- **D.** Tachykinesia
- **E.** Aggressiveness

_____ **25.** Parkinson's disease is caused by a reduced number of presynaptic terminals that release dopamine.
- **A.** True
- **B.** False

_____ **26.** Dopamine is given directly to the Parkinson's disease patient to help balance the dopamine/acetylcholine balance.
- **A.** True
- **B.** False

_____ **27.** Which nervous system works in opposition to the parasympathetic nervous system?
- **A.** Central
- **B.** Sympathetic
- **C.** Autonomic
- **D.** Somatic
- **E.** Antagonistic

_____ **28.** The agents that transport impulses through the synapse between neurons and between nerve cells and the target organs are called
- **A.** neuroeffectors.
- **B.** neurotransmitters.
- **C.** intrasynaptic agents.
- **D.** neuroleptic ions.
- **E.** transport cells.

_____ **29.** The cholinergic neurotransmitter is
- **A.** acetylcholine.
- **B.** epinephrine.
- **C.** norepinephrine.
- **D.** muscarinic antagonist.
- **E.** muscarinic agonist.

_____ **30.** Which neurotransmitter serves both the sympathetic and parasympathetic nervous systems?
- **A.** Acetylcholine
- **B.** Epinephrine
- **C.** Norepinephrine
- **D.** Dopamine
- **E.** None of the above

_____ **31.** A drug that stimulates the parasympathetic nervous system is called a(n)
- **A.** sympatholytic.
- **B.** sympathomimetic.
- **C.** parasympatholytic.
- **D.** parasympathomimetic.
- **E.** antiemetic.

_____ **32.** Which of the following is also a cholinergic drug?
- **A.** A sympatholytic
- **B.** A sympathomimetic
- **C.** A parasympatholytic
- **D.** A parasympathomimetic
- **E.** An antiemetic

_____ **33.** The acronym that describes the effects of cholinergic stimulation is
- **A.** SARIN.
- **B.** 2-PAM.
- **C.** SLUDGE.
- **D.** ALPHA.
- **E.** BETA.

_____ **34.** The effects of cholinergic stimulation include all of the following EXCEPT
- **A.** salivation.
- **B.** tachycardia.
- **C.** defecation.
- **D.** urination.
- **E.** emesis.

_____ **35.** The prototype anticholinergic drug is
- **A.** epinephrine.
- **B.** norepinephrine.
- **C.** acetylcholine.
- **D.** atropine.
- **E.** dopamine.

©2013 Pearson Education, Inc.
Paramedic Care: Principles & Practice, Vol. 2, 4th Ed.

36. Neuromuscular blockade produces paralysis and amnesia of the event.
    A. True
    B. False

37. Which of the following is NOT an action caused by nicotine?
    A. Tachycardia
    B. Increased salivation
    C. Vasoconstriction
    D. Hypotension
    E. Increased gastric secretion

38. The sympathetic nervous system originates from which regions of the spinal cord?
    A. Cranial and sacral
    B. Cranial and lumbar
    C. Cranial and thoracic
    D. Thoracic and lumbar
    E. Thoracic and sacral

39. Norepinephrine represents approximately what percentage of the hormones released by the stimulated adrenal medulla?
    A. 20 percent
    B. 40 percent
    C. 60 percent
    D. 80 percent
    E. 90 percent

40. Which of the following receptors is inhibitory?
    A. Alpha$_1$
    B. Alpha$_2$
    C. Beta$_1$
    D. Cholinergic
    E. Dopaminergic

41. Stimulation of which of the following receptors causes both vasodilation and bronchodilation?
    A. Alpha$_1$
    B. Alpha$_2$
    C. Beta$_1$
    D. Beta$_2$
    E. Dopaminergic

42. It has been long thought that stimulation of which of the following receptors caused dilation of the renal, coronary, and cerebral arteries?
    A. Alpha$_1$
    B. Apha$_2$
    C. Beta$_1$
    D. Beta$_2$
    E. Dopaminergic

43. Alpha$_1$ antagonist drugs are used almost exclusively to control hypertension.
    A. True
    B. False

44. What effect does alpha stimulation have on the heart?
    A. Increases heart rate
    B. Increases automaticity
    C. Increases contractile strength
    D. Increases oxygen consumption
    E. None of the above

45. Which type of drug decreases cardiac contractility and heart rate?
    A. Beta$_2$ agonists
    B. Beta$_1$ antagonists
    C. Beta$_1$ agonists
    D. Alpha$_1$ antagonists
    E. Alpha$_1$ agonists

46. Which type of drug causes bronchodilation?
    A. Beta$_2$ agonists
    B. Beta$_1$ antagonists
    C. Beta$_1$ agonists
    D. Alpha$_1$ antagonists
    E. Alpha$_1$ agonists

47. The prototype beta blocker is
    A. isoproterenol.
    B. dopamine.
    C. atropine.
    D. propranolol.
    E. none of the above.

48. Which of the following is NOT a naturally occurring catecholamine?
   A. Dopamine
   B. Epinephrine
   C. Norepinephrine
   D. Isoproterenol
   E. A and C

49. Which response contains the proper order of an electrical impulse as it travels through the cardiac conduction system?
   A. Bundle of His, SA node, AV node, Purkinje fibers, internodal pathways
   B. AV node, internodal pathways, SA node, bundle of His, Purkinje fibers
   C. Internodal pathways, AV node, SA node, Purkinje fibers, bundle of His
   D. SA node, internodal pathways, AV node, bundle of His, Purkinje fibers
   E. Bundle of His, SA node, internodal pathways, AV node, Purkinje fibers

50. The unique property of myocardial muscle tissue that permits it to generate an electrical impulse is
   A. inotropy.
   B. automaticity.
   C. contractility.
   D. autonomic firing.
   E. depolarization.

51. The heart's dominant pacemaker is the
   A. AV node.
   B. SA node.
   C. Purkinje fibers.
   D. bundle of His.
   E. internodal pathways.

52. Beta blockers and calcium channel blockers have similar effects on the heart.
   A. True
   B. False

53. Adenosine produces which of the following?
   A. Facial pallor
   B. Chest pain
   C. Bronchodilation
   D. Marked tachycardias
   E. All of the above

54. Hypertension affects about how many people in the United States?
   A. 10 million
   B. 25 million
   C. 50 million
   D. 100 million
   E. 250 million

55. Which of the following is an osmotic diuretic?
   A. Hydrochlorothiazide
   B. Furosemide
   C. Potassium chloride
   D. Mannitol
   E. Spironolactone

56. The renin-angiotensin-aldosterone system performs what function?
   A. Increasing hepatic function
   B. Decreasing blood volume
   C. Increasing vasoconstriction
   D. Causing severe bronchoconstriction
   E. All of the above

57. Which of the following drug types is used in the treatment of hypertension?
   A. Antihyperlipidemics
   B. Glucocorticoids
   C. Calcium channel blockers
   D. Cardiac glycosides
   E. All of the above

58. Which of the following is/are actions caused by the administration of digoxin?
   A. Decreases intracellular sodium levels
   B. Decreases intracellular calcium
   C. Increases the strength of cardiac muscle contraction
   D. Increases ventricular engorgement during left heart failure
   E. All of the above

©2013 Pearson Education, Inc.
Paramedic Care: Principles & Practice, Vol. 2, 4th Ed.

59. The primary action of nitroglycerin in angina is to
  A. reduce preload.
  B. reduce peripheral vascular resistance.
  C. dilate the coronary arteries.
  D. reduce the anginal pain.
  E. increase blood pressure.

60. The enzyme responsible for breaking down the fibrin of a clot once an injury has been repaired is
  A. adenosine diphosphate.
  B. thromboxane.
  C. vitamin K.
  D. plasmin.
  E. none of the above

61. Thrombi are the primary pathologies for which of the following?
  A. Stroke
  B. Myocardial infarction
  C. Pulmonary embolism
  D. Hypertension
  E. All of the above except D

62. Which of the following prevents thrombi by interrupting the clotting cascade?
  A. Antiplatelets
  B. Anticoagulants
  C. Fibrinolytics
  D. Hemostatic agents
  E. All of the above

63. All of the following are used to treat or prevent thrombi EXCEPT
  A. antiplatelets.
  B. antihyperlipidemic agents.
  C. fibrinolytics.
  D. oral anticoagulants.
  E. parenteral anticoagulants.

64. Warfarin is contraindicated in pregnant mothers because it is likely to cause
  A. uterine bleeding.
  B. birth defects.
  C. maternal hypertension.
  D. vitamin K toxicity.
  E. placenta previa.

65. Of the hemostatic agents, which can dissolve clots once they have formed?
  A. Aspirin
  B. Heparin
  C. Warfarin
  D. Streptokinase
  E. Thrombarin

66. Which of the following is of greatest help in reducing cholesterol levels in the blood?
  A. Low-density lipoproteins (LDL)
  B. Very-low-density lipoproteins (VLDL)
  C. High-density lipoproteins (HDL)
  D. Intermediate-density lipoproteins (IDL)
  E. Neutral-density lipoproteins (NDL)

67. Which of the following events occurs first in an asthma attack?
  A. Inflammatory response
  B. Mast cell rupture
  C. Release of histamine and leukotrienes
  D. Immediate bronchospasm
  E. Allergen binding to antibody on the mast cell

68. Which of the following groups is NOT used to treat asthma?
  A. Leukotriene antagonists
  B. Glucocorticoids
  C. Ganglionic blocking agents
  D. Methylxanthines
  E. Anticholinergics

69. Which of the following is the first line therapy for asthma?
  A. Selective beta$_2$ agonists
  B. Nonselective sympathomimetics
  C. Anticholinergics
  D. Glucocorticoids
  E. Leukotriene antagonists

_____ **70.** Nasal decongestants act by which of the following actions?
   A. Restricting histamine release
   B. Blocking histamine action
   C. Constricting nasal capillaries
   D. Thinning nasal mucus
   E. All of the above

_____ **71.** Histamine is a major agent in the severe anaphylactic reaction.
   A. True
   B. False

_____ **72.** Antihistamine drugs are NOT indicated for asthma patients because they thicken bronchial secretions.
   A. True
   B. False

_____ **73.** A drug that suppresses the urge to cough is a(n)
   A. expectorant.
   B. mucolytic.
   C. antitussive.
   D. surfactant.
   E. cannabinoid.

_____ **74.** Most peptic ulcer disease is caused by
   A. over-secretion of gastric acid.
   B. stress.
   C. alcohol consumption.
   D. decreased gastric circulation.
   E. a bacterium.

_____ **75.** Which of the following is a type of laxative?
   A. Bulk-forming
   B. Osmotic
   C. Surfactant
   D. Stimulant
   E. All of the above

_____ **76.** The drug chloramphenicol is used to treat what condition involving the ears?
   A. Bacterial infections
   B. Viral infections
   C. Impacted wax
   D. Inflammation/irritation
   E. All of the above

_____ **77.** Which of the following drugs has/have ototoxic properties?
   A. Aspirin
   B. Other nonsteroidal anti-inflammatory drugs
   C. Some antibiotics
   D. Furosemide
   E. All of the above

_____ **78.** The gland of the endocrine system that is regarded as the master gland is the
   A. pituitary.
   B. thyroid.
   C. parathyroid.
   D. pancreas.
   E. adrenal.

_____ **79.** The hormones produced by the thyroid play vital roles in growth, maturation, and
   A. acromegaly.
   B. electrolyte balance.
   C. metabolism.
   D. gastric secretion regulation.
   E. all of the above.

_____ **80.** Goiters are typically caused by an insufficiency in
   A. potassium.
   B. calcium.
   C. iodine.
   D. vitamin K.
   E. hemoglobin.

_____ **81.** The adrenal cortex is responsible for the production of hormones for all the following purposes EXCEPT
   A. to regulate salt balance.
   B. to regulate immunity.
   C. to regulate glucose production.
   D. to regulate water balance.
   E. to regulate sexual maturity.

74   PARAMEDIC CARE _Paramedicine Fundamentals_

©2013 Pearson Education, Inc.
Paramedic Care: Principles & Practice, Vol. 2, 4th Ed.

_____ 82. The type of diabetes that typically manifests during childhood is
    A. gestational.   **D.** type III.
    B. type I.   **E.** type IV.
    C. type II.

_____ 83. The pancreas secretes two hormones important to the regulation of glucose. They are insulin and
    A. glucagon.   **D.** cortisol.
    B. glycogen.   **E.** orinase.
    C. dextrose.

_____ 84. Which of the following forms of insulin is NOT likely to cause an allergic reaction?
    A. Lente   **D.** Recombinant
    B. Pork   **E.** Bovine
    C. Beef

_____ 85. The principal indication for estrogen replacement therapy in women is
    A. postmenopause replacement.   **D.** in delayed puberty.
    B. in contraception.   **E.** all of the above.
    C. to delay childbirth.

_____ 86. Serious hypotension may occur in a patient who takes sildenafil when also taking
    A. glucagon.   **D.** antibiotics.
    B. nitrates.   **E.** thyroxine.
    C. $D_{50}W$.

_____ 87. Antibiotics act by
    A. killing the bacteria outright.
    B. creating antigens to deactivate the bacteria.
    C. engulfing the bacteria.
    D. decreasing the bacteria's growth rate.
    E. A and D.

_____ 88. A solution containing whole antibodies for a specific pathogen is called a(n)
    A. vaccine.   **D.** rotovirus.
    B. serum.   **E.** none of the above.
    C. immunogen.

_____ 89. The best age for vaccination against disease is
    A. under 6 months.   **D.** over 5 years.
    B. under 2 years.   **E.** over 8 years.
    C. from 2 to 5 years.

_____ 90. The number associated with each B vitamin relates to
    A. its order of discovery.   **D.** its point of absorption.
    B. its molecular size.   **E.** none of the above.
    C. its importance to the body.

Special Project

Practicing as a paramedic involves the administration of numerous medications for patients with serious medical conditions. To be able to administer these medications safely, you must know each medication's indications, contraindications, precautions, routes of administration, and dosages. This information is not easy to commit to memory.

At the end of this workbook is a series of Emergency Drug Cards with indications, contraindications, precautions, routes of administration, and dosages for the drugs. Detach them and select those cards that represent drugs used by your EMS system or educational program. If there are drugs that your system or educational program uses that are not included in the drug cards, use index cards to create additional drug cards. Enter the important information for each drug under the listed categories and enter the drug name on the reverse side of the card. Review the material on each card from this workbook and on the cards that you create with your instructor and medical protocols. Ensure that they document the indications, dosages, and routes consistent with your protocols and with prehospital practice in your system. It is not unusual for systems to use slightly different indications, contraindications, and dosages. Also note that continuing research may change the types of medications and the way they are administered.

Once you have assembled the drug cards and they are consistent with your system protocols, review them to begin learning the important drug information. Once you feel comfortable with each drug's information, shuffle the cards and then check your ability to recognize the indications, contraindications, side effects, routes of administration, and dosages for each medication. Review these drugs from time to time during your education and with specific classroom sessions regarding medical emergencies and trauma emergencies. Ultimately, you should know all the information listed for each drug in your stack of cards.

©2013 Pearson Education, Inc.
Paramedic Care: Principles & Practice, Vol. 2, 4th Ed.

Intravenous Access and Medication Administration

Because Chapter 4 is lengthy, it has been divided into parts to aid your study. Read the assigned textbook pages; then, progress through the objectives and self-evaluation materials as you would with other chapters. When you feel secure in your grasp of the content, proceed to the next section.

Review of Chapter Objectives

After reading this chapter, you should be able to:

1. **Define key terms introduced in this chapter.**

   Knowing and being able to apply the key terms in each chapter is critical to understanding chapter concepts. Write the list of key terms. Then write the definition of each one in your own words. Check your understanding by confirming the definitions in the text glossary. Correct any misunderstandings. Create a study aid by writing each key term on the front of an index card and the definition on the back. Use the cards to quiz yourself or to have someone quiz you.

   (Objectives continue on the next page.)

Part 1: Principles and Routes of Medication Administration, p. 229

Review of Chapter Objectives

After reading this part of the chapter, you should be able to:

2. **Apply the six rights of medication administration when administering patient medications.**   p. 230

You can attain effective pharmacological therapy and eliminate medication errors by following the six rights of medication administration:

Right person. Ensure that the patient receiving the medication is the right person. Generally, you will provide one-on-one attention. In a clinical setting, however, keeping track of multiple patients proves more challenging.

Right medication. Ensure that you administer the proper medication. Many medications are contained in similar-appearing packages. To avoid inadvertently delivering the incorrect medication, read the label! Administering the incorrect medication can have disastrous consequences.

Right dose. Be certain that you administer the exact dosage of any medication. The correct dose may be standardized or require calculation. Never underdose or overdose a patient.

Right time. Timing their administration is important for many medications. Typically, in the emergent setting, you will quickly administer the necessary emergency medications. During transfers and critical care transports, you may have to administer other medications at preestablished intervals.

Right route. Specific medications require specific delivery routes. You must not only be familiar with the properties of individual medications but also with their different routes of administration.

Right documentation. Documenting medication administration is of paramount importance. You must record all appropriate information about every medication you administer. Pertinent information includes, but is not limited to, medication name(s), dose, route of delivery, person administering, time administered, and patient response to the medication—both good and bad.

3. **Identify the boundaries of your scope of practice pertaining to medication administration.**   p. 230

Paramedics do not practice autonomously. You will operate under the license of a medical director who is responsible for all of your actions. This responsibility extends to the administration of medications.

   The medical director (or the EMS system) determines which medications you will use and the routes by which you will deliver them. Some states have a "state medication list" whereby the medications a service carries are dictated by law or a legislative or regulatory agency.

4. **Recognize situations involving medication administration in which you should communicate directly with a medical direction physician.**   p. 230

While some medications can be administered via off-line medical direction (written standing orders), you may need specific authorization for others after consulting on-line or direct medical direction. You must strictly abide by all of your medical director's guidelines.

5. **Select the appropriate Standard Precautions for all medication administration situations.**   p. 231

During most patient care, you will wear gloves and eye protection. A mask is often required for procedures and patient-care conditions where there is an increased likelihood that splashes or sprays of blood, body fluids, or secretions may occur. This is especially important during suctioning, endotracheal intubation, and other airway procedures. Washing your hands before and after patient contact is one of the most effective ways to decrease your exposure to infectious material.

6. Demonstrate principles of medical asepsis in the administration of medications. p. 232

Medical asepsis describes a medical environment free of pathogens. Many paramedical procedures, especially those related to medication administration, place the patient at increased risk for infection. The external environment is full of microorganisms, many of them pathogenic. Techniques such as intravenous access or endotracheal intubation can allow pathogens to enter the patient's body, where they may cause local or systemic complications.

Medical asepsis practices, including the use of sterilization, disinfectants, and antiseptics, guard against this hazard. A sterile environment is free of all forms of life. Generally, environments are sterilized with extensive heat or chemicals. A sterile environment is difficult to attain in the prehospital setting. Consequently, you must practice medically clean techniques to minimize your patient's risk of infection. Medically clean techniques involve the careful handling of sterile equipment to prevent contamination.

When administering medications, you must use disinfectants and antiseptics to ensure local cleanliness. Disinfectants are toxic to living tissue. You will therefore use them only on nonliving surfaces or objects such as the inside of an ambulance or laryngoscope blades after use. Never use disinfectants on living tissue. Antiseptics are not toxic to living tissue. They destroy or inhibit pathogenic microorganisms that already exist on living surfaces and are generally used to cleanse the local area before a needle puncture.

7. Accurately and completely document the pertinent details of administering medication to a patient. pp. 232–233

When administering medications, proper and thorough documentation is extremely important. You must record all information concerning the patient and the medication, including indication for medication administration, dosage and route delivered, and patient response to the medication. You must also document the patient's condition and vital signs before medication administration as well as after.

8. Describe the procedures, precautions, risks, equipment, advantages, and disadvantages of each of the routes of percutaneous, pulmonary, enteral, and parenteral medication administration.

Percutaneous pp. 233–234

Percutaneous medications are those that are applied to and absorbed through the skin or the mucous membranes. They are easy to administer, and they bypass the digestive tract, making their absorption more predictable.

Medications given by the transdermal route promote slow, steady absorption.

The mucous membranes absorb medications at a moderate to rapid rate. Similar to transdermal administration, medication delivery through the mucous membranes avoids the digestive tract and complications associated with that route.

Pulmonary pp. 236–238

Special medications can be administered into the pulmonary system via inhalation or injection. Generally in the form of gases, powders, fine mists, or liquids, these medications include those that promote bronchodilation for respiratory emergencies. Other inhaled medications are mucolytics, antibiotics, and topical steroids. Inhalation can also be used for humidification and pulmonary decongestion.

Typically, medications administered by inhalation are delivered with the aid of a small volume nebulizer (SVN) or handheld nebulizer (HHN). A nebulizer uses pressurized oxygen or air to disperse a liquid into a fine aerosol spray or mist. Inhalation carries the aerosol into the lungs.

Inhaled medications may also be delivered through a metered dose inhaler (MDI). These small, handheld devices produce a medicated spray for inhalation. Patients with conditions such as asthma or COPD use metered dose inhalers to deliver a specific, or metered, dose of medication.

Although infrequently used, you can administer certain medications such as lidocaine (Xylocaine), vasopressin, epinephrine, atropine, and naloxone (Narcan) through an endotracheal tube if an intravenous line or intraosseous line is unavailable. Delivering liquid medications into the lungs theoretically permits rapid absorption through the pulmonary capillaries. However, recent research has shown that the administration of medications via an endotracheal tube is not as effective as once thought.

Enteral   pp. 238–240

The enteral route is the delivery of medication to be absorbed through the gastrointestinal tract. The gastrointestinal tract, or alimentary canal, travels from the mouth to the stomach and on through the intestines to the rectum. You can administer enteral medications orally, through a gastric tube, or rectally. Several advantages make the gastrointestinal tract the most common route for medication delivery. Aside from sheer convenience, it is the least expensive route, and its use requires little equipment and minimal training. Conversely, enteral medication administration poses several disadvantages. Physical activity, emotions, or food can significantly alter the gastrointestinal tract's chemical and physical environment, making absorption unreliable. In addition, as all blood from the stomach and small intestine must pass through the hepatic circulatory system (portal circulation), the liver's condition can reduce the medication's effectiveness.

Oral medication administration denotes any medication taken by mouth (oral) and swallowed into the gastrointestinal (GI) tract.

For patients who have difficulty swallowing or whose nutritional status is poor, you may place a gastric tube to support or completely supplement nutritional requirements. Gastric tubes are also used in instances of medication overdose, trauma, and upper gastrointestinal bleeding. They may be surgically inserted directly into the stomach through the abdomen or indirectly through the nose (nasogastric tube) or mouth (orogastric tube).

The rectum's extreme vascularity promotes rapid medication absorption. Additionally, because medications given rectally do not pass through the liver, they are not subject to hepatic alteration; thus, their absorption is more predictable.

Parenteral   pp. 242–254

The parenteral route denotes the administration of medication outside the gastrointestinal tract. Broadly, this encompasses pulmonary and some topical forms of medication delivery; however, additional, specific criteria apply to parenteral administration. Typically, the parenteral route involves the use of needles as medications are injected into the circulatory system or tissues. Consequently, some forms of parenteral medication delivery afford the most rapid medication delivery and absorption.

Using a syringe and hypodermic needle, intradermal injections deposit medication into the dermal layer of the skin. The amount of medication placed in the dermal layer is quite small, typically less than 1 mL.

Subcutaneous injections place medication into the subcutaneous tissue. The subcutaneous layer consists of loose connective tissue between the skin and muscle. The subcutaneous tissue has few blood vessels and thus promotes slow, sustained absorption, which prolongs a medication's effect on the body. Like intradermal injections, no more than 1.0 mL of medication is administered subcutaneously. Administering more than 1.0 mL of medication can cause irritation and, possibly, an abscess.

Intramuscular injections deposit medication into muscle. Muscle is extremely vascular and permits systemic delivery at a moderate absorption rate. Medication absorption through muscle is also relatively predictable. To reach the muscle, a needle must penetrate the dermal and subcutaneous tissue. The amount of medication that can be administered intramuscularly ranges from 2 to 5 mL depending upon the injection site.

Intravenous (IV) access, or cannulation, is a routine paramedic procedure. Circulating blood transports chemicals, proteins, and fluids throughout the body. Venous circulation can likewise deliver medications and fluids into the body and provides an invaluable tool for treating the sick and injured. The following situations indicate intravenous access: fluid and blood replacement, medication administration, and obtaining venous blood specimens for laboratory analysis.

Intraosseous (IO) infusions involve inserting a rigid needle into the cavity of a long bone or into the sternum. The bone marrow contains a network of venous sinusoids that drain into the nutrient and emissary veins. These sinusoids accept fluids and medications during intraosseous infusion and

©2013 Pearson Education, Inc.
Paramedic Care: Principles & Practice, Vol. 2, 4th Ed.

transport them to the venous system. Any solution or medication that can be administered intravenously, either by bolus or infusion, can be administered by the intraosseous route.

9. Demonstrate the safe administration of medications allowed in your scope of practice under the supervision of a lab instructor or clinical preceptor, including medications administered by percutaneous, pulmonary, enteral, and parenteral routes.

Transdermal   pp. 233–234

1. Use Standard Precautions and avoid contaminating the medication and inadvertently getting it on your skin.
2. Clean and dry your patient's skin at the administration site.
3. Apply medication to the site as specified by the manufacturer. Avoid overdosing or underdosing when using lotion, ointment, cream, or foam.
4. Leave the medication in place for the required time. Monitor the patient for desirable or adverse effects.

Sublingual   p. 234

1. Use Standard Precautions.
2. Confirm the indication, medication, dose, sublingual route, and expiration date.
3. Have your patient lift his tongue toward the top and back of his oral cavity.
4. Place the pill or direct spray between the underside of the tongue and the floor of the oral cavity. Have your patient relax his tongue and mouth. If administering a tablet, instruct the patient to let the tablet dissolve and not to swallow it.
5. Monitor the patient for desirable or adverse effects.

Buccal   pp. 234–235

1. Use Standard Precautions.
2. Confirm the indication, medication, dose, buccal route, and expiration date.
3. Place the medication between the patient's cheek and gum. Instruct the patient to allow the pill or other preparation to dissolve. Ensure that the patient does not swallow the medication.
4. Monitor the patient for desirable or adverse effects.

Ocular   p. 235

1. Use Standard Precautions.
2. Have your patient lie supine or lay his head back and look toward the ceiling.
3. Pull the lower eyelid downward to expose the conjunctival sac. Never touch the eye.
4. Use a medicine dropper to place the prescribed dosage on the conjunctival sac. Never administer medications directly on the eye unless specifically instructed.
5. Instruct the patient to hold his eye(s) shut for 1 to 2 minutes.

Nasal   pp. 235–236

1. Use Standard Precautions including face mask.
2. Have the patient blow his nose and tilt his head backwards.
3. Use a medicine dropper or squeezable nebulizer to administer the medication into the appropriate nare(s) according to the manufacturer's instructions.
4. Hold the nare(s) shut and/or tilt the head forward to distribute the medication.
5. Monitor the patient for desirable and undesirable effects.

Aural   p. 236

1. Use Standard Precautions.
2. Confirm the indication, medication, dose, and expiration date.
3. Determine the correct ear for administration.
4. Have the patient lie in the lateral recumbent position with the affected ear upward.
5. Manually open the ear canal: for adult patients, pull the ear up and back; for pediatric patients, pull it down and back.

6. Administer the appropriate dose of medication with a medicine dropper.
7. Have the patient continue to lie with his ear up for 10 minutes.
8. Monitor the patient for desirable and undesirable effects.

Nebulizer   pp. 236–237
1. Use Standard Precautions, including a mask.
2. Put the medication in the medication reservoir. If the medication is not diluted, combine it with 3 to 5 cc sterile saline solution. This will allow adequate aerosolization. Screw the reservoir in place.
3. Assemble the nebulizer.
4. Attach oxygen tubing to the oxygen port and oxygen source.
5. Set the oxygen source regulator for 5 to 8 liters per minute. Note: Never set the oxygen pressure outside of this range. Less than 5 liters per minute will not create enough pressure to aerosolize the medication. More than 8 liters per minute will create too much pressure and destroy the oxygen tubing or nebulizer at its weakest point. Furthermore, because of pressure restrictions, do not attach the nebulizer to an oxygen humidifier.
6. Place the nebulizer in the patient's mouth. Instruct him to exhale and then seal his lips around the mouthpiece. Now have him hold the nebulizer and slowly inhale as deeply as possible. On maximum inhalation, instruct the patient to hold in the medication for 1 to 2 seconds before exhaling. This permits maximum deposition and absorption. Continue this process until the medication is completely gone. Typically, this takes 3 to 5 minutes.

Metered Dose Inhaler   p. 238
1. Insert the medication canister into the plastic shell.
2. Remove the cap from the mouthpiece. Make sure the cap is clean.
3. Gently shake the MDI for 2 to 5 seconds.
4. Instruct the patient to maximally exhale.
5. Place the mouthpiece in the patient's mouth and have him form a seal with his lips.
6. As the patient inhales, press the canister's top downward to release the medication.
7. Have the patient hold his breath for several seconds.
8. Remove the inhaler from the patient's mouth and instruct him to breathe slowly.
9. If a second dose is necessary, wait according to the manufacturer's instructions. Then repeat.

Endotracheal   p. 238
Although infrequently used, you can administer certain medications such as lidocaine (Xylocaine), vasopressin, epinephrine, atropine, and naloxone (Narcan) through an endotracheal tube if an intravenous line or intraosseous line is unavailable. When using an endotracheal tube, you must increase conventional IV dosages from two to two-and-one-half times. You also should dilute the medication in normal saline to create 10 mL of solution and then quickly inject it down the endotracheal tube. Several ventilations must follow to aerosolize the medication and enhance its absorption. Ideally, you can pass a commercially manufactured catheter through the endotracheal tube and inject the medication through it.

Oral   pp. 239–240
1. Use Standard Precautions.
2. Note whether to administer the medication with food or on an empty stomach.
3. Gather any necessary equipment such as a soufflé cup or teaspoon; mix liquids or suspensions, or otherwise prepare medications as needed.
4. Have your patient sit upright (when not contraindicated).
5. Place the medication into your patient's mouth. Allow self-administration when possible; assist when needed.
6. Follow administration with 4 to 8 ounces of water or other liquid. Swallowing a liquid pushes the medication into the stomach.
7. Ensure that the patient has swallowed the medication and it is not hidden in his mouth. For some pediatric and psychiatric patients, you may have to visually confirm that the patient has swallowed the medication by inspecting the oral cavity.

1. Use Standard Precautions.
2. Confirm proper tube placement. Disconnect the tube from the drainage or suction unit or clamping device. Clamp the tube from the drainage or suction unit to avoid gastric contents' spilling from either device. Attach a cone-tipped syringe to the proximal end of the gastric tube. Gently inject air while auscultating over the stomach. Following this, withdraw the plunger while observing for the presence of gastric fluid or contents, which indicates appropriate placement. Leave the tube disconnected from the drainage or suction unit.
3. Irrigate the gastric tube. To irrigate the gastric tube, draw up 50 to 100 mL of normal saline into a cone-tipped syringe. Insert the syringe into the open end of the gastric tube. With the syringe tip pointed at the floor, gently inject the saline into the tube. If the saline encounters resistance, look for problems such as tube kinking. Also, have the patient lie on his left side and reattempt injection. If the saline still meets resistance, reattach the tube to the drainage or suction unit and contact medical direction for further directives.
4. Prepare the medication(s) for delivery. Crush tablets or empty capsules into 30 cc of warm water. Ensure that all particles are small so that they will not occlude the tube. You may administer liquid medications without further preparation.
5. Draw the medication into a 30- to 50-mL cone-tipped syringe and place the tip into the open gastric tube. Gently administer the medication into the gastric tube. Forceful application may create considerable distention and patient discomfort.
6. Draw 50 to 100 mL of warm normal saline into a cone-tipped syringe and attach it to the open end of the gastric tube. Gently inject the saline. This facilitates the medication's passage into the stomach and rinses the tube, ensuring that the patient receives the entire dose. Repeated administrations may be necessary.
7. Clamp off the distal tube. Use a commercially manufactured device or hemostat to clamp shut the distal portion of the gastric tube for approximately 30 minutes after you administer the medication. Do not reattach to the drainage or suction unit. This will prevent the medication's inadvertent removal from the stomach.

Rectal   p. 242

1. Use Standard Precautions.
2. Confirm the indication for administration and dose, and draw the correct quantity of medication into a syringe.
3. Place the hub of a 14-gauge Teflon catheter (removed from the IV catheter) on the end of a needleless syringe.
4. Insert the Teflon catheter into the patient's rectum and inject the medication. Try to keep the medication in the lower part of the rectum. Administration higher in the rectum may result in the medication's being absorbed by veins that deliver the medication to the portal circulation.
5. Withdraw the catheter and hold the patient's buttocks together, thus permitting retention and absorption.

Enema   p. 242

1. Use Standard Precautions and confirm the need for administration via a small volume enema.
2. Place the patient on his left side. Flex his right leg to expose the anus.
3. Insert the prelubricated rectal tip into the anus and advance 3 to 4 inches.
4. Gently squeeze the medicated solution of the bottle into the rectum and colon.
5. Hold the buttocks together to enhance absorption into the rectal and intestinal tissue.

Intradermal Injection   p. 249

1. Assemble and prepare the needed equipment.
2. Use Standard Precautions and confirm the medication, indication, dosage, and need for intradermal injection.
3. Draw up medication as appropriate.
4. Prepare the site with antiseptic solution. The intended site must be cleansed of pathogens, therein decreasing the likelihood of infection. Generally, you will use alcohol or similar antiseptics.

To appropriately cleanse the site, start at the site itself and work outward with an expanding circular motion. This motion will push pathogens away from the intended site of puncture.

5. Pull the patient's skin taut with your nondominant hand.
6. Insert the needle, bevel up, just under the skin, at a 10° to 15° angle.
7. Slowly inject the medication; look for a small bump or wheal to form as medication is deposited and collects in the intradermal tissue.
8. Remove the needle and dispose of it in the sharps container.
9. Place the adhesive bandage over the site; use the gauze for hemorrhage control if needed.

Subcutaneous Injection   p. 251

1. Assemble and prepare equipment.
2. Use Standard Precautions and confirm the medication, indication, dosage, and need for subcutaneous injection.
3. Draw up the medication as appropriate.
4. Prepare the site with antiseptic solution.
5. Gently pinch a 1-inch fold of skin.
6. Insert the needle just into the skin at a 45° angle with the bevel up.
7. Pull the plunger back to aspirate tissue fluid.
8. If blood appears, the hypodermic needle is in a blood vessel and absorption will be too rapid. Start the procedure over with a new syringe.
9. If no blood appears, proceed with step 10.
10. Slowly inject the medication.
11. Remove the needle and dispose of it in a sharps container.
12. Place an adhesive bandage over the site; use the gauze for hemorrhage control if needed.
13. Monitor the patient.

Intramuscular Injection   pp. 253–254

1. Assemble and prepare the needed equipment.
2. Use Standard Precautions and confirm the medication, indication, dosage, and need for intramuscular injection.
3. Draw up the medication as appropriate.
4. Prepare the site with antiseptic solution.
5. Stretch the skin taut over the injection site with your nondominant hand.
6. Insert the needle just into the skin at a 90° angle with the bevel up.
7. Pull back the plunger to aspirate tissue fluid. If blood appears, the hypodermic needle is in a blood vessel, and absorption of the medication will be too rapid. Start the procedure over with a new syringe. If no blood appears, proceed with step 8.
8. Slowly inject the medication.
9. Remove the needle and dispose of it in the sharps container.
10. Place an adhesive bandage over the site; use gauze for hemorrhage control if needed.
11. Monitor the patient.

Intravenous Access (Hand, Arm, and Leg)   p. 262

1. Confirm indication and type of IV setup needed. Gather and arrange all supplies and equipment beforehand to make the process easy and accessible: IV fluid, administration set, intravenous cannula, tape or commercial securing device, venous blood drawing equipment, venous constricting band, and antiseptic solution. When appropriate, explain the entire process to the patient. Apply the proper Standard Precautions— gloves, mask, and protective eyewear goggles—as IV access is invasive and presents the potential for blood exposure.
2. Prepare all needed equipment. Examine the IV fluid for clarity and expiration date. Insert the administration tubing spike in the IV solution bag's administration set port. Squeeze fluid from the IV fluid container into the drip chamber until it reaches the fill line. Open the clamp and/or flow regulator to flush the solution through the administration tubing and expel trapped air bubbles. Shut down the flow regulator and replace the cap over the needle adapter. Remember that the IV administration set is sterile; if any contamination occurs, you must replace the set with a new one.

©2013 Pearson Education, Inc.
Paramedic Care: Principles & Practice, Vol. 2, 4th Ed.

3. Select the venipuncture site. Acceptable sites have clearly visible veins and are free of bruising or scarring. Straight veins are easier to cannulate than crooked ones.
4. Place the constricting band proximal to the intended site of puncture. Tighten it enough to impede venous blood flow without restricting arterial blood passage. Never leave the constricting band in place more than 2 minutes, as intrinsic changes will occur in the slowed venous blood.
5. Cleanse the venipuncture site. You must cleanse the intended site of pathogens to decrease the likelihood of infection. Alcohol and similar antiseptic solutions are the most commonly used. Start at the site itself and work outward in an expanding circle. This pushes pathogens away from the puncture site.
6. Insert the intravenous cannula into the vein. With your nondominant hand, pull all local skin taut to stabilize the vein and prevent it from rolling. With the distal bevel of the metal stylet up, insert the cannula into the vein at a 10° to 30° angle. Continue until you feel the cannula "pop" into the vein or see blood in the flashback chamber. The metal stylet is now in the vein; however, the Teflon catheter is not. To place the catheter into the vein, carefully advance the cannula approximately 0.5 cm further. (If you are using a butterfly cannula, it has no Teflon catheter, and you must carefully advance the needle itself.)
7. Holding the metal stylet stationary, slide the Teflon catheter over the needle into the vein. Place a finger over the vein at the catheter tip and tamponade (press gently downward to occlude the vein), thus preventing blood from flowing from the catheter and/or air from entraining into the circulatory system. Carefully remove the metal stylet, retract the needle, and promptly dispose of it in the sharps container. Remove the venous constricting band.
8. Obtain venous blood samples as discussed in the section on venous blood sampling.
9. Attach the administration tubing to the cannula. Remove the protective cap from the needle adapter and tightly secure the needle adapter into the cannula hub. Open the flow regulator and allow the fluid to run freely for several seconds. Adjust the flow rate. Do not let go of the cannula and administration tubing until you have secured them as explained in step 10.
10. Cover the catheter and puncture site with an adhesive bandage or other commercial device. Loop the distal tubing and secure with tape. This makes the medication administration port more accessible and attaches the device to the patient more securely. Continue by taping the administration tubing to the patient, proximal to the venipuncture site.
11. Label the intravenous solution bag with the following information: date and time initiated, and person initiating the intravenous access.
12. Continually monitor the patient and flow rate.

Intravenous Access (External Jugular)   pp. 263–265
1. Prepare all equipment as for peripheral IV access in an arm, hand, or leg. In addition, fill the 10-mL syringe with 3 to 5 mL of sterile saline. Attach the distal part of the syringe to the flashback chamber of a large bore, over-the-needle catheter. Use Standard Precautions.
2. Place the patient supine and/or in the Trendelenburg position. This position will increase blood flow to the chest and neck, thus distending the vein and making it easier to see. In addition, the supine-Trendelenburg position decreases the chance of air entering the circulatory system during cannulation.
3. Turn the patient's head to the side opposite of access. This maneuver makes the site easier to see and reach; do not perform it if the patient has traumatic head and/or neck injuries.
4. Cleanse the site with antiseptic solution. Start at the site of intended puncture and work outward 1 to 2 inches in ever-increasing circles.
5. Occlude venous return by placing a finger on the external jugular just above the clavicle. This should distend the vein, again allowing greater visualization and ease of puncture. Never apply a venous constricting band around the patient's neck.
6. Position the intravenous cannula parallel with the vein, midway between the angle of the jaw and the clavicle. Point the catheter at the medial third of the clavicle and insert it, bevel up, at a 10° to 30° angle.
7. Enter the external jugular while withdrawing on the plunger of the attached syringe. You will see blood in the syringe or feel a pop as the cannula enters the vein. Once inside the vein, advance the entire catheter another 0.5 cm so the tip of the Teflon catheter lies within the lumen of the vein.

Then slide the Teflon catheter into the vein and remove the metal stylet as previously described and retract the needle. Immediately dispose of the metal stylet.

8. Obtain venous blood samples as discussed in the section on venous blood sampling.
9. Attach the administration tubing to the IV catheter. Allow the intravenous solution to run freely for several seconds. Set the flow rate and secure as appropriate.
10. Monitor the patient for complications.

Intravenous Access (Measured Volume Administration Set)   p. 265

1. Prepare the tubing by closing all clamps, and insert the flanged spike into the IV solution bag's spike port.
2. Open the airway handle. Open the uppermost clamp and fill the burette chamber with approximately 20 mL of fluid. Squeeze the drip chamber until the fluid reaches the fill line. Open the bottom flow regulator to purge air through the tubing. When all air is purged, close the bottom flow regulator.
3. Continue to fill the burette chamber with the designated amount of solution.
4. Close the uppermost clamp and open the flow regulator until you reach the desired drip rate. Leave the airway handle open, so that air replaces the displaced fluid.

Intravenous Access (Blood Tubing)   p. 265

1. Prepare the tubing by closing all clamps, and insert the flanged spike into the spike port of the blood and/or normal saline solution (Y-configured tubing).
2. Squeeze the drip chamber until it is one-third full and blood covers the filter. Repeat for the normal saline if you are using Y tubing.
3. If you are using straight tubing, piggyback a secondary line of normal saline into the blood tubing, unless you plan to piggyback the straight blood tubing into a large-bore primary line.
4. Flush all tubing with normal saline and blood as appropriate.
5. Attach blood tubing to the intravenous cannula or into a previously established IV line.
6. Ensure patency by infusing a small amount of normal saline. Shut down when you have confirmed patency.
7. Open the clamp(s) and/or flow regulator(s) that allows blood to move from the bag to the patient. Adjust the flow rate accordingly.
8. When blood therapy is complete or must be discontinued, shut down the flow regulator from the blood supply and open the regulator(s) for the normal saline solution.

Intravenous Bolus   p. 269

1. Ensure that the primary IV line is patent.
2. Confirm the medication, indication, dosage, and need for an IV bolus. Confirm that the medication is compatible with the solution being infused.
3. Draw up the medication or prepare a prefilled syringe as appropriate.
4. Cleanse the medication port nearest the IV site with an antiseptic preparation.
5. Insert a hypodermic needle through the port membrane.
6. Pinch the IV line above the medication port. This prevents the medication from traveling toward the fluid bag, forcing it instead toward the patient.
7. Inject the medication as appropriate.
8. Remove the hypodermic needle and syringe and release the tubing.
9. Open the flow regulator to allow a 20-cc fluid flush. The fluid will push the medication into the patient's circulatory system.
10. Dispose of the hypodermic needle and syringe as appropriate. Monitor the patient for desired or undesired effects.

Intravenous Infusion   pp. 269–272

1. Establish a primary IV line and ensure patency.
2. Confirm administration indications and patient allergies.
3. Prepare the infusion bag or bottle. (If the infusion is premixed, continue to step 4.)
   a. Draw up the appropriate quantity of medication from its source with a syringe.
   b. Cleanse the IV bag or bottle's medication port with an antiseptic wipe.

©2013 Pearson Education, Inc.
Paramedic Care: Principles & Practice, Vol. 2, 4th Ed.

    c. Insert the hypodermic needle into the medication port and inject the medication.

    d. Gently agitate the bag or bottle to mix its contents.

    e. Label the bag or bottle.

4. Connect administration tubing to the medication bag or bottle and fill the drip chamber to the fluid line. Most infusions require microdrip tubing. If you use a mechanical infusion pump, you may need to use special tubing.

5. Place the hypodermic needle on the administration tubing's needle adapter and flush the tubing with solution. (The needle adapter typically accepts a 20-gauge needle.)

6. Cleanse the medication administration port on the primary line with alcohol and insert the secondary line's hypodermic needle. Secure the hypodermic needle and the secondary administration line with tape or another securing device.

7. Reconfirm the indication, medication, dose, and route of administration.

8. Shut down the primary line so that no fluid will flow from the primary solution bag.

9. Adjust the secondary line to the desired drip rate. If you are using a mechanical infusion pump, set it accordingly.

10. Properly dispose of the needle and syringe.

Heparin/Saline Lock Access   pp. 272–273

1. Select the venipuncture site.

2. Place the constricting band proximal to the puncture site.

3. Cleanse the venipuncture site with antiseptic solution.

4. Insert the intravenous cannula into the vein.

5. Slide the Teflon catheter into the vein.

6. Carefully remove the metal stylet, retract or protect the stylet, and promptly dispose of it into the sharps container. Remove the venous constricting band.

7. Obtain venous blood samples.

8. Attach the heparin lock tubing to the catheter hub.

9. Cleanse the medication port and inject 3 to 5 mL of sterile saline into the lock. Easy flow of the saline without edema at the puncture site indicates patency. If you encounter resistance or if edema forms, restart the procedure with new equipment. If a heparin lock is desired, fill the port with the designated heparin flush solution.

10. Apply an adhesive bandage or other commercial device. Secure the tubing to the patient.

Heparin/Saline Lock Access (Medication Administration)   p. 273

1. Confirm the medication, indication, dosage, and need for an IV bolus.

2. Draw up the medication or prepare a prefilled syringe as appropriate.

3. Cleanse the medication port nearest the IV site with an antiseptic solution.

4. Ensure that the plastic clamp is open.

5. Insert the hypodermic needle through the port membrane.

6. Inject the medication as appropriate.

7. Remove the hypodermic needle and dispose of it in the sharps container.

8. Follow the medication administration with a 10- to 20-mL saline flush from another syringe.

9. Properly dispose of the hypodermic needle and syringe. Monitor the patient for desired or undesired effects.

Venous Access Device   pp. 273–274

1. Use Standard Precautions.

2. Fill a 10-mL syringe with approximately 7 mL of normal saline.

3. Place a 21- or 22-gauge Huber needle (or other specialized needle) on the end of the syringe.

4. Cleanse the skin over the injection port with an antiseptic solution.

5. Stabilize the site with one hand while inserting the Huber needle at a 90° angle. Gently advance it until it meets resistance. This signals that the needle has contacted the floor of the injection port.

6. Pull back on the plunger and observe for blood return. The presence of blood confirms placement.

7. Slowly inject the normal saline to ensure patency.

Venous Access Device (Medication Administration)   p. 274

1. Prepare the medication, fluid, or blood for administration.
2. Attach a 21- or 22-gauge Huber needle (or other specialized needle) to the end of the syringe.
3. Cleanse the skin over the injection port with an antiseptic solution.
4. Insert the needle into the injection port at a 90° angle until the needle cannot be further advanced. Pull back on the plunger of the syringe and observe for the return of blood. The presence of blood confirms proper placement.
5. Inject the medication as appropriate.
6. Remove and dispose of the syringe appropriately.
7. With another syringe and attached specialized needle, administer a bolus of heparinized saline to clear the catheter of any blood clots or other obstruction.

Venous Access Device (IV Fluid Administration)   p. 274

1. Prepare a primary IV line. Be sure to prime or flush the air from the administration tubing.
2. Attach a 21- or 22-gauge Huber needle (or other specialized needle) to the primary IV administration tubing. Insert a 10-mL syringe and hypodermic needle filled with 7 mL of normal saline solution into the tubing medication delivery port nearest the venous access device.
3. Cleanse the skin over the injection port with an antiseptic solution.
4. Insert the needle into the injection port at a 90° angle until it encounters resistance.
5. Pinch the administration tubing above the medication administration port and pull back on the syringe plunger. Observe for the return of blood. The presence of blood confirms proper placement.
6. Gently inject the 7 mL of normal saline solution.
7. Set the primary line to the appropriate flow rate.

Venous Access Device (Medication Infusion)   p. 274

1. Prepare a secondary line containing the fluid, blood, or medicated solution for infusion.
2. Attach a hypodermic needle to the needle adapter of the secondary line. Insert the secondary line into a medication administration port on the primary tubing.
3. Shut down the primary line and infuse the medicated solution as appropriate. Look for ease of administration as a sign of patency.
4. When infusion is complete, administer a bolus of heparinized saline to clear the catheter of any blood clots or other obstruction.

Intraosseous Access   pp. 280–283

1. Determine the indication for intraosseous access.
2. Assemble and check all equipment.
3. Position the patient. Rotate the leg toward the outside to expose the medial, proximal aspect of the tibia.
4. Locate the access site. Palpate the tibia and use all landmarks.
   a. Pediatric. Locate the tibial tuberosity. Move from one to two fingerbreadths below the tibial tuberosity and find the flat expanse medial to the anterior tibial crest.
   b. Adult or geriatric. Find the medial locations (based on the device you are using). These can include the tibial tuberosity, sternum, or humeral head. Be familiar with the accepted access sites as well as the operation of the particular IO device you are using.
5. Cleanse the site with an antiseptic solution. Start at the puncture site and work outward in an expanding circular motion.
6. Perform the puncture. Holding the needle perpendicular to the puncture site, insert it with a twisting motion until you feel a decrease in resistance or a "pop." When this occurs, the needle is in the medullary canal. Do not advance it any further. Generally, you will need to insert the needle only 2 to 4 mm for entry.
7. Remove the trocar and attach the syringe. Slowly pull back the plunger to attempt aspiration into the syringe. Easy aspiration of bone marrow and blood confirms correct medullary placement.
8. Once you have confirmed placement, rotate the plastic disk toward the skin to secure the needle.
9. Remove the syringe and attach the prepared administration tubing and solution. Set the appropriate flow rate.

©2013 Pearson Education, Inc.
Paramedic Care: Principles & Practice, Vol. 2, 4th Ed.

10. Secure the intraosseous needle as if securing an impaled object by surrounding it with bulky dressings and taping them securely in place. Commercial devices for securing an intraosseous needle are available.

10. Prepare medications for administration from a variety of types of packaging, including vials, nonconstituted vials, ampules, prefilled syringes, and packaging for intravenous solutions.

Vials   pp. 245–246
To obtain medication from a vial, follow these steps:
1. Confirm medication indications and patient allergies.
2. Confirm the vial label (name, dose, and expiration).
3. Determine the volume of medication to be administered.
4. Prepare the syringe and hypodermic needle. Because the vial is vacuum packed, you will have to replace the volume of medication removed with air in order to maintain equilibrium in the vial. Withdraw the plunger to draw a volume of air into the syringe equal to the volume of medication to be administered. This technique permits easy medication retrieval from the vial.
5. Cleanse the vial's rubber top with an antiseptic alcohol preparation.
6. Insert the hypodermic needle into the rubber top and inject the air from the syringe into the vial. Then withdraw the appropriate volume of medication.
7. Reconfirm the indication, medication, dose, and route of administration.
8. Administer appropriately via the indicated route.
9. Properly dispose of the needle, syringe, and vial.

Nonconstituted Vials   pp. 246–248
To prepare a medication from a nonconstituted medication vial, use the following technique:
1. Confirm medication indications and patient allergies.
2. Confirm the vial's label (name, dose, expiration date).
3. Remove all solution from the vial containing the mixing solution, using the same procedure as you would to withdraw medication from a single or multidose vial.
4. With an alcohol preparation, cleanse the top of the vial containing the powdered medication and inject the mixing solution.
5. Gently agitate or shake the vial to ensure complete mixture.
6. Determine the volume of newly constituted medication to be administered.
7. Prepare the syringe and hypodermic needle. Because the vial is vacuum packed, you will have to replace the volume of medication removed with air in order to retain equilibrium in the vial. By withdrawing the plunger, place into the syringe a volume of air equal to the volume of medication that will be removed. This technique permits easy medication retrieval from the vial.
8. Cleanse the medication vial's rubber top with an antiseptic alcohol preparation.
9. Insert the hypodermic needle into the rubber top and withdraw the appropriate volume of medication.
10. Reconfirm the indication, medication, dose, and route of administration.
11. Administer appropriately via the indicated route.
12. Monitor the patient for the desired effects.
13. Properly dispose of the needle and syringe.

Ampules   pp. 244–245
To obtain medication from a glass ampule you will need a syringe and needle. Use the following technique:
1. Confirm medication indications and patient allergies.
2. Confirm the ampule label (medication name, dose, and expiration).
3. Hold the ampule upright and tap its top to dislodge any trapped solution.
4. Place gauze around the thin neck and snap it off with your thumb.
5. Place the tip of the hypodermic needle inside the ampule and withdraw the medication into the syringe.
6. Reconfirm the indication, medication, dose, and route of administration.

7. Administer the medication appropriately via the indicated route.
8. Properly dispose of the needle, syringe, and broken glass ampule.

Prefilled Syringes p. 247

Follow these steps to administer a medication from a prefilled syringe:
1. Confirm medication indications and patient allergies.
2. Confirm the prefilled syringe label (name, dose, and expiration date).
3. Assemble the prefilled syringe. Remove the pop-off caps and screw together.
4. Reconfirm the indication, medication, dose, and route of administration.
5. Administer appropriately via the indicated route.
6. Properly dispose of the needle and syringe.

IV Fluid p. 262

1. Use proper Standard Precautions.
2. Examine the IV fluid for clarity and expiration date.
3. Insert the administration tubing spike in the IV solution bag's administration set port.
4. Squeeze fluid from the IV fluid container into the drip chamber until it reaches the fill line.
5. Open the clamp and/or flow regulator to flush the solution through the administration tubing and expel trapped air bubbles.
6. Shut down the flow regulator and replace the cap over the needle adapter. Remember that the IV administration set is sterile. If any contamination occurs, you must replace the set with a new one.

Case Study Review

Reread the case study on pages 228–229 in Paramedic Care: Paramedicine Fundamentals; *then, read the following discussion.*

Susan and Todd are presented with a typical emergency patient in this scenario. While Susan anticipated asthma from the patient's wheezing, her positioning, and her general appearance (all determined during the first impression of the patient), she is meticulous in her complete patient evaluation and determination of baseline vital signs, ECG, pulse oximetry, and patient (SAMPLE) history. This information is essential to identify the pathology affecting the patient and to identify and document the indications, and rule out possible contraindications, for medication administration.

Susan and Todd identify that the patient attempted to use a metered dose inhaler for relief from the asthma attack. Because of their knowledge of various medication administration techniques and their respective advantages and disadvantages, they know that in severe attacks of respiratory distress, the ventilatory exchange is poor and limits the effectiveness of the inhaler. They employ albuterol nebulization because the prolonged and humidified inhalation may be more effective in delivering the drug to the deeper respiratory tissue. Susan administers methylprednisolone via an intravenous line as an anti-inflammatory agent to combat that component of the severe asthma condition. This drug comes in a special two-part vial that permits an increased shelf life but requires that Susan be familiar with special aspects of the drug's preparation and administration. Reassessment reveals minimal improvement and Susan places the patient on CPAP.

For each of these drug routes, Susan must be familiar with the specific equipment used, the location for injections, and the technique of drug injection and must recognize what common complications may be associated with a particular route of administration. Susan must also be able to calculate the proper dose of the drug and the volume of drug on hand that contains that dose.

During each medication administration, Susan must follow the proper protocol, identify the six rights of drug administration, and employ the appropriate technique to draw up and deliver the medication. She must also observe Standard Precautions measures and aseptic and medically clean techniques; dispose of sharps, drug containers, and other biohazards properly; and document the indications, administration, and effects of each drug she used. While this is a complicated process, it will become second nature to you once you begin your career as a paramedic.

©2013 Pearson Education, Inc.
Paramedic Care: Principles & Practice, Vol. 2, 4th Ed.

Content Self-Evaluation

MULTIPLE CHOICE

_____ 1. Medication administration is an important part of the medical care provided by paramedics.
  A. True
  B. False

_____ 2. Which of the following is NOT one of the six rights of drug administration?
  A. The right dosage   D. The right documentation
  B. The right indication   E. The right patient
  C. The right time

_____ 3. The process you use to ensure you hear and correctly understand the medical direction physician's order to administer a medication is
  A. protocol compliance.
  B. order confirmation with your partner.
  C. redundant physician orders.
  D. echoing the order back to the physician.
  E. asking the physician to repeat the order.

_____ 4. Which of the following must you know about the drugs you are authorized to administer?
  A. Their usual dosages
  B. Their contraindications
  C. Their common side effects
  D. Their routes of administration
  E. All of the above

_____ 5. When you administer drugs, which of the following Standard Precautions measures should you always employ?
  A. Gloves   D. Gown
  B. Mask   E. A and D
  C. Goggles

_____ 6. The condition in which a medical environment is free of all pathogens is described as
  A. asepsis.   D. disinfection.
  B. uncontaminated.   E. none of the above.
  C. medically clean.

_____ 7. The environment that paramedics should strive to maintain while delivering prehospital emergency care is
  A. aseptic.   D. disinfected.
  B. sterile.   E. none of the above.
  C. medically clean.

_____ 8. To cleanse the site of a parenteral injection, you would use a(n)
  A. aseptic.   D. antiseptic.
  B. disinfectant.   E. dilutant.
  C. detergent.

_____ 9. When possible, you should recap needles
  A. as a last resort, using the "one-handed-scoop" method.
  B. when in a moving ambulance only.
  C. except when in a moving ambulance.
  D. only when they have not been used on a patient.
  E. when directed by a physician.

10. Documentation regarding the administration of a drug should include all of the following EXCEPT the
    A. time of administration.
    B. route of administration.
    C. class of drug administered.
    D. positive patient responses.
    E. negative patient responses.

11. Transdermal medications are provided in which of the following forms?
    A. Ointments
    B. Wet dressings
    C. Foams
    D. Lotions
    E. All of the above

12. Which of the following factors can decrease the absorption rate with transdermal medication administration?
    A. Thin skin
    B. Overdose
    C. Penetrating solvents
    D. Peripheral vascular disease
    E. All of the above

13. Which of the following is a common emergency drug administered sublingually?
    A. Sodium bicarbonate
    B. Epinephrine
    C. Nitroglycerin
    D. Aspirin
    E. Magnesium

14. The route in which a drug is administered between the cheek and gum is
    A. transdermal.
    B. sublingual.
    C. buccal.
    D. aural.
    E. inhalation.

15. Ocular medications are given for which conditions?
    A. Eye pain
    B. Eye infection
    C. Increased intraocular pressure
    D. Lubricating the eyelid
    E. All of the above

16. Ocular medications are most commonly administered
    A. over the pupil.
    B. over the iris.
    C. over the sclera.
    D. into the conjunctival sac.
    E. all of the above.

17. Nasal administration of medication is used frequently because of its rapid absorption rate and systemic effects.
    A. True
    B. False

18. The small-volume nebulizer often used in prehospital emergency medical service administers what volume of medication?
    A. 1 to 2 mL
    B. 3 to 5 mL
    C. 5 to 10 mL
    D. 10 to 15 mL
    E. 15 to 20 mL

19. The small volume nebulizer can be attached to a mouthpiece, mask, CPAP device, or endotracheal tube.
    A. True
    B. False

20. The metered dose inhaler is activated to release its medication
    A. just before the patient seals his lips to the mouthpiece.
    B. as the patient exhales.
    C. as the patient inhales.
    D. during both inhalation and exhalation.
    E. between inhalation and exhalation.

_____ **21.** Nebulizers and metered dose inhalers are advantageous in respiratory emergencies because they deliver their medication to the exact site of action.
   - **A.** True
   - **B.** False

_____ **22.** Endotracheal medication administration calls for drugs to be diluted to what volume?
   - **A.** 1 mL
   - **B.** 2 mL
   - **C.** 3 mL
   - **D.** 5 mL
   - **E.** 10 mL

_____ **23.** Which of the following drugs is NOT administered via the endotracheal route?
   - **A.** Meperidine
   - **B.** Naloxone
   - **C.** Atropine
   - **D.** Vasopressin
   - **E.** Epinephrine

_____ **24.** Enteral medications are absorbed through the
   - **A.** liver.
   - **B.** gastrointestinal tract.
   - **C.** mucous membranes.
   - **D.** portal system.
   - **E.** accessory organs.

_____ **25.** Liver function is an important factor in the effectiveness of enteral drug administration.
   - **A.** True
   - **B.** False

_____ **26.** When using a medicine cup to measure an oral dose of medication, you should use what aspect of fluid level to determine the fluid volume?
   - **A.** The highest point of the meniscus
   - **B.** The lowest point of the meniscus
   - **C.** Between the high and low point of the meniscus
   - **D.** One calibration below the lowest level of the meniscus
   - **E.** None of the above

_____ **27.** The normal teaspoon holds about what volume of fluid?
   - **A.** 2 mL
   - **B.** 3 mL
   - **C.** 5 mL
   - **D.** 10 mL
   - **E.** 12 mL

_____ **28.** The advantage of rectal administration over the other enteral drug routes is that
   - **A.** the rectal route is easier to administer drugs through.
   - **B.** there is no hepatic alteration of the drug.
   - **C.** the rectal route can absorb more medication.
   - **D.** rectal irritation is rare.
   - **E.** all of the above.

_____ **29.** To inject a drug rectally, you may use
   - **A.** a large catheter with needle removed.
   - **B.** a special enema container with a rectal tip.
   - **C.** a small endotracheal tube attached to a syringe.
   - **D.** all of the above.
   - **E.** none of the above.

_____ **30.** A syringe should be chosen for drug administration that is slightly smaller than the volume of drug to be administered.
   - **A.** True
   - **B.** False

_____ **31.** The smaller the gauge of a hypodermic needle, the smaller the diameter of its lumen.
   - **A.** True
   - **B.** False

32. What is the total dose of a drug contained in an ampule with 5 mL of a drug in a 0.3-mg/mL concentration?
   A. 0.3 mg
   B. 1.5 mg
   C. 5 mg
   D. 15 mg
   E. None of the above

33. Which of the following drug containers may contain multiple doses of a drug?
   A. Vial
   B. Ampule
   C. Mix-O-Vial
   D. Preloaded syringe
   E. Medicated solutions

34. Prior to drawing medication from a vial, you must first inject an equal volume of air into the vial.
   A. True
   B. False

35. Which of the following must be cleansed with an alcohol swab before the drug is withdrawn?
   A. Vial
   B. Ampule
   C. Mix-O-Vial
   D. Preloaded syringe
   E. A and C

36. The drug route that calls for insertion of the needle at 10° to 15° is
   A. intradermal.
   B. subcutaneous.
   C. intramuscular.
   D. intraosseous.
   E. none of the above.

37. Through which of the following routes should you inject no more than 1 mL of a drug?
   A. Intradermal
   B. Subcutaneous
   C. Intramuscular
   D. A and B
   E. All of the above

38. For intradermal and subcutaneous injections, the needle is inserted with the bevel down.
   A. True
   B. False

39. Which of the following is most likely to be an acceptable site for subcutaneous injection?
   A. Forearms
   B. Calves
   C. Abdomen
   D. Buttocks
   E. All of the above are acceptable

40. At which of the following intramuscular injection sites should you administer a maximum of 2 mL of a drug?
   A. Deltoid
   B. Gluteal
   C. Vastus lateralis
   D. Rectus femoris
   E. B and C

41. When you pull back on the syringe plunger during subcutaneous or intramuscular injection and blood appears, you should:
   A. inject the drug.
   B. inject the drug followed by a small bubble of air.
   C. insert the needle 1 cm further.
   D. attempt the injection at another site.
   E. consider the appearance of blood insignificant.

42. The drug route that calls for use of a 21- to 23-gauge needle is
   A. intradermal.
   B. subcutaneous.
   C. intramuscular.
   D. intraosseous.
   E. none of the above.

_____ **43.** The drug route that calls for use of a needle $^3/_8$ to 1 inch long is
  A. intradermal.
  B. subcutaneous.
  C. intramuscular.
  D. all of the above.
  E. none of the above.

_____ **44.** The recommended angle of insertion for the needle when administering an intramuscular injection is
  A. 10°.
  B. 15°.
  C. 45°.
  D. 90°.
  E. between 10° and 15°.

_____ **45.** After injecting an intramuscular drug, massaging the site is contraindicated because it will slow absorption.
  A. True
  B. False

Special Project

MATCHING

Match the following routes with the primary medication administration route.

  A. percutaneous

  B. pulmonary

  C. enteral

  D. parenteral

_____ **1.** Intramuscular

_____ **2.** Sublingual

_____ **3.** Endotracheal

_____ **4.** Subcutaneous

_____ **5.** Ocular

_____ **6.** Aural

_____ **7.** Intravenous

_____ **8.** Nebulizer

_____ **9.** Oral

_____ **10.** Rectal

_____ **11.** Transdermal

_____ **12.** Intradermal

_____ **13.** Buccal

_____ **14.** Intraosseous

_____ **15.** Metered dose inhaler

Part 2: Intravenous Access, Blood Sampling, and Intraosseous Infusion, p. 254

Review of Chapter Objectives

After reading this part of the chapter, you should be able to:

11. **Describe the indications, contraindications, procedure, equipment, and risks associated with peripheral intravenous access.** pp. 254–261

Intravenous (IV) access, or cannulation, is a routine paramedic procedure. Circulating blood transports chemicals, proteins, and fluids throughout the body. Venous circulation can likewise deliver medications and fluids into the body and provides an invaluable tool for treating the sick and injured. The following situations indicate intravenous access: fluid and blood replacement, medication administration, and obtaining venous blood specimens for laboratory analysis. Since veins are easier to locate and penetrate, venous access is preferable to arterial access. Additionally, venous circulation pressure is lower than arterial and presents fewer hemorrhage control complications.

To establish intravenous access, you will need the following specialized equipment and supplies: intravenous fluids, administration tubing, intravenous cannulas, and venous constricting band. Intravenous access is an invasive procedure; therefore, you must use medically clean techniques, including antiseptic preparations, to prevent infection. Applying a sterile, impermeable dressing after venipuncture decreases the chance of infection. Once you have established an IV, you must secure it to avoid losing the access. Medical tape and an adhesive bandage are inexpensive and easy to apply. You can also apply clear membranes over the site. Commercial devices manufactured specifically for this task are also available. Have gauze on hand for hemorrhage control if IV cannulation is unsuccessful or if blood leaks from around the site.

Intravenous access procedure:

1. Confirm indication and type of IV setup needed. Gather and arrange all supplies and equipment beforehand to make the process easy and accessible: IV fluid, administration set, intravenous cannula, tape or commercial securing device, venous blood drawing equipment, venous constricting band, and antiseptic solution. When appropriate, explain the entire process to the patient. Apply the proper Standard Precautions—gloves, mask, and protective eyewear goggles—as IV access is invasive and presents the potential for blood exposure.

2. Prepare all needed equipment. Examine the IV fluid for clarity and expiration date. Insert the administration tubing spike in the IV solution bag's administration set port. Squeeze fluid from the IV fluid container into the drip chamber until it reaches the fill line. Open the clamp and/or flow regulator to flush the solution through the administration tubing and expel trapped air bubbles. Shut down the flow regulator and replace the cap over the needle adapter. Remember that the IV administration set is sterile; if any contamination occurs, you must replace the set with a new one.

3. Select the venipuncture site. Acceptable sites have clearly visible veins and are free of bruising or scarring. Straight veins are easier to cannulate than crooked ones.

4. Place the constricting band proximal to the intended site of puncture. Tighten it enough to impede venous blood flow without restricting arterial blood passage. Never leave the constricting band in place more than 2 minutes, as intrinsic changes will occur in the slowed venous blood.

5. Cleanse the venipuncture site. You must cleanse the intended site of pathogens to decrease the likelihood of infection. Alcohol and similar antiseptic solutions are the most commonly used. Start at the site itself and work outward in an expanding circle. This pushes pathogens away from the puncture site.

6. Insert the intravenous cannula into the vein. With your nondominant hand, pull all local skin taut to stabilize the vein and prevent it from rolling. With the distal bevel of the metal stylet up, insert the cannula into the vein at a 10° to 30° angle. Continue until you feel the cannula "pop" into the vein or see blood in the flashback chamber. The metal stylet is now in the vein; however, the Teflon

catheter is not. To place the catheter into the vein, carefully advance the cannula approximately 0.5 cm further. (If you are using a butterfly cannula, it has no Teflon catheter, and you must carefully advance the needle itself.)

7. Holding the metal stylet stationary, slide the Teflon catheter over the needle into the vein. Place a finger over the vein at the catheter tip and tamponade (press gently downward to occlude the vein), thus preventing blood from flowing from the catheter and/or air from entraining into the circulatory system. Carefully remove the metal stylet, retract the needle, and promptly dispose of it in the sharps container. Remove the venous constricting band.

8. Obtain venous blood samples as discussed in the section on venous blood sampling.

9. Attach the administration tubing to the cannula. Remove the protective cap from the needle adapter and tightly secure the needle adapter into the cannula hub. Open the flow regulator and allow the fluid to run freely for several seconds. Adjust the flow rate. Do not let go of the cannula and administration tubing until you have secured them as explained in step 10.

10. Cover the catheter and puncture site with an adhesive bandage or other commercial device. Loop the distal tubing and secure with tape. This makes the medication administration port more accessible and attaches the device to the patient more securely. Continue by taping the administration tubing to the patient, proximal to the venipuncture site.

11. Label the intravenous solution bag with the following information: date and time initiated, and person initiating the intravenous access.

12. Continually monitor the patient and flow rate.

12. **Describe devices used for central venous access.**   pp. 255–256

Central venous access utilizes veins located deep within the body. These include the internal jugular, subclavian, and femoral veins. Central IV lines are placed near the heart for long-term use. Typically, they are used when medical conditions require repeated access for medication and/or fluid delivery. They also are used for transvenous pacing or for monitoring central venous pressure. A special type of central line is the peripherally inserted central catheter, or PICC, line. PICC lines are most often used in infants and children requiring long-term care. Central venous access is typically restricted to the hospital setting because of its invasive nature and high risk of complications such as arterial puncture, pneumothorax, and air embolism.

13. **Describe the characteristics of various intravenous fluids, including colloids, crystalloids, and oxygen-carrying solutions.**   pp. 256–257

Colloidal solutions contain large proteins that cannot pass through the capillary membrane. Consequently, they remain in the circulatory system for a long time. In addition, colloids have osmotic properties that attract water into the circulatory system. A small quantity of colloid can significantly increase intravascular volume (volume of blood and fluid contained within the blood vessels). Common colloids include the following: plasma protein fraction (Plasmanate), albumin, dextran, and hetastarch (Hespan).

Crystalloids are the primary prehospital IV solutions. Crystalloids contain electrolytes and water but lack colloids' larger proteins and larger molecules. The many preparations of crystalloid solutions are classified by their tonicity (number of particles per unit volume) relative to that of body plasma. The three most commonly used IV fluids in prehospital are are: lactated Ringer's, normal saline, and 5 percent dextrose in water (D_5W).

Considerable research has been devoted to the development of solutions that carry oxygen. There are two general classes of oxygen-carrying solutions: perfluorocarbons and hemoglobin-based oxygen-carrying solutions (HBOCs). These agents provide a significant advantage over standard colloids and crystalloids because, as their name indicates, in addition to replacing volume they can transport oxygen.

14. **Given a variety of scenarios, select an appropriate intravenous fluid, infusion set, catheter, and infusion rate.**

Intravenous Fluids

pp. 256–257

Colloids. Colloidal solutions contain large proteins that cannot pass through the capillary membrane. Consequently, they remain in the circulatory system for a long time. Common colloids include the following:

   a. **Plasma protein fraction (Plasmanate).** Plasmanate is a protein-containing colloid. Its principal protein, albumin, is suspended with other proteins in a saline solvent.

   b. **Albumin.** Albumin contains only human albumin. Each gram of albumin will retain approximately 18 milliliters of water in the bloodstream.

   c. **Dextran.** Dextran is not a protein but a large sugar molecule with osmotic properties similar to those of albumin. It comes in two molecular weights: 40,000 and 70,000 Daltons. Dextran 40 has from two to two-and-a-half times the colloidal osmotic pressure of albumin. Anaphylactic reaction is a possible side effect.

   d. **Hetastarch (Hespan).** Like Dextran, hetastarch is a sugar molecule with osmotic properties similar to those of protein. Hetastarch does not appear to share dextran's side effects.

Crystalloids. Crystalloids are the primary prehospital IV solutions. Crystalloids contain electrolytes and water but lack colloids' larger proteins and larger molecules. The particular type of IV solution you select depends on your patient's needs. The three most commonly used IV fluids in prehospital care are:

   a. **Lactated Ringer's.** Lactated Ringer's solution, also called Hartman's solution, is an isotonic electrolyte solution. It contains sodium chloride, potassium chloride, calcium chloride, and sodium lactate in water.

   b. **Normal saline solution.** Normal saline is an isotonic electrolyte solution containing 0.9 percent sodium chloride in water.

   c. **5 percent dextrose in water (D_5W).** D_5W is a hypotonic glucose solution used to keep a vein patent and to supply calories needed for cellular metabolism. While D_5W initially increases circulatory volume, glucose molecules rapidly diffuse across the vascular membrane and increase the free water.

Both lactated Ringer's and normal saline solution are used for fluid replacement because of their immediate ability to expand the circulating volume. However, due to the movement of electrolytes and water, two-thirds of either solution will be lost to the extravascular space within 1 hour.

Blood. The most desirable fluid for replacement is whole blood. Unlike colloids and crystalloids, the hemoglobin in blood carries oxygen.

Oxygen-Carrying Solutions. There are two general classes of oxygen-carrying solutions: perfluorocarbons and hemoglobin-based oxygen-carrying solutions (HBOCs). These agents provide a significant advantage over standard colloids and crystalloids because, as their name indicates, in addition to replacing volume they can transport oxygen.

   a. **Perfluorocarbons.** Perfluorocarbon agents are denser than water and have a high capacity to dissolve large quantities of gases such as oxygen.

   b. **Hemoglobin-based oxygen-carrying solutions (HBOCs).** HBOCs differ from other intravenous fluids in that they have the capability to transport oxygen. HBOCs contain long chains of polymerized hemoglobin. This hemoglobin is obtained from either expired donated human blood or bovine (cow) blood. HBOCs are compatible with all blood types and do not require blood typing, testing, or cross-matching.

Infusion Set

pp. 257–259

Intravenous administration tubing connects the solution bag to the IV cannula that is inserted into the patient's vein. Administration tubing is made of very flexible clear plastic. You must select from several types of administration tubing according to your patient's need.

   a. **Microdrip.** Microdrip administration tubing delivers relatively small amounts of fluid to the patient. It is more appropriate when you need to restrict the overall fluid volume a patient will receive.

©2013 Pearson Education, Inc.
Paramedic Care: Principles & Practice, Vol. 2, 4th Ed.

b. **Macrodrip.** Macrodrip administration tubing delivers relatively large amounts of fluid. It is more appropriate when volume replacement is necessary, as in shock, fluid replacement, or hypotension.

c. **Electromechanical Pump Tubing.** Mechanical infusion devices may require specially manufactured pump tubing. Typically, pump tubing has special components that attach directly to the pump. Additionally, bladders and relief points permit you to void possible air bubbles.

d. **Blood Tubing.** Administering whole blood or blood components requires blood tubing, which contains a filter that prevents clots and other debris from entering the patient.

Catheter   pp. 260–261

The intravenous cannula permits actual puncture and access into a patient's vein. The distal portion of the administration tubing connects to the IV cannula, thus completing the bridge between the solution bag and patient. The three basic types of IV cannulas are:

a. **Over-the-Needle Catheter.** Often called an IV catheter or cannula, an over-the-needle catheter comprises a semiflexible catheter enclosing a sharp metal stylet (needle) that is hollow and beveled at the distal end.

b. **Hollow-Needle Catheter.** For pediatrics or other patients with tiny, delicate veins, use hollow-needle catheters. These catheters do not have a Teflon tube; rather, the metal stylet itself is inserted into the vein and secured there. These hollow-needle catheters are referred to as winged catheters or butterfly catheters.

c. **Catheter Inserted Through the Needle.** The catheter inserted through the needle is also called an intracatheter. It consists of a Teflon catheter inserted through a large metal stylet. Used in the hospital setting to implement central lines, its proper placement requires great skill.

The size of an intravenous cannula is expressed as its gauge. The larger the gauge, the smaller the diameter of the stylet and catheter. For example, a 22-gauge cannula is smaller than a 14-gauge cannula. The larger-diameter, 14-gauge catheter allows greater flow rates than the smaller-diameter, 22-gauge cannula. When establishing venous access, choose the cannula size most appropriate for the patient's condition. Typical uses for the various sizes of cannulas are:

a. **22 gauge.** Small gauges are used for fragile veins such as those of the elderly or children.

b. **20 gauge.** Moderate gauges are used for the average adult who does not need fluid replacement.

c. **18 gauge, 16 gauge, or 14 gauge.** Larger-gauge cannulas are used to increase volume or to administer viscous medications such as dextrose. Blood can be administered only through a cannula that is 16 gauge or larger.

The largest gauge cannula that will fit into a vein is not always appropriate. A cardiac patient with large veins should not receive a 14-gauge cannula for medication administration, just as a multisystems trauma patient with good veins should not receive a 22-gauge cannula for fluid administration.

Infusion Rate   pp. 261, 289–290

Infusion rates are based on patient needs. As an example, a cardiac patient who needs IV access maintained for possible medication administration will usually have a TKO (To Keep Open) or KVO (Keep Vein Open) rate, whereas a critical trauma patient may have boluses of fluid (usually 20 mL/kg) repeated to maintain a systolic blood pressure of 90–100 mmHg (follow your local protocol). Pediatric patients may need smaller amounts titrated to maintain adequate perfusion. Paramedics may also receive specific orders for a set amount of fluid to be administered for a specific amount of time. In these cases, the paramedic will need to calculate the drip rate based on the amount, time, and administration tubing being used.

15. Assemble an intravenous infusion line.   p. 262

Examine the IV fluid for clarity and expiration date. Insert the administration tubing spike in the IV solution bag's administration set port. Squeeze fluid from the IV fluid container into the drip chamber until it reaches the fill line. Open the clamp and/or flow regulator to flush the solution through the administration tubing and expel trapped air bubbles. Shut down the flow regulator and replace the cap over the needle adapter. Remember that the IV administration set is sterile; if any contamination occurs, you must replace the set with a new one.

16. Establish a peripheral intravenous line under the supervision of a lab instructor or clinical preceptor.   **p. 262**

To establish a peripheral IV in the hand, arm, or leg, use the following technique:

1. Confirm indication and type of IV setup needed. Gather and arrange all supplies and equipment before-hand to make the process easy and accessible: IV fluid, administration set, intravenous cannula, tape or commercial securing device, venous blood drawing equipment, venous constricting band, and antiseptic solution. When appropriate, explain the entire process to the patient. Apply the proper Standard Precautions:—gloves, mask, and protective eyewear goggles—as IV access is invasive and presents the potential for blood exposure.

2. Prepare all needed equipment. Examine the IV fluid for clarity and expiration date. Insert the administration tubing spike in the IV solution bag's administration set port. Squeeze fluid from the IV fluid container into the drip chamber until it reaches the fill line. Open the clamp and/or flow regulator to flush the solution through the administration tubing and expel trapped air bubbles. Shut down the flow regulator and replace the cap over the needle adapter. Remember that the IV administration set is sterile; if any contamination occurs, you must replace the set with a new one.

3. Select the venipuncture site. Acceptable sites have clearly visible veins and are free of bruising or scar-ring. Straight veins are easier to cannulate than crooked ones.

4. Place the constricting band proximal to the intended site of puncture. Tighten it enough to impede venous blood flow without restricting arterial blood passage. Never leave the constricting band in place more than 2 minutes, as intrinsic changes will occur in the slowed venous blood.

5. Cleanse the venipuncture site. You must cleanse the intended site of pathogens to decrease the likelihood of infection. Alcohol and similar antiseptic solutions are the most commonly used. Start at the site itself and work outward in an expanding circle. This pushes pathogens away from the puncture site.

6. Insert the intravenous cannula into the vein. With your nondominant hand, pull all local skin taut to stabilize the vein and prevent it from rolling. With the distal bevel of the metal stylet up, insert the cannula into the vein at a 10° to 30° angle. Continue until you feel the cannula "pop" into the vein or see blood in the flashback chamber. The metal stylet is now in the vein; however, the Teflon catheter is not. To place the catheter into the vein, carefully advance the cannula approximately 0.5 cm further. (If you are using a butterfly cannula, it has no Teflon catheter, and you must carefully advance the needle itself.)

7. Holding the metal stylet stationary, slide the Teflon catheter over the needle into the vein. Place a finger over the vein at the catheter tip and tamponade (press gently downward to occlude the vein), thus preventing blood from flowing from the catheter and/or air from entraining into the circulatory system. Carefully remove the metal stylet, retract the needle, and promptly dispose of it in the sharps container. Remove the venous constricting band.

8. Obtain venous blood samples as discussed in the section on venous blood sampling.

9. Attach the administration tubing to the cannula. Remove the protective cap from the needle adapter and tightly secure the needle adapter into the cannula hub. Open the flow regulator and allow the fluid to run freely for several seconds. Adjust the flow rate. Do not let go of the cannula and administration tubing until you have secured them as explained in step 10.

10. Cover the catheter and puncture site with an adhesive bandage or other commercial device. Loop the distal tubing and secure with tape. This makes the medication administration port more accessible and attaches the device to the patient more securely. Continue by taping the administration tubing to the patient, proximal to the venipuncture site.

11. Label the intravenous solution bag with the following information: date and time initiated, and person initiating the intravenous access.

12. Continually monitor the patient and flow rate.

17. Troubleshoot an intravenous infusion.   **pp. 265–266**

Constricting band. Has the venous constricting band been removed? This is probably the most common mistake both in and out of the hospital. Additionally, ensure that the patient is not wearing restrictive clothing that interferes with venous blood flow.

Edema at the puncture site. Swelling at the IV site indicates fluid collection caused by infiltration. This extravasation occurs if you accidentally puncture the vein more than once, thus allowing IV solution and blood to escape from the second puncture and accumulate in the surrounding tissue. An infiltrated IV site is not usable.

Cannula abutting the vein wall or valve. If the distal tip of the cannula butts against a wall or valve, carefully reposition it. You may have to untape and retape the cannula once you have achieved an adequate flow rate. Additionally, you may need to use an arm board to keep the patient's extremity straight, as flexion may kink the vein at the site and impede the solution's flow.

Administration set control valves. Ensure that the flow regulator is open. Be sure to check the flow regulator and clamps of both the primary and any secondary or extension tubing.

IV bag height. When you move the patient, you may raise the cannulation site above the IV solution bag. This interrupts the solution's gravitational flow from the bag into the patient.

Completely filled drip chamber. Is the drip chamber completely filled? You can easily correct this by inverting the bag and squeezing the fluid from the drip chamber back into the bag.

Catheter patency. A blood clot at the end of the Teflon catheter or needle may obstruct the flow of solution from the IV solution bag into the body. If the flow slows, increase the IV drip rate to keep the catheter or needle clear. If the flow stops completely, cleanse the medication administration port closest to the IV entry site with alcohol preparations and insert a syringe and hypodermic needle. Gently aspirate back on the syringe until the blood clot is pulled into the syringe. Never flush an IV that has stopped running because of a clot. Flushing will force the clot into the circulatory system and can cause occlusions in the heart or lungs.

18. **Recognize complications of intravenous infusion.** pp. 266–268

Pain. Pain at the puncture site occurs during needle penetration or with extravasation. To minimize pain, use a smaller-gauge catheter or use a 1 percent lidocaine solution (without epinephrine) to anesthetize the overlying skin before insertion.

Local Infection. Local infection occurs if you do not properly cleanse the site and thus introduce pathogens through the puncture. This complication does not become apparent until after the IV has been established for several hours. You must cleanse the intended site of pathogens to decrease the likelihood of infection. Alcohol and similar antiseptic solutions are the most commonly used. Start at the site itself and work outward in an expanding circle. This pushes pathogens away from the puncture site.

Pyrogenic Reaction. Pyrogens (foreign proteins capable of producing fever) in the administration tubing or IV solution can cause a pyrogenic reaction. The abrupt onset of fever (100°F to 106°F), chills, backache, headache, nausea, and vomiting characterize these reactions. Cardiovascular collapse may also result. Typically, a pyrogenic reaction will occur within 1/2 to 1 hour after you initiate an IV. If you suspect a pyrogenic reaction, immediately terminate the IV and reestablish access in the opposite side with new equipment and fluid. Typically, pyrogenic reactions occur secondary to the use of intravenous solutions that have been contaminated with a microorganism or other foreign matter.

Allergic Reaction. A patient receiving IV therapy may develop an allergic reaction. Most often, allergic reactions accompany the administration of blood or colloidal (protein-containing) solutions. In addition, some patients may react to the latex in some types of IV administration tubing. The sudden onset of hives (urticaria), itching (pruritus), localized or systemic edema, or shortness of breath may signify an allergic reaction. If you suspect an allergic reaction, stop the IV infusion and remove the IV catheter.

Catheter Shear. A catheter shear can occur if you pull the Teflon catheter through or over the needle after you have advanced it into the vein. The soft plastic catheter will easily snag on the metal stylet's sharp point and shear off, thus forming a plastic embolus. Therefore, never draw the Teflon catheter over the metal stylet after you have advanced it.

Inadvertent Arterial Puncture. Because arteries may lie close to veins, accidental arterial puncture may occur. Arterial blood is bright red and characteristically spurts with each contraction of the heart.

When an arterial puncture occurs, immediately remove the catheter and apply direct pressure to the site for at least 5 minutes. Do not release the pressure until the hemorrhage has stopped.

Circulatory Overload. Circulatory overload occurs if you administer too much fluid for the patient's condition. You must monitor flow rates carefully, especially for patients with medical conditions such as kidney failure or heart failure who are intolerant of excessive fluid. Continually examine the patient for signs of circulatory overload (crackles, tachypnea, dyspnea, and jugular venous distension. If you encounter circulatory overload, adjust the flow rate.

Thrombophlebitis. Thrombophlebitis, or inflammation of the vein, is particularly common in long-term intravenous therapy. Redness and edema at the puncture site are typical signs of thrombophlebitis. This complication may also present as pain along the course of the vein, sometimes accompanied by inflammation and tenderness. Typically, thrombophlebitis does not occur until several hours after IV initiation. When you suspect thrombophlebitis, terminate the IV and apply a warm compress to the site.

Thrombus Formation. A thrombus, or blood clot, can form if IV access injures the vessel wall. A thrombus may form around the catheter and occlude the movement of fluid between the IV and the blood vessel. If you suspect a thrombus, restart the IV using new equipment. Do not attempt to dislodge the clot with a fluid bolus, as this may create an embolus that causes neurologic or pulmonary complications.

Air Embolism. Air embolism occurs when air enters the vein. Air embolus is most likely to occur during central venous access or when administration tubing has not been properly flushed. Failure to tamponade larger veins during cannulation may allow air into the vein.

Necrosis. Necrosis, or the sloughing off of dead tissue, occurs later in IV therapy as medication (e.g., norepinephrine, epinephrine, dopamine, dobutamine) has extravasated into the interstitial space.

Anticoagulants. Anticoagulant medications such as aspirin, platelet aggregate inhibitors, warfarin (Coumadin), or heparin increase the chance of bleeding and impede hemorrhage control during IV establishment. They drastically increase the complications of hematoma or infiltration.

19. **Change an intravenous solution bag or bottle.** pp. 268–269

You may sometimes have to change an IV bag or bottle. This generally occurs when only 50 mL of solution remain and you must continue therapy after those 50 mL are depleted. Changing the solution bag or bottle is a sterile process. If the equipment becomes contaminated you should dispose of it. To change the IV solution bag or bottle, use the following technique:
   1. Prepare the new IV solution bag or bottle by removing the protective cover from the IV tubing port.
   2. Occlude the flow of solution from the depleted bag or bottle by moving the roller clamp on the IV administration tubing.
   3. Remove the spike from the depleted IV bag or bottle. Be careful not to drop or contaminate the spike in any way.
   4. Insert the spike into the new IV bag or bottle. Ensure that the drip chamber is filled appropriately.
   5. Open the roller clamp to the appropriate flow rate.

   If air becomes entrained within the administration tubing during this process, cleanse the medication administration port below the trapped air and insert a hypodermic needle and syringe. Pull the plunger back to aspirate the trapped air into the syringe. After you have removed the air, adjust the IV flow rate as needed.

20. **Establish a heparin or saline lock under the supervision of a lab instructor or clinical preceptor.** pp. 272–273

A heparin lock is a peripheral IV port that does not use a bag of fluid. Like a typical IV start, it places an IV cannula into a peripheral vein; however, instead of IV administration tubing, it has attached short tubing with a clamp and a distal medication port.

   To place a heparin lock, follow these steps:
   1. Select the venipuncture site.
   2. Place the constricting band proximal to the puncture site.
   3. Cleanse the venipuncture site with antiseptic solution.
   4. Insert the intravenous cannula into the vein.

©2013 Pearson Education, Inc.
Paramedic Care: Principles & Practice, Vol. 2, 4th Ed.

5. Slide the Teflon catheter into the vein.
6. Carefully remove the metal stylet, retract or protect the stylet, and promptly dispose of it into the sharps container. Remove the venous constricting band.
7. Obtain venous blood samples.
8. Attach the heparin lock tubing to the catheter hub.
9. Cleanse the medication port and inject 3 to 5 mL of sterile saline into the lock. Easy flow of the saline without edema at the puncture site indicates patency. If you encounter resistance or if edema forms, restart the procedure with new equipment. If a heparin lock is desired, fill the port with the designated heparin flush solution.
10. Apply an adhesive bandage or other commercial device. Secure the tubing to the patient.

21. If permitted in your scope of practice, access an implanted venous access device under the supervision of a lab instructor or clinical preceptor. pp. 273–274

To administer fluids, medication, or blood through a venous access device, you must first prepare the site using the following technique:
1. Use Standard Precautions.
2. Fill a 10-mL syringe with approximately 7 mL of normal saline.
3. Place a 21- or 22-gauge Huber needle (or other specialized needle) on the end of the syringe.
4. Cleanse the skin over the injection port with an antiseptic solution.
5. Stabilize the site with one hand while inserting the Huber needle at a 90° angle. Gently advance it until it meets resistance. This signals that the needle has contacted the floor of the injection port.
6. Pull back on the plunger and observe for blood return. The presence of blood confirms proper placement.
7. Slowly inject the normal saline to ensure patency.

To administer the medication by intravenous bolus, use the following technique:
1. Prepare the medication, fluid, or blood for administration.
2. Attach a 21- or 22-gauge Huber needle (or other specialized needle) to the end of the syringe.
3. Cleanse the skin over the injection port with an antiseptic solution.
4. Insert the needle into the injection port at a 90° angle until the needle cannot be further advanced. Pull back on the plunger of the syringe and observe for the return of blood. The presence of blood confirms proper placement.
5. Inject the medication as appropriate.
6. Remove and dispose of the syringe appropriately.
7. With another syringe and attached specialized needle, administer a bolus of heparinized saline to clear the catheter of any blood clots or other obstruction. If the venous access device is not patent or access proves difficult, contact medical direction for further directives.

To administer IV fluids, use the following technique:
1. Prepare a primary IV line. Be sure to prime or flush the air from the administration tubing.
2. Attach a 21- or 22-gauge Huber needle (or other specialized needle) to the primary IV administration tubing. Insert a 10-mL syringe and hypodermic needle filled with 7 mL of normal saline solution into the tubing medication delivery port nearest the venous access device.
3. Cleanse the skin over the injection port with an antiseptic solution.
4. Insert the needle into the injection port at a 90° angle until it encounters resistance.
5. Pinch the administration tubing above the medication administration port and pull back on the syringe plunger. Observe for the return of blood. The presence of blood confirms proper placement.
6. Gently inject the 7 mL of normal saline solution.
7. Set the primary line to the appropriate flow rate.

If administering a secondary medicated infusion, continue as follows:
1. Prepare a secondary line containing the fluid, blood, or medicated solution for infusion.
2. Attach a hypodermic needle to the needle adapter of the secondary line. Insert the secondary line into a medication administration port on the primary tubing.
3. Shut down the primary line and infuse the medicated solution as appropriate. Look for ease of administration as a sign of patency.

4. When infusion is complete, administer a bolus of heparinized saline to clear the catheter of any blood clots or other obstruction.

Using a venous access device is a very sterile procedure. You must take care to clean the site before delivering medications.

22. Demonstrate venous blood sampling under the supervision of a lab instructor or clinical preceptor.
pp. 276–277

To obtain blood directly from the IV catheter, use the following procedure:

1. Assemble and prepare all equipment. Inspect the blood tubes for expiration or damage and insert the multidraw needle into the vacutainer. Note: Never place blood tubes into the assembled vacutainer and multidraw needle until you are ready to draw blood. This will destroy the vacuum and render the blood tube useless.
2. Establish IV access with the IV catheter. Do not connect IV administration tubing.
3. Attach the end of the multidraw needle adapter to the hub of the cannula.
4. In correct order, insert the blood tubes so that the rubber-covered needle punctures the self-sealing rubber top. Blood should be pulled into the blood tube.
5. Fill all blood tubes completely, as the amount of anticoagulant is proportional to the tube's volume. Gently agitate the tubes to mix the anticoagulant evenly with the blood.
6. Tamponade the vein and remove the vacutainer and multidraw needle. Attach the IV and ensure patency.
7. Properly dispose of all sharps.
8. Label all blood tubes with the following information:
   a. Patient's first and last name
   b. Patient's age and gender
   c. Date and time drawn
   d. Name of the person drawing the blood

To obtain blood directly from a vein, use the following procedure:

1. Assemble and prepare all equipment. Inspect the blood tubes for expiration or damage, and insert the multidraw needle into the vacutainer.
2. Apply the constricting band and select an appropriate puncture site.
3. Cleanse the site with antiseptic solution.
4. Insert the end of the multi-sampling needle or the Luer sampling needle into the vein and remove the constricting band.
5. In the correct order, insert each blood tube so that the rubber-covered needle punctures the self-sealing rubber top. Blood should be pulled into the tube.
6. Gently agitate the tube to evenly mix the anticoagulant with the blood. Completely fill all blood tubes, as the anticoagulant is proportional to the volume of the tube.
7. Place sterile gauze over the site and remove the sampling needle. Properly dispose of all sharps.
8. Cover the puncture site with gauze and tape or an adhesive bandage.
9. Label all blood tubes with the following information:
   a. Patient's first and last name
   b. Patient's age and gender
   c. Date and time drawn
   d. Person drawing the blood

23. Discontinue a peripheral intravenous infusion.
p. 277

You should remove any IV that will not flow or has fulfilled its need. To do so, completely occlude the tubing with the flow regulator and/or clamp. Remove all tape or other securing devices from the tubing and patient. Place a sterile gauze pad over the puncture site. Apply pressure to the gauze with the fingers or thumb of your nondominant hand. With your dominant hand, grasp the cannula at its hub and swiftly remove it, pulling straight back. The site may bleed, so apply direct pressure with the gauze for 5 minutes. Immediately dispose of all materials in the appropriate biohazard container. Apply an adhesive bandage or tape clean gauze over the site to protect against infection. Document that the catheter was removed intact.

©2013 Pearson Education, Inc.
Paramedic Care: Principles & Practice, Vol. 2, 4th Ed.

24. **Establish an intraosseous infusion in adult and pediatric patients under the supervision of a lab instructor or clinical preceptor.**   pp. 280–283

To place an intraosseous line, use the following technique:

1. Determine the indication for intraosseous access.
2. Assemble and check all equipment.
3. Position the patient. Rotate the leg toward the outside to expose the medial, proximal aspect of the tibia.
4. Locate the access site. Palpate the tibia and use all landmarks.
   a. Pediatric. Locate the tibial tuberosity. Move from one to two fingerbreadths below the tibial tuberosity and find the flat expanse medial to the anterior tibial crest.
   b. Adult or geriatric. Find the medial locations (based on the device you are using). These can include the tibial tuberosity, sternum, or humeral head. Be familiar with the accepted access sites as well as the operation of the particular IO device you are using.
5. Cleanse the site with an antiseptic solution. Start at the puncture site and work outward in an expanding circular motion.
6. Perform the puncture. Holding the needle perpendicular to the puncture site, insert it with a twisting motion until you feel a decrease in resistance or a "pop." When this occurs, the needle is in the medullary canal. Do not advance it any further. Generally, you will need to insert the needle only 2 to 4 mm for entry.
7. Remove the trocar and attach the syringe. Slowly pull back the plunger to attempt aspiration into the syringe. Easy aspiration of bone marrow and blood confirms correct medullary placement.
8. Once you have confirmed placement, rotate the plastic disk toward the skin to secure the needle.
9. Remove the syringe and attach the prepared administration tubing and solution. Set the appropriate flow rate.
10. Secure the intraosseous needle as if securing an impaled object by surrounding it with bulky dressings and taping them securely in place. Commercial devices for securing an intraosseous needle are available.

25. **Troubleshoot an intraosseous infusion.**   pp. 283, 267–268

Fractures. Be sure to use the appropriate-size needle and avoid being too forceful when inserting.

Infiltration. Immediately discontinue infusion and restart on the other leg.

Growth Plate Damage. Locating the site with proper technique is the most effective way to avoid this complication.

Complete Insertion. To avoid complete puncture, stop advancing the needle once you feel the pop. If complete puncture occurs, remove the intraosseous needle with a reverse twisting motion and start again on the other leg. Apply direct pressure and a sterile dressing over the site(s) for at least 5 minutes.

Pulmonary Embolism. Proper technique and vigilance for signs associated with pulmonary embolism (sudden onset of chest pain or shortness of breath) are important to establishing and maintaining intraosseous access.

Local infection. Occurs if you do not properly cleanse the site and thus introduce pathogens through the puncture. This complication does not become apparent until after the IV has been established for several hours.

26. **Recognize complications of an intraosseous infusion.**   p. 283

Fractures. Too large a needle or too forceful an insertion can fracture the tibia, particularly in very young children.

Infiltration. Infiltration occurs when IV solution collects in the local tissues instead of in the intramedullary canal. Infiltration may occur if you run fluids through an incorrectly placed needle or if a fracture has occurred. An infusion that does not run freely or the formation of an edema at the puncture site indicates infiltration.

Growth Plate Damage. An improperly located puncture may damage the growth plate and result in long-term growth complications.

Complete Insertion. Complete insertion occurs when the needle passes through both sides of the tibia, rendering the site useless.

Pulmonary Embolism. If bone, fat, or marrow particles make their way into the circulatory system, pulmonary embolism may result. Proper technique and vigilance for signs associated with pulmonary embolism (sudden onset of chest pain or shortness of breath) are important to establishing and maintaining intraosseous access.

Local Infection. Other complications of intraosseous access are similar to those of peripheral intravenous access. They include local infection, thrombophlebitis, air embolism, circulatory overload, and allergic reaction.

27. **Identify indications and contraindications for intraosseous infusion.**   pp. 277–278, 283

While intravenous lines remain the preferred route of vascular access, IOs provide a rapid and reliable method for administering medications and fluids when an IV cannot be established. The most frequent need for IO access will be with patients in shock and cardiac arrest. IO access may be needed in pediatric hypovolemia. Victims of multiple trauma may benefit from IO therapy, although the prevailing evidence shows that prehospital fluids in trauma patients are of questionable benefit.

   Do not attempt intraosseous placement in the following situations: fracture to the tibia or femur on the side of access, osteogenesis imperfect (a congenital bone disease that results in fragile bones), osteoporosis, or establishment of a peripheral IV line.

Content Self-Evaluation

MULTIPLE CHOICE

_____ 1. Which of the following is an indication for intravenous administration?
  A. Fluid replacement
  B. Blood replacement
  C. Drug administration
  D. Need of blood for analysis
  E. All of the above

_____ 2. Which of the following is a likely site for intravenous cannulation?
  A. The hands
  B. The arms
  C. The legs
  D. The neck
  E. All of the above

_____ 3. Which of the following is NOT a central venous vessel?
  A. The internal jugular
  B. The subclavian
  C. The femoral
  D. The antecubital
  E. All of the above are central venous vessels

_____ 4. Both central venous and peripheral venous cannulation are common in prehospital care.
  A. True
  B. False

_____ 5. The solution that contains large proteins is
  A. colloid.
  B. crystalloid.
  C. isotonic.
  D. hypotonic.
  E. hypertonic.

Paramedic Care: Principles & Practice, Vol. 2, 4th Ed.

6. The solution that contains an electrolyte concentration close to that of plasma is
   A. colloid.
   B. crystalloid.
   C. isotonic.
   D. hypotonic.
   E. hypertonic.

7. The solution that contains an electrolyte concentration greater than that of plasma is
   A. colloid.
   B. crystalloid.
   C. isotonic.
   D. hypotonic.
   E. hypertonic.

8. One example of a hypotonic solution is
   A. normal saline.
   B. lactated Ringer's solution.
   C. plasmanate.
   D. 5 percent dextrose in water.
   E. dextran.

9. The most desirable replacement for blood lost during trauma is
   A. normal saline.
   B. lactated Ringer's solution.
   C. plasmanate.
   D. 5 percent dextrose in water.
   E. none of the above.

10. Which intravenous fluid bag would you discard?
   A. One that is cloudy
   B. One that is discolored
   C. One that is leaking
   D. One that is expired
   E. All of the above

11. The administration set most appropriate for administration of intravenous solutions for fluid replacement is the
   A. macrodrip administration set.
   B. microdrip administration set.
   C. measured volume administration set.
   D. blood tubing set.
   E. none of the above.

12. For optimal fluid delivery, the drip chamber should be how full?
   A. One-fourth
   B. Three-eighths
   C. One-half
   D. Two-thirds
   E. None of the above

13. The greatest microdrip setting equaling 1 mL is
   A. 10 drops.
   B. 20 drops.
   C. 45 drops.
   D. 60 drops.
   E. none of the above.

14. The administration set most appropriate for administration of a very specific volume of intravenous solution or drug is the
   A. macrodrip administration set.
   B. microdrip administration set.
   C. measured volume administration set.
   D. blood tubing set.
   E. none of the above.

15. The major difference between blood tubing and a standard intravenous administration set is that blood tubing has a filter to remove clots and particulate matter.
   A. True
   B. False

16. Blood is not administered with fluids like lactated Ringer's solution because such solutions increase blood's potential for coagulation.
   A. True
   B. False

_____ 17. Many patients are prone to develop hypothermia during fluid administration.
  A. True
  B. False

_____ 18. The most common intravenous cannula(s) used in the prehospital setting is/are the
  A. over-the-needle.
  B. through-the-needle.
  C. hollow needle.
  D. angiocatheter.
  E. A and D.

_____ 19. A needle gauge of 18 is smaller than a needle gauge of 22.
  A. True
  B. False

_____ 20. A venous constricting band should be left in place no longer than
  A. 1 minute.
  B. 2 minutes.
  C. 3 minutes.
  D. 5 minutes.
  E. 10 minutes.

_____ 21. Leaving the constricting band on for too long is likely to cause
  A. collapse of the vein.
  B. damage to the distal blood vessels.
  C. damage to the vessels under the band.
  D. changes in the distal venous blood.
  E. all of the above.

_____ 22. When cleansing the site for intravenous cannulation, you should make one swipe over the intended site with a povidone-iodine or alcohol swab.
  A. True
  B. False

_____ 23. The angle of insertion for intravenous cannulation is
  A. 10°.
  B. 10° to 30°.
  C. 45°.
  D. 60°.
  E. 60° to 90°.

_____ 24. After you feel the "pop" associated with intravenous cannulation, you should
  A. advance the catheter.
  B. advance the needle 0.5 cm, then advance the catheter.
  C. advance the needle 1 cm, then advance the catheter.
  D. advance the needle 2 cm, then advance the catheter.
  E. withdraw the needle, then advance the catheter.

_____ 25. You should consider using the external jugular vein as an IV access site only after you have exhausted other means of peripheral access or when the patient needs immediate fluid administration.
  A. True
  B. False

_____ 26. During external jugular vein cannulation, the patient's head should be
  A. moved to the sniffing position.
  B. turned toward the side of access.
  C. turned away from the side of access.
  D. hyperextended.
  E. hyperflexed.

_____ 27. To fill the jugular access site and make the vessel easier to both locate and cannulate, you should
  A. apply a venous constricting band tightly.
  B. apply a venous constricting band loosely.
  C. occlude the vein gently with a finger.
  D. perform the procedure without occluding the vein.
  E. have the patient take a deep breath and hold it.

©2013 Pearson Education, Inc.
Paramedic Care: Principles & Practice, Vol. 2, 4th Ed.

_____ 28. When establishing an IV with blood tubing, you must be careful to
    A. fill the drip chamber one-third full.
    B. completely cover the blood filter with blood.
    C. fill the set with normal saline first.
    D. fill the drip chamber three-fourths full.
    E. A and B.

_____ 29. Which of the following is a factor that may affect intravenous flow rates?
    A. Failure to remove a venous constricting band
    B. Edema at the access site
    C. The cannula tip up against a vein valve
    D. A clogged catheter
    E. All of the above

_____ 30. The complication of peripheral venous access in which a plastic embolus can form is
    A. pyrogenic reaction.   **D.** catheter shear.
    B. pain.   **E.** all of the above.
    C. thrombophlebitis.

_____ 31. The most common cause of catheter shear is
    A. cannulating thick veins.
    B. cannulating underneath the constricting band.
    C. withdrawing the needle from within the catheter.
    D. withdrawing the catheter from the needle.
    E. faulty catheter construction.

_____ 32. If a blood clot appears to stop or slow intravenous fluid flow, forcefully inject a small amount of heparin into the catheter and continue the infusion.
    A. True
    B. False

_____ 33. You should change a large (500- to 1,000-mL) infusion bag when the volume remaining in the bag is
    A. 10 mL.
    B. 20 mL.
    C. 30 mL.
    D. 50 mL.
    E. 100 mL.

_____ 34. If air becomes entrained in the administration set when you are changing an IV bag or bottle, you should
    A. continue the infusion, because the volume of air is negligible.
    B. discard the set and use a new one.
    C. use a syringe placed between the bubbles and patient to withdraw the air.
    D. reverse the fluid flow until the bubbles enter the fluid bag or drip chamber.
    E. squeeze the tubing to push the bubbles into the drip chamber or bag.

_____ 35. Never administer an intravenous drug infusion as the primary IV line.
    A. True
    B. False

_____ 36. A heparin lock decreases the risk of accidental fluid overload and electrolyte derangement.
    A. True
    B. False

_____ 37. Which of the following is NOT true regarding infusion pumps?
    A. They deliver fluids under pressure.
    B. They are large and difficult to carry.
    C. Most pumps contain alarms for occlusion.
    D. Most pumps contain alarms for fluid source depletion.
    E. They deliver fluids at precise rates.

38. The laboratory analysis of blood can provide valuable information about
- **A.** electrolytes.
- **B.** gases.
- **C.** hormones.
- **D.** other chemicals.
- **E.** all of the above.

39. Do not use a blood tube after its expiration date because the anticoagulant and vacuum may have become ineffective.
- **A.** True
- **B.** False

40. Drawing blood and injecting it into the blood tubes in the wrong order may result in
- **A.** leaving the wrong volume of blood in a tube.
- **B.** cross-contamination of the blood with anticoagulants.
- **C.** depletion of the vacuum in the tubes at too early a stage.
- **D.** coagulation in the last tubes to be filled.
- **E.** all but C.

41. The device that accepts the blood tube to permit its filling is
- **A.** the Luer Lot.
- **B.** the Huber needle.
- **C.** the vacutainer.
- **D.** the Luer sampling needle.
- **E.** A or C.

42. You should fill the blood tube to between a third and a half of its volume because the anticoagulant is measured for this amount of blood.
- **A.** True
- **B.** False

43. When using a syringe to fill your blood tubes, you should draw a volume of blood of about
- **A.** 5 mL.
- **B.** 10 mL.
- **C.** 20 mL.
- **D.** 35 mL.
- **E.** 50 mL.

44. Hemoconcentration occurs during drawing blood
- **A.** when the constricting band is left in place too long.
- **B.** when blood is drawn back through a needle that is too small.
- **C.** with premature mixing of the anticoagulant.
- **D.** with too vigorous a mixing of the blood and anticoagulant.
- **E.** with too forceful an aspiration of blood into the syringe.

45. The complication from drawing blood in which red blood cells are destroyed is
- **A.** hematocrit.
- **B.** hemoconcentration.
- **C.** hemolysis.
- **D.** hemoptysis.
- **E.** hematuria.

46. When an IV catheter is withdrawn, place pressure on the venipuncture site with a sterile gauze pad for about 5 minutes.
- **A.** True
- **B.** False

47. The bone most commonly used for pediatric and adult intraosseous access is the
- **A.** proximal tibia.
- **B.** humeral head.
- **C.** medial malleolus
- **D.** distal tibia.
- **E.** sternum.

48. The IO device that uses a small drill to place the needle into the bone is the
- **A.** Bone Injection Gun (B.I.G.).
- **B.** FAST1.
- **C.** EZ-IO.
- **D.** Illinois sternal/iliac aspiration needle.
- **E.** none of the above.

©2013 Pearson Education, Inc.
Paramedic Care: Principles & Practice, Vol. 2, 4th Ed.

_____ **49.** Confirmation that you are in the medullary space is achieved by
    A. feeling the bone "pop."
    B. pushing the needle 2 to 4 mm.
    C. aspirating bone marrow and blood.
    D. feeling resistance to the twisting of insertion.
    E. none of the above.

_____ **50.** Complications of intraosseous cannulation include all of the following EXCEPT
    A. pulmonary embolism.
    B. fracture.
    C. growth plate damage.
    D. aspiration of bone marrow.
    E. complete insertion.

Special Project

Medication Administration: Personal Benchmarking

To administer medications to the patient experiencing a trauma or medical emergency, you must be familiar with the subcutaneous, intramuscular, and intravenous administration sites located around the body. By locating these various sites on your own body, you can become accustomed to the texture and feel of the various sites used for administration of medications and fluids. This personal benchmarking can help you identify these locations as you begin to treat patients.

Subcutaneous Injection Sites: Medications such as epinephrine are injected subcutaneously because of the slow, steady, and dependable absorption associated with that method. The hypodermic needle is inserted into a "pinch" of skin located on the proximal arm, lateral thigh, and, in some cases, the abdomen (as shown in the illustration on page 251 of the textbook). Examine each of these areas on yourself or a friend and locate possible administration sites where you can easily pinch the skin and feel it separate from the muscular tissue below. Inspect the tissue to ensure it is free of superficial blood vessels, nerves, and tendons, and avoid areas of bruising, scar tissue, or tattoos.

Intramuscular Injection Sites: Medications such as glucagon and morphine are administered into the muscular tissue because it has both the ability to accept a relatively large (2 to more than 5 mL) amount of the drug and a moderate and predictable absorption rate. A hypodermic needle is inserted directly (at an angle of 90° to the skin surface) through the skin and subcutaneous tissue and into the muscle mass directly beneath. Muscle masses for IM medication administration are chosen carefully to reduce the risk of injecting the drug into a blood vessel or nerve. Common IM sites include the deltoid muscle, the dorsal gluteal muscle, the vastus lateralis muscle, and the rectus femoris muscle. These muscle locations are diagrammed on page 253 of your textbook. Palpate each muscle on yourself and a friend to identify the proper locations for IM needle insertions and medication administration. You should be able to feel the firm muscle mass as pictured on page 253 and locate the safe regions to inject medications. Avoid areas of scar tissue and bruises and try to select ones that are free of superficial blood vessels.

Intravenous Injection Sites: Most medications during prehospital care are administered through the intravenous route. This route allows rapid introduction of a drug into the bloodstream, where it is mixed with blood and then distributed throughout the body. The most common venipuncture sites include the veins of the back of the hand, the arm, the antecubital fossa, and the legs and the external jugular vein (see page 255 of the textbook). It is preferable to initiate an IV cannulation with the smallest vein needed at the most distal site, because infiltration or blood vessel injury limits the usefulness of the vein distal to the injury. Obtain a venous constricting band and place it just proximal to the area you will examine for veins. Wait a few seconds until the veins engorge with blood and become more prominent. Then look at the skin below the band for a prominent bump along the course of the vein and a possible bluish discoloration due to the accumulation of blood. Palpate the vessel and appreciate the spongy feel of the blood-filled tube. As you collapse the vessel with your finger pressure, you should feel it compress easily and form a hollow depression beneath your finger. Close your eyes and palpate a region, trying to locate veins by touch. In many patients you will not see the prominence of veins and may only have the characteristic feel of the skin's surface to go by. Palpate the antecubital fossa to locate the antecubital vein. Note that it is rather central in the fold of the elbow and has the spongy feel. This vessel may be the only one you can locate on the patient with severe hypovolemia.

Stand in front of a mirror and look for the external jugular vein. Turn your head to the side and place digital pressure on the jugular vein just above the clavicle. The vein should initially be collapsed and difficult to see in a standing patient, but occluding the vein should cause it to rapidly engorge and become prominent. Notice the course the vein takes as it travels down from the angle of the jaw to the clavicle.

Intraosseous Injection Sites: When other injection sites are unavailable in pediatric, geriatric, and adult patients, an alternative site is the tibia (intraosseous). This site has the advantages of permitting the injection of any intravenous drug or fluid and of being easily located when the patient is otherwise in vascular collapse and the veins are very difficult to find. It is only used when another intravenous site cannot be established. Four sites are used, the proximal tibial site, the distal tibial site, the sternum, and the humeral head (see page 278 of the textbook). Locate the proximal tibial site by identifying the prominent bump at the top of the tibia (the tibial tuberosity) and then locating the flat surface one to two finger widths below and medial to it. Locate the distal tibial site by locating the medial malleolus (the medial prominence of the ankle) and then the flat surface one to two finger widths above and anterior to it (medial to the anterior tibial crest).

Part 3: Medical Mathematics, p. 284

Review of Chapter Objectives

After reading this part of the chapter, you should be able to:

28. **Given a variety of scenarios involving medication orders and patient factors, precisely calculate intravenous infusion rates and drug dosages.** pp. 284–290

The basic units used for most of medicine are metric: the gram for weight, the liter for volume, and the meter for distance. The metric system is a decimal system that uses suffixes and prefixes to delineate larger and smaller quantities, most commonly kilo (1,000), milli (1/1,000), and micro (1/1,000,000). Pharmacology math involves working with addition, subtraction, multiplication, and division, as well as working extensively with ratios, fractions, and formulas.

The centigrade (officially known as Celsius) scale graduates the temperature between the point at which ice melts and the point at which water boils, at 100°. The Fahrenheit scale graduates the range between the lowest temperature at which a salt-water mixture would remain a liquid (0°) and the boiling point of water, at 212°. The Celsius scale is used in medicine, and the conversion between the two is demonstrated by the following formulas:

$$°F = 9/5 \ °C + 32 \quad °C = 5/9 \ (°F - 32)$$

Weight. Weight conversion between household and metric measures is accomplished by dividing a weight in pounds by 2.2 to find the equivalent metric weight in kilograms. Conversely, if you know a weight in kilograms, multiply it by 2.2 to get the weight in pounds

$$kg = lb/2.2 \quad lb = kg \times 2.2$$

Volume. Volume conversion between household and metric measures is based on the recognition that 1 quart is about equal to 1 liter, 1 cup to 250 milliliters, and so on.

The major formula for determining the amount of a drug to be administered is as follows:

$$Dh = \frac{Vh \times Dd}{Va}$$

The formula is mathematically manipulated so that the unknown element can be computed using the known values.

Other elements of drug calculation call for determining the volume flowing through an intravenous administration set by monitoring the number of drops falling in a drip chamber per minute. Conversion is based upon the number of drops that equal 1 milliliter of fluid.

©2013 Pearson Education, Inc.
Paramedic Care: Principles & Practice, Vol. 2, 4th Ed.

$$\text{Dose on hand} = \frac{\text{Volume on hand} \times \text{Desired dose}}{\text{Volume to be administered}}$$

You may also be required to convert pounds to kilograms (if the patient dosing is in weight of drug per kilogram of body weight). To do this you should know that:

$$1 \text{ pound} = 2.2 \text{ kilograms}$$

In some cases, it is important to administer a volume of medication over time, and the associated formula for such administration is:

$$\text{Drops / Minute} = \frac{\text{Volume to be administered} \times \text{Drip factor}}{\text{Time in minutes}}$$

Content Self-Evaluation

MULTIPLE CHOICE

_____ 1. The metric system's fundamental unit relating to mass is the
A. meter.
B. watt.
C. liter.
D. gram.
E. micron.

_____ 2. The metric system's fundamental unit relating to distance is the
A. meter.
B. watt.
C. liter.
D. gram.
E. micron.

_____ 3. The metric system's fundamental unit relating to volume is the
A. meter.
B. watt.
C. liter.
D. gram.
E. micron.

_____ 4. All of the following are commonly used prefixes in pharmacology EXCEPT
A. kilo-
B. centi-
C. milli-
D. deka-
E. micro-

_____ 5. A patient weighing 275 pounds is equivalent to a patient weighing
A. 125 kilograms.
B. 137.5 kilograms.
C. 250 kilograms.
D. 275 kilograms.
E. 605 kilograms.

_____ 6. In the Celsius temperature system, the freezing point of water is
A. 0°.
B. 32°.
C. 70°.
D. 100°.
E. 212°.

_____ 7. In the Fahrenheit temperature system, the boiling point of water is
A. 0°.
B. 32°.
C. 70°.
D. 100°.
E. 212°.

_____ 8. The specific quantity of medication needed is called the
A. unit on hand.
B. dosage on hand.
C. concentration.
D. desired dose.
E. volume on hand.

_____ 9. A liquid medication's concentration is the medication's weight (grams, milligrams, or micrograms) per volume of liquid (mL) in which it is dissolved.
   A. True
   B. False

_____ 10. Because infants and children differ drastically from adults in size and internal development, their dosages often depend on weight.
   A. True
   B. False

Special Project

Pharmacology (Drip and Drug) Math

Guide to Easier Drug Calculations

Although there might be more rapid systems to calculate drip rates and concentrations, the following step-wise approach is designed to help you understand the math so you are able to solve almost any problem. Math is an essential skill for the paramedic, and most drip calculations are simple, standard, and easy to perform once you become familiar with the drugs and drip rates used in your system.

Step I: Identify all known elements.

Elements for most drug dose calculations:

   C = Concentration (g, mg, or mcg per mL)
   Dd = Desired dose
   Va = Volume to be administered
   Dh = Weight (Dose on hand) (g, mg, or mcg)
   Vh = Volume on hand (convert to mL)

Elements for most drip calculations:

   R = Rate (either in drops/min, drops/mcg, or mL/min)
   V = Volume (convert to mL)
   T = Time (convert to minutes)
   D = Drip conversion (drops per mL)

Step II: Select the proper formula.

The element that you don't know (and need to find) should be equal to the remainder of the formula.

Concentration = Dose on hand/Volume on hand $C = Dh/Vh$
Dose on hand = Volume on hand × Concentration $Dh = Vh \times C$
Volume on hand = Dose on hand/Concentration $Vh = Dh/C$

$$\text{Volume to be adminstered} = \frac{\text{Volume on hand} \times \text{Desired dose}}{\text{Dosage on hand}} \qquad Va = \frac{Vh \times Dd}{Dh}$$

$$\text{Dose on hand} = \frac{\text{Volume on hand} \times \text{Desired dose}}{\text{Volume to be administered}} \qquad Dh = \frac{Vh \times Dd}{Va}$$

$$\text{Desired dose} = \frac{\text{Volume to be administered} \times \text{Dosage on hand}}{\text{Volume on hand}} \qquad Dd = \frac{Va \times Dh}{Vh}$$

$$\text{Volume on hand} = \frac{\text{Volume to be administered} \times \text{Dosage on hand}}{\text{Desired dose}} \qquad Vh = \frac{Va \times Dh}{Dd}$$

Rate = Volume/Time (R = V/T)

©2013 Pearson Education, Inc.
Paramedic Care: Principles & Practice, Vol. 2, 4th Ed.

Volume = Rate × Time (V = R × T)

Time = Volume/Rate (T = V/R)

Step III: Convert all variables into common terms.

Use the drip conversion figure or other conversion formula to convert all values to metric and standard values.

Rate—into milliliters or milligrams/minute

Volume—into milliliters

Concentration—into milligrams/milliliter

Time—into minutes

Weight—into milligrams

Step IV: Plug in the known values.

Complete the formula, inserting the values identified in Step I.

Step V: Cancel out labels.

Cross multiply labels to cancel them out. The result should leave you with the label in terms of the unknown value.

$$\text{Volume} = \frac{\text{Rate} \times \text{Time}}{\text{min}} = \frac{X \text{ ml} \times Y \text{ min}}{\text{min}} = X \text{ mL} \times Y = X \times Y \text{ mL}$$

Step VI: Do the mathematical operations.

Multiply, divide, add, or subtract as necessary.

$3 \times 7 = 21 \quad 3/7 = 0.43 \quad 7 + 3 = 10 \quad 7 - 3 = 4$

Step VII: Apply any needed conversions.

Use the mathematical conversions needed, such as the drip conversion, to give you the final answer. Ensure that your answer is provided in the form and label the question asks for.

$$\frac{X \text{ mL} / \text{min}}{\text{min}} \text{ using a } \frac{Y \text{ drops} / \text{mL}}{\text{mL}} = X \text{ mL} \times \text{drops} = \frac{X \times Y \text{ drops}}{\text{min}} = X \times Y \text{ drops} / \text{min}$$

There are two particular types of math used in prehospital care. One deals with continuous intravenous infusions (drip math) and the other deals with parenteral bolus or enteral administration (drug math). Included within this and the following workbooks are exercises for drip and drug math.

Drip Math Worksheet I

Formulas

Rate = Volume/Time mL/min = drops per min/drops per mL

Volume = Rate × Time drops/min = mL per min × drops per mL

Time = Volume/Rate mL = drops/drops per mL

Please complete the following drip math problems.

1. You are running a D_5W drip (60 drops/mL) into a patient at 15 drops/min. During a 25-minute trip to the hospital, how much fluid would you infuse? _____

2. Medical direction requests that you infuse 250 mL of a solution during a 1-hour transport. What rate do you need to set:

    A. for a 60-drops/mL infusion set? _____

    B. for a 10-drops/mL infusion set? _____

3. If a 50-mL bag of normal saline is hung and running through a 45-drops/mL administration set at 32 drops per minute, how long will the fluid last? _____

4. If you are running a macro drip (10 drops/mL) at 4 drops per second, how much fluid could you infuse in 45 minutes? _____

5. Medical direction orders you to infuse 1.5 mL of a solution every minute. What drip rate would you set:

    A. with a 60-drops/mL set? _____

    B. with a 45-drops/mL set? _____

    C. with a 10-drops/mL set? _____

Drug Math Worksheet 2

Formulas

Concentration = Dose on hand/Volume on hand $C = Dh/Vh$

Dose on hand = Volume on hand × Concentration $Dh = Vh \infty C$

Volume on hand = Dose on hand/Concentration $Vh = Dh/C$

$$\text{Volume to be adminstered} = \frac{\text{Volume on hand} \times \text{Desired dose}}{\text{Dosage on hand}} \qquad Va = \frac{Vh \times Dd}{Dh}$$

$$\text{Dose on hand} = \frac{\text{Volume on hand} \times \text{Desired dose}}{\text{Volume to be administered}} \qquad Dh = \frac{Vh \times Dd}{Va}$$

$$\text{Desired dose} = \frac{\text{Volume to be administered} \times \text{Dosage on hand}}{\text{Volume on hand}} \qquad Dd = \frac{Va \times Dh}{Vh}$$

$$\text{Volume on hand} = \frac{\text{Volume to be administered} \times \text{Dosage on hand}}{\text{Desired dose}} \qquad Vh = \frac{Va \times Dh}{Dd}$$

Please complete the following drug math problems.

1. What volume of atropine, provided as 1 mg in 5 mL, would you administer to provide 0.5 mg of drug to the patient? _____

2. The medical direction physician asks you to administer 40 mg of furosemide to a patient. It comes in an ampule with 80 mg in 4 mL. What volume will you administer? _____

3. What volume of epinephrine would you administer to provide a patient with 1 mg of the drug:

    A. if provided as a 1:1,000 solution? (1 g/1,000 mL) _____

    B. if provided as a 1:10,000 solution? (1 g/10,000 mL) _____

4. Protocol calls for the administration of 0.2 mg/kg of adenosine for a pediatric patient. Your patient weighs 6 kilograms, and the drug is supplied in a vial with 6 mg in 2 mL. What volume would you administer to your patient? _____

©2013 Pearson Education, Inc.
Paramedic Care: Principles & Practice, Vol. 2, 4th Ed.

5

Airway Management and Ventilation

Because Chapter 5 is lengthy, it has been divided into parts in this workbook to aid your study. Read the assigned textbook pages, then progress through the objectives and self-evaluation materials as you would with other chapters. When you feel secure in your grasp of the content, proceed to the next section.

Review of Chapter Objectives

After reading this chapter, you should be able to:

1. **Define key terms introduced in this chapter.**

   Knowing and being able to apply the key terms in each chapter is critical to understanding chapter concepts. Write the list of key terms. Then write the definition of each one in your own words. Check your understanding by confirming the definitions in the text glossary. Correct any misunderstandings. Create a study aid by writing each key term on the front of an index card and the definition on the back. Use the cards to quiz yourself or to have someone quiz you.

Part 1: Respiratory Anatomy, Physiology, and Assessment, p. 298

Review of Chapter Objectives

After reading this part of the chapter, you should be able to:

2. **Explain the importance of immediate recognition and management of problems with a patient's airway, breathing, or oxygenation.**   **p. 298**

   Airway management and ventilation are the first and most critical steps in the primary assessment of every patient you will encounter (unless the patient is in cardiac arrest, when chest compressions will come first). Airway management and ventilation go hand in hand. You must immediately establish and maintain an open airway while providing adequate oxygen delivery and carbon dioxide elimination for all patients. Without adequate airway maintenance and ventilation, the patient will succumb to brain injury or even death in as little as 4 minutes. Early detection and intervention of airway and breathing problems, including dispatcher-guided interventions by bystanders, are vital to patient survival.

3. **Explain the importance of nonlinear thinking and action in assessment and management of problems with the airway and ventilation.** p. 298

Airway management and ventilation have always been taught to occur in a stepwise (linear) process. Recommended sequences include the standard ABC (airway, breathing, circulation) sequence, as well as the CAB (compressions, airway, breathing) sequence recommended by the American Heart Association for a patient who appears to be in cardiac arrest when chest compression must come first. These established sequences (ABC and CAB) can help rescuers remember what to do in emergency situations. With regard to airway and/or ventilation problems, paramedics should approach the patient more globally and consider the whole picture, rather than blindly following predetermined steps. You cannot assess an airway if the patient is not breathing. You cannot assess breathing if there is no airway. Therefore, airway and ventilation need to be considered and managed together. Stated another way, airway and ventilation problems must be approached in a nonlinear fashion with a number of factors considered simultaneously.

4. **Describe the legal liability associated with poor assessment and management of airway and ventilation.** pp. 298, 320, 380

Airway management and ventilation are the first and most critical steps in the primary assessment of every patient you will encounter. As such, failure to appropriately assess and manage your patient's airway and breathing can open the paramedic up to liability issues. Misplaced endotracheal tubes represent a significant area of liability in EMS and the documentation provided by this technology can provide irrefutable evidence of proper endotracheal tube placement. A significant percentage of claims and lawsuits that are filed against prehospital providers involve airway issues, and often these cases are won or lost based on the field documentation.

5. **Recognize the anatomical structures of the upper and lower airway.** pp. 298–302

The upper airway consists of the nasal cavity, the oral cavity, the pharynx, and the larynx. The lower airway consists of the trachea, the bronchi, the alveoli, the lung parenchyma, and the pleura.

Nasal cavity. The nasal cavity is the most superior part of the airway. The maxillary, frontal, nasal, ethmoid, and sphenoid bones comprise the lateral and superior walls of the nasal cavity. The hard palate forms the floor of the nasal cavity. The cartilaginous and highly vascular nasal septum separates the right and left nasal cavities. Several structures connect with the nasal cavity. These include the sinuses, the eustachian tubes, and the lacrimal ducts. Air enters the nasal cavity through the external nares (nostrils).

Oral cavity. The cheeks, the hard and soft palates, and the tongue form the mouth, or oral cavity. The lips that surround the mouth's opening are fleshy folds of skin. Behind the lips lie the gums and teeth, normally numbering 32 in the adult. The hard palate anteriorly and the soft palate posteriorly form the top of the oral cavity and separate it from the nasal cavity. The tongue, a large muscle on the bottom of the oral cavity, is the most common airway obstruction. It attaches to the mandible and the hyoid bone through a series of muscles and ligaments. The U-shaped hyoid bone is located just beneath the chin. The hyoid bone is unique. It is the only bone in the axial skeleton that does not articulate with any other bone. Instead, it is suspended by ligaments from the styloid process of the temporal bone and serves to anchor the tongue and larynx, as well as to support the trachea.

Pharynx. The pharynx is a muscular tube that extends vertically from the back of the soft palate to the superior aspect of the esophagus. The pharynx is divided into three regions: the nasopharynx, the oropharynx, and the laryngopharynx (hypopharynx). The nasopharynx is the uppermost region, extending from the back of the nasal opening to the plane of the soft palate. The oropharynx extends from the plane of the soft palate to the hyoid bone. The adenoids, lymphatic tissue in the mouth and nose, filter bacteria. The laryngopharynx extends posteriorly from the hyoid bone to the esophagus and anteriorly to the larynx. The laryngopharynx is especially important in airway management. Located anteriorly in the hypopharynx is the epiglottis, a leaf-shaped cartilage that prevents food from entering the respiratory tract during swallowing. Just anterior and superior to the epiglottis is the vallecula, a fold formed by the base of the tongue and the epiglottis. A series of ligaments and muscles connect the epiglottis to the hyoid bone and mandible. Immediately behind the hypopharynx are the fourth and fifth cervical vertebral bodies.

Larynx. The larynx is the complex structure that joins the pharynx with the trachea. Lying midline in the neck, it is attached to and lies just inferior to the hyoid bone and anterior to the esophagus. It consists of the thyroid and cricoid cartilage (both considered tracheal cartilage), glottic opening, vocal cords, arytenoid cartilage, pyriform fossae, and cricothyroid membrane.

The main laryngeal cartilage is the shield-shaped thyroid cartilage. Larger in males than in females, the thyroid cartilage forms the anterior prominence called the Adam's apple. The arytenoid cartilage, which forms a pyramid-shaped attachment for the vocal cords posteriorly, is an important landmark for endotracheal intubation. Posteriorly, smooth muscle closes a gap in the thyroid cartilage. Directly behind the Adam's apple, the thyroid cartilage houses the glottic opening, the narrowest part of the adult trachea, which is bordered by the vocal cords. On either side of the glottic opening are the pyriform fossae, recesses that form the lateral borders of the larynx. The thyrohyoid membrane attaches the upper end of the thyroid cartilage to the hyoid bone. Within the laryngeal cavity lie the true vocal cords, white bands of cartilage that regulate the passage of air through the larynx and produce voice by contraction of the laryngeal muscles. Beneath the thyroid cartilage is the cricoid cartilage, which forms the inferior border of the larynx. Often it is considered the first tracheal ring. Unlike the thyroid and other tracheal cartilages, whose posterior surfaces are open and not fused, the cricoid cartilage forms a complete ring. The fibrous cricothyroid membrane connects the inferior border of the thyroid cartilage with the superior aspect of the cricoid cartilage.

Trachea. As air enters the lower airway from the upper airway, it first enters and then passes through the trachea. The trachea is a 10- to 12-centimeter-long tube that connects the larynx to the two mainstem bronchi. It contains cartilaginous, C-shaped, open rings that form a frame to keep it open. The trachea is lined with respiratory epithelium containing cilia and mucous producing cells.

Bronchi. At the carina, the trachea divides, or bifurcates, into the right and left mainstem bronchi. The right mainstem bronchus is almost straight, while the left mainstem bronchus angles more acutely to the left. Mainstem bronchi enter the lung tissue at the hilum and then divide into the secondary and tertiary bronchi. The secondary and tertiary bronchi ultimately branch into the bronchioles, or small airways. The bronchioles are encircled with smooth muscle that contains beta-2 (β_2) adrenergic receptors. After approximately 22 divisions, the bronchioles turn into the respiratory bronchioles. These structures contain only muscular connective tissue and have a limited capacity for gas exchange. The respiratory bronchioles terminate at the alveoli.

Alveoli. The respiratory bronchioles divide into the alveolar ducts, which terminate in balloon-like clusters of alveoli called alveolar sacs. The alveoli contain an alveolar membrane that is only one or two cell layers thick. Because of this, the alveoli comprise the key functional unit of the respiratory system. The alveoli's surface area is massive, totaling more than 40 square meters. These hollow structures resist collapse largely because of the presence of surfactant, a chemical that decreases their surface tension and makes it easier for them to expand.

Lung parenchyma. The alveoli are the terminal ends of the respiratory tree and the functional units of the lungs. As such, they are the core of the lung parenchyma. The lung parenchyma is arranged in two pulmonary lobules that form the anatomic division of the lungs. These lobules are further organized into lobes. The right lung has three lobes, the upper lobe, the middle lobe, and the lower lobe. The left lung, which shares thoracic space with the heart, has only two lobes, the upper lobe and the lower lobe.

Pleura. Membranous connective tissue, called pleura, covers the lungs. The pleura consist of two layers, visceral and parietal. The visceral pleura envelop the lungs and does not contain nerve fibers. In contrast, the parietal pleura lines the thoracic cavity and does contain nerve fibers. The potential space between these two layers, called the pleural space, usually holds a small amount of fluid that reduces friction between the pleural layers during respiration.

6. Describe the functions of the upper and lower airway structures. pp. 298–302

Nasal cavity. The sinuses, named for the bone where they are contained, help reduce the overall weight of the head and are thought to assist in heating, purifying, and moistening the inhaled air. The sinuses help trap bacteria and other substances entering the nasal cavity. The eustachian tubes, or auditory tubes, connect the ear with the nasal cavity and allow for equalization of pressure on each side of the tympanic membrane. The nasolacrimal ducts drain tears and debris from the eyes into the nasal cavity. Nasal hairs just inside the external nares initially filter the incoming air. The air then proceeds into the nasal cavity, where it strikes three bony projections called turbinates, or conchae. These shelf-like structures, which are parallel to the nasal floor, serve as conduits into the sinuses, increase the surface area of the nasal cavity, and cause turbulent airflow. This turbulence helps to filter the air by depositing airborne particles on the mucous membrane lining the nasal cavity. Hair-like fibers called cilia propel those trapped particles to the back of the pharynx, where they are swallowed. Because the mucous membrane is covered with mucus and has a rich blood supply, it also immediately warms and humidifies the air entering the nose. By the time the air reaches the lower airway, it is at body temperature (37 °C), 100 percent humidified, and virtually free of airborne particles.

Oral cavity. The oral cavity allows air to flow into and out of the respiratory tract and food and liquids to pass into the digestive system.

Pharynx. The pharynx allows air to flow into and out of the respiratory tract and food and liquids to pass into the digestive system. The adenoids, lymphatic tissue in the mouth and nose, filter bacteria. Either hypertrophy or swelling of the adenoids from infection may make them large enough to obscure your view. Because the mouth and pharynx serve dual purposes for respiration and digestion, a number of mechanisms help prevent accidental blockage. To prevent foreign material from entering the trachea and lungs, sensitive nerves activate the body's cough and swallowing mechanisms as well as the gag reflex. The epiglottis, a leaf-shaped cartilage, prevents food from entering the respiratory tract during swallowing.

Larynx. The arytenoid cartilage, which forms a pyramid-shaped attachment for the vocal cords posteriorly, is an important landmark for endotracheal intubation. Within the laryngeal cavity lie the true vocal cords, white bands of cartilage that regulate the passage of air through the larynx and produce voice by contraction of the laryngeal muscles. The vocal cords can also close together to prevent foreign bodies from entering the airway. A mucous membrane lines most of the larynx. Rich with nerve endings from the vagus nerve, it is so sensitive that any irritation sparks a cough, or forceful exhalation of a large volume of air. First, air is drawn into the respiratory passageways. Next, the glottic opening shuts tightly, trapping the air within the lungs. Then the abdominal and thoracic muscles contract, pushing against the diaphragm and increasing intrathoracic pressure. The vocal cords suddenly open, and a burst of air forces foreign particles out of the lungs. The laryngeal mucous membrane is so sensitive that its stimulation by a laryngoscope or endotracheal tube can cause bradycardia (slow pulse rate), hypotension (low blood pressure), and decreased respiratory rate.

Trachea. The trachea is lined with respiratory epithelium containing cilia and mucous-producing cells. The mucus traps particles that the upper airway did not filter. The cilia then move the trapped particulate matter up into the mouth, where it is swallowed or expelled.

Bronchi. The bronchioles are encircled with smooth muscle that contains beta-2 (β_2) adrenergic receptors. When stimulated, these beta-2 receptors relax the bronchial smooth muscle, thus increasing the airway's diameter. This bronchodilation can increase the amount of air transported through the bronchiole; conversely, parasympathetic receptors, when stimulated, cause the bronchial smooth muscles to contract, thus reducing the diameter of the bronchiole. This bronchoconstriction can inhibit the movement of air through the bronchiole.

Alveoli. The alveoli contain an alveolar membrane that is only one or two cell layers thick. Because of this, the alveoli comprise the key functional unit of the respiratory system. Most oxygen and carbon dioxide gas exchanges take place here, although limited gas exchange may occur in the alveolar ducts and respiratory bronchioles. Alveolar collapse (atelectasis) can occur if surfactant is insufficient or if the alveoli are not inflated. No gas exchange takes place in atelectatic alveoli.

Pleura. The potential space between these two layers, called the pleural space, usually holds a small amount of fluid that reduces friction between the pleural layers during respiration.

7. **Apply knowledge of differences in pediatric airway and respiratory anatomy to managing a pediatric patient's airway and ventilation.**   **p. 302**

The pediatric airway is fundamentally the same as an adult's. In the pharynx, the jaw is smaller and the tongue relatively larger, resulting in greater potential airway encroachment. The epiglottis is much floppier and rounder ("omega" shaped). The dental (alveolar) ridge and teeth are softer and more fragile than an adult's and potentially more subject to damage from airway maneuvers. The larynx lies more superior and anterior in children and is funnel-shaped because the cricoid cartilage is undeveloped. Before the age of 10, the cricoid cartilage is the narrowest part of the airway. The ribs and the cartilage of the pediatric thoracic cage are softer and more pliable. This lack of rigidity lessens the thoracic wall's and accessory muscles' ability to assist lung expansion during inspiration. As a result, infants and children tend to rely more on their diaphragms for breathing.

8. **Explain the physiology of respiration and ventilation.**   **pp. 302–304**

Mechanics of ventilation. Respiration is the exchange of gases between a living organism and its environment. Ventilation is the mechanical process that moves air into and out of the lungs. Ventilation is necessary for respiration to occur. The volume of the thorax expands as the diaphragm contracts and displaces downward. The intercostal muscles contract, pulling the rib cage upward and outward. The muscles of the neck enhance this action as they lift the sternum. The lungs expand with the chest as the pleural seal secures the exterior of the lung to the interior of the thorax. The expansion of the lungs reduces the air pressure within them, and air flows into the alveoli. Gravity and the intrinsic elasticity of the lungs then cause the thorax to settle, the pressure within the lungs to increase, and air to be exhaled.

Pulmonary circulation. The right ventricle pumps blood depleted of its oxygen into the pulmonary artery. The blood is directed to the respective lungs through the right and left pulmonary arteries that then divide, ultimately, into the pulmonary capillaries. In the capillaries, the blood releases carbon dioxide and the hemoglobin becomes saturated with oxygen. The blood then returns through the pulmonary veins to the left atrium.

Gas exchange in the lungs. The air brought into the lungs contains 21 percent oxygen and very little carbon dioxide. Oxygen diffuses through the alveolar and capillary walls and is bound to the hemoglobin, while carbon dioxide diffuses in the opposite direction. The air exhaled contains about 16 percent oxygen and 5 percent carbon dioxide.

Diffusion of the respiratory gases. The oxygen from inspired air diffuses from the alveolar space through the alveolar wall and the pulmonary capillary membrane, where it attaches to the hemoglobin of the blood. Carbon dioxide, mostly transported as bicarbonate, diffuses from the blood plasma across the capillary membrane and through the alveolar wall.

9. **Describe the etiologies and pathophysiology of the upper airway and inadequate ventilation.**   **pp. 308–309**

Airway obstruction may be either partial or complete. Partial obstruction allows either adequate or poor air exchange. Patients with adequate air exchange can cough effectively; those with poor air exchange cannot.

The tongue is the most common cause of airway obstruction. Normally, the submandibular muscles directly support the tongue and indirectly support the epiglottis. However, without sufficient muscle tone, the relaxed tongue falls back against the posterior pharynx, thus occluding the airway. This may produce snoring respiratory noises. Foreign bodies, such as large, poorly chewed pieces of food, can obstruct the upper airway by becoming lodged in the hypopharynx. The patient may clutch his neck between the thumb and fingers, a universal distress signal. Children, especially toddlers, often aspirate foreign objects, as they have the tendency to put objects into their mouths.

In trauma, particularly when the patient is unresponsive, loose teeth, facial bone fractures, and avulsed or swollen tissue may obstruct the airway. Secretions such as blood, saliva, and vomitus may compromise the airway and risk aspiration. Additionally, penetrating or blunt trauma may obstruct the airway by fracturing or displacing the larynx, allowing the vocal cords to collapse into the tracheal lumen (channel).

Since the glottis is the narrowest part of an adult's airway, edema (swelling) or spasm (spasmodic closure) of the vocal cords is potentially lethal. Even moderate edema can severely obstruct airflow and cause asphyxia.

Vomitus is the most commonly aspirated material. Patients most at risk for this are those who are so obtunded (drowsy) that they cannot adequately protect their airways. This can occur with hypoxia, central nervous system toxins, or brain injury, among other causes.

10. Recognize the signs and symptoms of upper airway obstruction and inadequate ventilation. pp. 308–309

Partial obstruction allows either adequate or poor air exchange. Patients with adequate air exchange can cough effectively; those with poor air exchange cannot. They often emit a high-pitched noise while inhaling (stridor), and their skin may have a bluish appearance (cyanosis). They also may have increased breathing difficulty, which can manifest as choking, gagging dyspnea, or dysphonia (difficulty speaking). When you cannot feel or hear airflow from the nose and mouth, or when the patient cannot speak (aphonia), breathe, or cough, his airway is completely obstructed. He will quickly become unconscious and die if you do not relieve the obstruction. In the absence of breathing, difficulty ventilating the patient will indicate complete airway obstruction.

Insufficient minute volume respirations can compromise adequate oxygen intake and carbon dioxide removal. Additionally, oxygenation may be insufficient when conditions increase metabolic oxygen demand or decrease available oxygen. A reduction of either the rate or the volume of inhalation leads to a reduction in minute volume. In some cases, the respiratory rate may be rapid but so shallow that little air exchange takes place. Among the causes of such decreased ventilation are depressed respiratory functions as from impairment of respiratory muscles or nervous system, bronchospasm from intrinsic disease, fractured ribs, pneumothorax, hemothorax, drug overdose, renal failure, spinal or brainstem injury, or head injury. In some conditions, such as sepsis, the body's metabolic demand for oxygen can exceed the patient's ability to supply it. Additionally, the environment may contain a decreased amount of oxygen, as in high altitude conditions or a house fire, which also produces toxic gases such as cyanide and carbon monoxide. These situations of inadequate ventilation can lead to hypercarbia and hypoxia.

11. Demonstrate management of upper airway obstruction and inadequate ventilation. pp. 308–309, 321, 330

The patient's tongue can block his airway whether he is lateral, supine, or prone; however, the blockage depends on the position of the patient's head and jaw, so simple airway maneuvers such as the jaw-thrust can usually open his airway.

Laryngeal spasm may sometimes be partially overcome by strengthening ventilatory effort, forceful upward pull of the jaw, or the use of muscle relaxants, although the success of these maneuvers is quite variable.

Basic airway management and ventilation includes most airway maneuvers that have been shown to be lifesaving, including proper positioning, suctioning, oxygen administration, and bag-valve-mask (BVM) ventilation.

Advanced airway management includes endotracheal intubation, surgical airways, and other invasive airways that do not pass through the vocal cords, such as extraglottic airways.

12. Identify problems with the airway, breathing, and oxygenation through primary and secondary patient assessment and noninvasive respiratory monitoring. pp. 309–320

The purpose of the primary assessment is to identify any immediate threats to the patient's life, specifically airway, breathing, and circulation problems (ABCs). Snoring or gurgling may indicate potential airway problems. The absence of breath sounds on one side may indicate a pneumothorax or hemothorax in the trauma patient. Irregular breathing suggests a significant problem and usually requires ventilatory support. Observe the chest wall for any asymmetrical movement. This condition, known as paradoxical breathing, may suggest a flail chest.

During the secondary assessment you will obtain a patient history and conduct a physical exam. The patient's past medical history will put his present complaints into perspective and help to identify the risk factors for a variety of likely diagnoses. Your physical examination of a patient with respiratory problems should continue the evaluation of his airway, breathing, and circulation begun during your primary assessment. Now you will use the physical examination techniques of inspection, auscultation, and palpation to evaluate his injury or illness in more detail and determine your plan of action.

During inspection, note modified forms of respiration, such as coughing, sneezing, hiccoughing, sighing, or grunting, that may be indicative of airway problems. Respiratory patterns may also give clues to underlying conditions: Kussmaul's respirations (diabetic ketoacidosis), Cheyne-Stokes respirations (brainstem injury), Biot's respirations (increases intracranial pressure), central neurogenic hyperventilation (increased intracranial pressure), and agonal respirations (brain anoxia).

During auscultation, various sounds indicate airflow compromise (snoring, gurgling, stridor, wheezing, and quiet) or compromise of gas exchange (crackles and rhonchi).

Several available devices will help you measure the effectiveness of oxygenation and ventilation and maintain parameters at the appropriate levels. Those measurements used most commonly in prehospital care are pulse oximetry, CO-oximetry, and capnography. Peak expiratory flow testing can also be useful in the prehospital setting for some respiratory diseases, although it is not widely employed. These measurements use various devices and methodologies that, when used alone, have their limitations. However, when used together they can provide a fairly comprehensive and reliable picture of the patient's respiratory status.

13. Differentiate between patients for whom supplemental oxygen administration is indicated and those for whom it is not indicated. p. 322

Providing supplemental oxygen to patients who are frankly hypoxemic will diminish the hypoxia's secondary effects on organs such as the brain and the heart and lessen subjective respiratory distress.

In some circumstances, oxygen administration is also indicated even though the patient's oxygen saturation may be normal. Oxygen administration is also very important prior to intubation, regardless of the oxygen saturation. Ill or injured pregnant patients may benefit from supplemental oxygen administration, regardless of their oxygen saturation, to enhance oxygen delivery to the fetus.

Never withhold oxygen from any patient for whom it is indicated. Caution is advised in patients with COPD, who may have developed a hypoxic drive to breathe (in which reduced oxygen levels trigger breathing), as opposed to a normal hypercarbic drive to breathe (in which breathing is triggered by chronic hypercarbia, or elevated levels of carbon dioxide). In these patients there is a theoretical risk of depressing respirations as the body senses plentiful oxygen.

14. Describe the risks and benefits of supplemental oxygen administration. p. 322

Oxygen may be carried both on hemoglobin and dissolved in the blood. Under normal circumstances, the dissolved portion of oxygen is relatively insignificant. When supplemental oxygen is administered, the dissolved portion of oxygen may increase many fold. This relatively small amount of extra oxygen may be important to patients with tissue hypoxemia from any cause such as septic shock, myocardial infarction, cardiogenic shock, or severe trauma.

Patients with COPD may have developed a hypoxic drive to breathe as opposed to a normal hypercarbic drive to breathe. In these patients there is a theoretical risk of depressing respirations as the body senses plentiful oxygen. This is rarely a clinical issue during all but the longest EMS transports. Thus, you should feel comfortable giving as much oxygen as necessary to maintain adequate oxygen saturations. Remember, however, that you do not necessarily need to return these patients to normal oxygen saturations, as their bodies are generally used to lower oxygen levels. Of course, you should monitor your patient closely for evidence of respiratory depression.

There is now evidence that high oxygen levels (hyperoxia) may be as dangerous as low levels (hypoxia) because of the possible formation of oxygen free radicals. This has been demonstrated in post–cardiac arrest patients, stroke patients, neonates, and head trauma patients. Therefore, oxygen saturation should always be maintained in the normal range, using the lowest necessary oxygen flow.

Case Study Review

Reread the case study on pages 296–297 in Paramedic Care: Paramedicine Fundamentals; *then, read the following discussion.*

Kathy, Bill, and Sharon attend a trauma patient with a mechanism of injury suggesting serious internal injuries. They are immediately obligated to employ spinal precautions, requiring that they position the patient's head and neck in the neutral position and maintain that positioning. As they move to the airway evaluation portion of the initial assessment, Kathy hears gurgling and attempts to clear the airway with positioning (displacing the jaw forward while maintaining the spinal immobilization) and suction. Airway maintenance is more difficult in this trauma patient because of the inability to extend his head and neck due to the potential for spine injury. The landmarks for endotracheal intubation are also more difficult to visualize because the head cannot be brought to the sniffing position and because there is likely to be some blood in the airway.

While the clenched teeth (trismus) prevent insertion of the oral airway, a nasopharyngeal airway could help maintain the airway. However, with the possibility of severe head injury and basilar skull fracture, Sharon must be very careful with its insertion, directing it straight back and along the floor of the nasal cavity.

The Glasgow Coma Score of 5 for this patient mandates field intubation. The rapid sequence procedure is required because of the clenched jaw. Etomidate is a great agent for induction since it rarely causes any rise or drop in blood pressure or pulse. It also works extremely fast with a relatively consistent dose response. Succinylcholine is a smooth muscle relaxant that relaxes the clenched jaw and permits opening of the mouth for intubation. It also relaxes the muscles of the airway and makes intubation somewhat easier to perform. Succinylcholine may increase intracranial pressure (a possible contraindication for this patient) and may increase the likelihood of vomiting. The greatest benefit to using succinylcholine is its short duration of action. If the rapid sequence intubation fails, it will only be a few minutes until the paralytic effects of the drug wear off. During the time until the jaw relaxes, Kathy ventilates her patient with full breaths at a rate of about 10 times per minute. Any faster would blow off too much carbon dioxide and possibly increase intracranial pressure.

Kathy is unsuccessful at intubation and the patient's oxygen saturations are falling. The decision was made to place an LMA-Supreme.

Once the LMA-Supreme is placed, both Bill and Kathy must carefully ensure it is properly located. All signs demonstrate that the ventilations are effective, including bilateral and equal lung sounds with each breath, increasing oxygen saturation, and waveform change on the capnometer. Bill, Kathy, or Sharon will carefully secure the tube in place. A real danger in prehospital care is the unnoticed dislodging of an airway device during C-collar placement, immobilization to the long spine board, movement of the patient to the long spine board, or while loading or unloading the patient from the ambulance. Bill, Kathy, and Sharon will check the breath sounds, oximetry, and the capnometer after each move and frequently during their care and transport.

Content Self-Evaluation

MULTIPLE CHOICE

_____ **1.** The sinuses help trap bacteria and can become infected.
   A. True
   B. False

_____ **2.** The nasal cavity is responsible for all of the following functions EXCEPT
   A. warming the air.
   B. deoxygenating the air.
   C. humidifying the air.
   D. cleansing the air.
   E. the sense of smell.

_____ **3.** Which of the following is the only bone in the axial skeleton that does not articulate with another bone?
   A. The mandible
   B. The maxilla
   C. The hyoid bone
   D. The thyroid
   E. The zygomatic bone

©2013 Pearson Education, Inc.
Paramedic Care: Principles & Practice, Vol. 2, 4th Ed.

_____ **4.** The space located between the base of the tongue and the epiglottis is called the
- **A.** vallecula.
- **B.** cricoid.
- **C.** arytenoid fold.
- **D.** epiglottic fossa.
- **E.** glottic opening.

_____ **5.** Which of the following correctly lists the order in which air passes through airway structures during inspiration?
- **A.** Trachea, larynx, laryngopharynx, nasopharynx, nares
- **B.** Nares, nasopharynx, trachea, laryngopharynx, larynx
- **C.** Nares, nasopharynx, laryngopharynx, larynx, trachea
- **D.** Laryngopharynx, nares, nasopharynx, larynx, trachea
- **E.** Trachea, nares, laryngopharynx, larynx, nasopharynx

_____ **6.** The narrowest part of the adult airway is the
- **A.** cricoid ring.
- **B.** thyroid ring.
- **C.** glottis.
- **D.** carina.
- **E.** tracheal stricture.

_____ **7.** Which of the following can be caused by stimulation with a laryngoscope during an intubation attempt?
- **A.** Coughing
- **B.** Bradycardia
- **C.** Hypotension
- **D.** Decreased respiratory rate
- **E.** All of the above

_____ **8.** The point at which the trachea divides into the two mainstem bronchi is called the
- **A.** hilum.
- **B.** parenchyma.
- **C.** vallecula.
- **D.** carina.
- **E.** pleura.

_____ **9.** The mainstem bronchus that leaves the trachea at almost a straight angle is the right mainstem bronchus.
- **A.** True
- **B.** False

_____ **10.** Beta-2 stimulation will cause the bronchioles to
- **A.** constrict.
- **B.** dilate.
- **C.** shorten.
- **D.** stiffen.
- **E.** none of the above.

_____ **11.** The tissue covering each lung and the interior of the thorax is the
- **A.** hilum.
- **B.** parenchyma.
- **C.** vallecula.
- **D.** carina.
- **E.** pleura.

_____ **12.** Which of the following is NOT one of the differences in respiration between pediatric patients and adults?
- **A.** The pediatric airway is smaller in all aspects.
- **B.** Pediatric ribs are softer and contribute less to respiration than those of adults.
- **C.** Children rely more on their diaphragms for breathing than adults do.
- **D.** The glottis is the narrowest point of the pediatric airway, whereas the cricoid cartilage is the narrowest point in adults.
- **E.** Children's teeth are softer and more prone to damage than those of adults.

_____ **13.** Internal respiration occurs in the
- **A.** peripheral capillaries.
- **B.** airway.
- **C.** alveoli.
- **D.** pulmonary capillaries.
- **E.** C and D.

14. Which aspect of the respiratory cycle is passive?
    A. Inspiration
    B. Expiration
    C. Neither A nor B
    D. Both A and B
    E. Both A and B, but only during stress

15. The oxygenated circulation that provides perfusion for the lung tissue itself flows through the
    A. pulmonary arteries.
    B. pulmonary veins.
    C. bronchial arteries.
    D. bronchial veins.
    E. none of the above.

16. The amount of nitrogen in the air is approximately
    A. 79 percent.
    B. 4 percent.
    C. 0.4 percent.
    D. 0.04 percent.
    E. 0.10 percent.

17. The normal oxygen saturation of hemoglobin in blood as it leaves the lungs is about
    A. 75 percent.
    B. 85 percent.
    C. 90 percent.
    D. 95 percent.
    E. 97 percent.

18. The majority of the carbon dioxide carried by the blood is
    A. carried by the hemoglobin.
    B. dissolved in the plasma.
    C. transported as bicarbonate.
    D. found as free gas in the blood.
    E. carried as free radicals.

19. Which of the following will reduce the carbon dioxide levels in the blood?
    A. Administration of bicarbonate
    B. Administration of antacids
    C. Hyperventilation
    D. High-flow oxygen
    E. Hypoventilation

20. Which of the following would NOT increase the production of carbon dioxide?
    A. Fever
    B. Airway obstruction
    C. Shivering
    D. Metabolic acids
    E. Exercise

21. The primary center controlling respiration is located in the
    A. medulla.
    B. pons.
    C. spinal cord.
    D. cerebrum.
    E. cerebellum.

22. Chemoreceptors are stimulated by:
    A. decreased PaO_2, decreased $PaCO_2$, and increased pH.
    B. decreased PaO_2, increased $PaCO_2$, and increased pH.
    C. increased PaO_2, increased $PaCO_2$, and decrease pH.
    D. decreased PaO_2, increased $PaCO_2$, and increased pH.
    E. decreased PaO_2, increased $PaCO_2$, and decrease pH.

23. The amount of air moved with one normal respiratory cycle is called
    A. minute volume.
    B. alveolar air.
    C. tidal volume.
    D. dead air space.
    E. total lung capacity.

24. The volume of air contained in a normal inspiration is about
    A. 150 mL.
    B. 350 mL.
    C. 500 mL.
    D. 6,000 mL.
    E. none of the above.

©2013 Pearson Education, Inc.
Paramedic Care: Principles & Practice, Vol. 2, 4th Ed.

_____ 25. Which of the following is the most common cause of upper airway obstruction?
   A. The tongue
   B. Foreign bodies
   C. Trauma
   D. Laryngeal swelling
   E. Aspiration of blood or vomitus

_____ 26. All of the following conditions may cause reduced inspiratory volumes EXCEPT
   A. pneumothorax.
   B. renal failure.
   C. high inspired oxygen concentrations.
   D. respiratory muscle paralysis.
   E. emphysema.

_____ 27. The normal respiratory rate for an adult at rest is
   A. 8 to 12.
   B. 12 to 20.
   C. 18 to 24.
   D. 24 to 32.
   E. 40 to 60.

_____ 28. Which of the following is a breathing pattern associated with flail chest?
   A. Abdominal breathing
   B. Paradoxical breathing
   C. Diaphragmatic breathing
   D. Intercostal retraction
   E. A and C

_____ 29. Severe tissue hypoxia is not possible without cyanosis.
   A. True
   B. False

_____ 30. Which modified form of respiration is designed to expand alveoli that may have collapsed during periods of inactivity or rest?
   A. Coughing
   B. Sneezing
   C. Hiccoughing
   D. Grunting
   E. Sighing

_____ 31. The respiratory pattern that presents with deep and rapid respirations is
   A. apneustic respirations.
   B. Cheyne-Stokes respirations.
   C. Biot's respirations.
   D. central neurogenic hyperventilation.
   E. agonal respirations.

_____ 32. Stridor is most commonly associated with
   A. laryngeal constriction or edema.
   B. the tongue blocking the airway.
   C. narrowing of the bronchioles.
   D. fluids within the airway.
   E. foreign bodies in the lower airway.

_____ 33. The feeling of flexibility or stiffness associated with the lungs and ventilation is
   A. back pressure.
   B. resiliency.
   C. compliance.
   D. effusion.
   E. Hering-Breuer reflex.

_____ 34. Pulse oximetry measures the amount of oxygen dissolved in the plasma of the blood.
   A. True
   B. False

_____ 35. Pulse CO-oximeters are devices that detect normal hemoglobins such as carboxyhemoglobin (from carbon monoxide poisoning) and methemoglobin (as seen in methemoglobinemia).
   A. True
   B. False

_____ 36. The normal partial pressure of CO_2 in exhaled air is
  A. 5 mmHg.
  B. 25 mmHg.
  C. 38 mmHg.
  D. 45 mmHg.
  E. 86 mmHg.

_____ 37. The disposable device that records the level of exhaled CO_2 using pH-sensitive chemically impregnated paper is a
  A. capnometer.
  B. capnograph.
  C. capnogram.
  D. colormetric device.
  E. non-waveform $ETCO_2$ device.

_____ 38. If the colormetric $ETCO_2$ detector becomes contaminated with gastric contents, further readings may be unreliable.
  A. True
  B. False

_____ 39. During CPR, the $ETCO_2$ reflects cardiac output and coronary perfusion pressure.
  A. True
  B. False

_____ 40. The value of capnography is that it can assess which of the following?
  A. The effectiveness of CPR
  B. Proper initial endotracheal tube placement
  C. Proper continued endotracheal tube placement
  D. Patient responses to medications
  E. All of the above

©2013 Pearson Education, Inc.
Paramedic Care: Principles & Practice, Vol. 2, 4th Ed.

Special Project

Label the Diagram

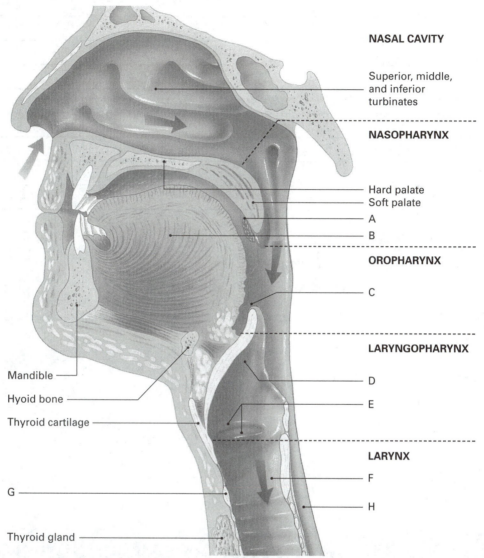

NASAL CAVITY

Superior, middle, and inferior turbinates

NASOPHARYNX

Hard palate
Soft palate
A
B

OROPHARYNX

C

LARYNGOPHARYNX

D
E

Mandible
Hyoid bone
Thyroid cartilage

LARYNX

F
H

G

Thyroid gland

Write the names of the components of the upper airway marked A, B, C, D, E, F, G, and H on the above diagram in the spaces provided.

A. _____

B. _____

C. _____

D. _____

E. _____

F. _____

G. _____

H. _____

Airway Obstruction

List the five causes of airway obstruction and identify the mechanism that causes each problem.

1. _____
   _____

2. _____
   _____

3. _____
   _____

4. _____
   _____

5. _____
   _____

Normal Respiratory Values:

Identify the normal values for each of the items listed below.

	Inspired Air	**Expired Air**	
% Oxygen	_____	_____	PaO_2 _____
% Carbon dioxide	_____	_____	$PaCO_2$ _____

Normal Respiratory Rates/Volumes:

Infant: _____ to _____
Child: _____ to _____
Adult: _____ to _____
Tidal volume: _____
Alveolar volume: _____
Dead space volume: _____
Minute volume: _____

Part 2: Basic Airway Management and Ventilation, p. 321

Review of Chapter Objectives

After reading this part of the chapter, you should be able to:

15. **Recognize the indications and contraindications for basic airway interventions, including the following:**

    a. **various positioning techniques**   **p. 321**
       Trauma patients are often confined to the supine position as a result of spinal immobilization. However, some circumstances may warrant flexibility, if permitted by local protocols. For example, the

©2013 Pearson Education, Inc.
Paramedic Care: Principles & Practice, Vol. 2, 4th Ed.

patient with facial and airway trauma who is able to maintain his airway as long as he is sitting up may be placed in a cervical collar in a seated position rather than restricted to a supine position.

Conscious medical patients should be maintained in their position of comfort if they are not placed in cervical immobilization. Unconscious medical patients who do not require other interventions, such as BVM ventilation, should be placed on their side with the head elevated (if not contraindicated) to minimize the risk of aspiration.

Unconscious patients who do require airway and ventilation interventions, such as BVM ventilation or intubation, are usually best maintained in an ear-to-sternal-notch position, in which the supine patient's head is elevated to the point where the ear and the sternal notch are horizontally aligned. This position is often referred to as the sniffing position in non-obese patients and the ramped position in obese patients. With both the sniffing and ramped positions, the ear-to-sternal notch alignment is maintained. This positioning maximizes upper airway patency allowing for effective ventilation and, if required, endotracheal intubation. It also improves the mechanics of ventilation, both with spontaneous breathing and with BVM ventilation.

b. administering supplemental oxygen by a variety of devices pp. 323–324

The nasal cannula is a catheter placed at the nares. It provides an optimal oxygen supplementation of up to 40 percent when set at 6 L/min flow. At flow rates above 6 L/min, the nasal mucous membranes become very dry and easily break down. It is indicated for low-to-moderate oxygen requirements and long-term oxygen therapy.

The Venturi mask is a high-flow face mask that uses a Venturi system to deliver relatively precise oxygen concentrations, regardless of the patient's rate and depth of breathing. It can deliver concentrations of 24 percent, 28 percent, 35 percent, or 40 percent oxygen. The liter flow depends on the oxygen concentration desired. The Venturi mask is particularly useful for COPD patients, who benefit from careful control of inspired oxygen concentration.

The simple face mask is indicated for patients requiring moderate oxygen concentrations. Flow rates generally range from about 6 to 10 L/min, providing 40 to 60 percent oxygen at the maximum rate, depending on the patient's respiratory rate and depth. Delivery of volumes beyond 10 L/min does not enhance oxygen concentration.

The partial rebreather mask is indicated for patients requiring moderate-to-high oxygen concentrations when satisfactory clinical results are not obtained with the simple face mask.

Minimal dilution occurs with inspiration of residual expired air along with the supplemental oxygen. Maximal flow rate is 10 L/min.

The nonrebreather mask provides the highest oxygen concentration of all oxygen delivery devices available, or about 80 percent when set at 15 L/min of oxygen and the mask is fit tightly to the face. Any patient who requires a nonrebreather should be closely monitored for refractory hypoxemia that requires invasive or noninvasive positive pressure ventilation.

Small volume nebulizers with a chamber containing 3 to 5 cc of fluid are attached to a face mask, or other delivery device, which allows for delivery of medications in an aerosol form (nebulization) that is more likely to pass through the upper airway to the lower airways.

Positive airway pressure (PAP) is delivered via a face mask to maintain a constant level of pressure within the airway, which assists a patient in breathing by preventing collapse of the airway during inhalation. Continuous positive airway pressure (CPAP) maintains a steady level of pressure during both inhalation and exhalation. Bilevel positive airway pressure (BiPAP) maintains a higher level of pressure during inhalation and a lower level of pressure during exhalation. CPAP and BiPAP devices can be used to administer oxygen in conjunction with increased airway pressures.

c. manual airway maneuvers p. 324

Manual maneuvers are the simplest airway management techniques. They require no specialized equipment, are safe, and are noninvasive. They are highly effective but are often neglected in prehospital care. The head-tilt/chin-lift and the jaw-thrust are safe and dependable maneuvers for relieving this obstruction. You should perform one of these techniques on all unconscious patients, but do not perform them on responsive patients. If you suspect cervical spine injury, perform the modified jaw-thrust with in-line stabilization of the cervical spine.

d. inserting basic airway adjuncts pp. 325–327

The nasopharyngeal airway (NPA), or "nasal trumpet," is an uncuffed tube made of soft rubber or plastic. The nasopharyngeal airway follows the natural curvature of the nasopharynx, passing through the nose and extending from the nostril to the posterior pharynx just below the base of the tongue. They are well tolerated in most patients and are very effective at maintaining the airway. Specific indications for the use of the nasopharyngeal airway include obtunded patients (those with reduced mental acuity, with or without a suppressed gag reflex) and unconscious patients. If the patient does not tolerate the nasopharyngeal airway, you should remove it.

The oropharyngeal airway (OPA) is a noninvasive semicircular plastic or rubber device designed to follow the palate's curvature. It holds the base of the tongue away from the posterior oropharynx, thus preventing it from obstructing the glottis. Its use is indicated in patients with no gag reflex. Do not use an oropharyngeal airway in conscious or semiconscious patients who have a gag reflex, because it may cause vomiting (by stimulating the posterior tongue gag reflexes) or laryngospasm.

Oral and/or nasal airways should be considered in all obtunded older pediatric and adult patients and are mandatory whenever the patient has signs of airway obstruction ("noisy breathing is obstructed breathing") or bag-valve-mask ventilation is difficult.

16. **Demonstrate techniques of basic airway management, including positioning, administering supplemental oxygen by a variety of devices, manual airway maneuvers, and inserting basic airway adjuncts.**   pp. 323–327

To use oxygen delivery devices:
1. Explain the need for supplemental oxygen to the patient.
2. Turn on the oxygen source and adjust the flow rate to match the delivery device.
   a. Nasal cannula: 6 L/min
   b. Venturi mask: match the liter flow indicated based on the percentage of oxygen desired
   c. Simple face mask: 6–10 L/min
   d. Partial rebreather mask: up to 10 L/min
   e. Nonrebreather mask: 15 L/min
   f. CPAP/BiPAP: follow local protocol and manufacturer's instructions for the type of device you use.
3. Place the delivery device on the patient.
4. Adjust liter flow, as needed, to maintain proper oxygen delivery.

To insert a nasopharyngeal airway:
1. Ensure or maintain effective ventilation with supplemental oxygen.
2. Lubricate the exterior of the tube with a water-soluble gel to decrease trauma during insertion. Lidocaine gel may be used to increase tolerance of the device after insertion.
3. Select the nare that appears largest. Push gently up on the tip of the nose and pass the tube gently into the nostril with the bevel oriented toward the septum and the airway directed straight back along the nasal floor, parallel to the mouth. Avoid pushing against any resistance, because this may cause tissue trauma and airway kinking.
4. Verify the appropriate position of the airway. Resolution of noisy breathing and improved compliance during bag-valve-mask ventilation support correct positioning. Also, feel at the airway's proximal end for airflow on expiration.
5. Provide supplemental oxygen and/or ventilate the patient as indicated.

To insert the oropharyngeal airway:
1. Open the mouth and remove any visible obstructions.
2. Ensure or maintain effective ventilation with supplemental oxygen.
3. Grasp the patient's jaw and lift anteriorly.
4. With your other hand, hold the airway device at its proximal end and insert it into the patient's mouth. Make sure the curve is reversed, with the tip pointing toward the roof of the mouth.
5. Once the tip reaches the level of the soft palate, gently rotate the airway 180° until it comes to rest over the tongue.
   a. An alternative insertion method useful in both pediatric and adult patients is to press the tongue upward and forward with a tongue blade. Then, the airway can be advanced until the flange is seated at the teeth. This is the preferred method of airway insertion in infants and children.
6. Verify appropriate position of the airway. Clear breath sounds and chest rise indicate correct placement.
7. Apply supplemental oxygen and/or positive pressure ventilation if indicated.

©2013 Pearson Education, Inc.
Paramedic Care: Principles & Practice, Vol. 2, 4th Ed.

17. Differentiate between adequate and inadequate breathing in a patient.
                                                                        pp. 304, 307, 309, 311–312

A patient with adequate breathing would have a normal respiratory rate (12–20 breaths per minute in adults; 18–24 breaths per minute in children, and 40–60 breaths per minute in infants) and normal tidal volume (5–7 cc/kg). Lab values should show normal levels of oxygen ($PaO_2 = 80–100$ torr) and carbon dioxide ($PaCO_2 = 35–45$ torr).

A patient with inadequate breathing would display one or more signs of respiratory impairment. The respiratory rate may be above (hyperventilation) or below (hypoventilation) normal parameters. The tidal volume may be above or below normal. The patient may be displaying modified forms of respiration (coughing, sneezing, hiccoughing, sighing, or grunting) or abnormal respiratory patterns (Kussmaul's, Cheyne-Stokes, Biot's, central neurogenic hyperventilation, or agonal). You might auscultate sounds of airflow compromise (snoring, gurgling, stridor, wheezing, or quiet) or sounds that may indicate compromised gas exchange (crackles or rhonchi).

18. Recognize the need for artificial ventilation of a patient.   p. 327

Many of your cases in the field will call for ventilatory support. These situations range from apneic (non-breathing) patients to less obvious instances when patients are experiencing depressed respiratory function. An unconscious patient's respiratory center may not function adequately. A significant decrease in the patient's rate or depth of breathing will lead to decreased respiratory minute volume with subsequent hypercarbia and respiratory acidosis. This will result in further decreases in mental status, creating a vicious cycle. Hypoxemia may also result if the decrease in breathing is significant or oxygen demand is substantial. Acidosis and/or hypoxemia may eventually lead to respiratory or cardiac arrest. Any patient presenting with signs or symptoms of inadequate breathing will need some level of assistance.

19. Demonstrate techniques of ventilation, including:

a. mouth-to-mouth/mouth-to-nose ventilation (in an apneic patient in the absence of equipment)   p. 327
Ventilation by mouth-to-mouth or mouth-to-nose is an easy technique that requires no equipment, though it risks disease transmission. The rescuer seals his mouth over the patient's mouth or nose (or both with the small child or infant), closes the nostrils or mouth with his fingers, takes a deep breath, and inflates the patient's lungs. When possible, mouth-to-mask or bag-valve-mask ventilation is recommended.

b. mouth-to-mask ventilation   pp. 327–328
To perform the mouth-to-mask technique, position the head to open the airway by the head-tilt/chin-lift or jaw-thrust, position the mask to obtain a good seal, and provide adequate ventilatory volumes. As with mouth-to-mouth and mouth-to-nose methods, hyperinflation of the patient's lungs, gastric distension in the patient, and hyperventilation in the rescuer are potential complications.

c. bag-valve-mask ventilation   pp. 328–329
Bag-valve-mask devices are mechanical devices that provide positive pressure ventilation. The mask is sealed to the patient's face with one hand while the other hand squeezes the bag, pushing air into the patient's lungs. The device is best used for the intubated patient because the volume of air and the pressure delivered to the patient is low. If the patient is not intubated, the air exchange achieved by one person may not be enough to sustain life. With two or more persons, one rescuer seals the mask to the face and maintains head positioning while another uses both hands to squeeze the bag. Since the volume of the bag is limited, it is essential to obtain a good seal on the face when using the bag-valve-mask. Any time the bag-valve-mask is used, it should have the oxygen reservoir attached and oxygen flowing at 12 to 15 L/min.

d. use of cricoid pressure in conjunction with techniques of ventilation   pp. 329–329
To locate the cricoid cartilage, palpate the thyroid cartilage (Adam's apple) and feel the depression just below it (cricothyroid membrane). The prominence just inferior to this depression is the ring of cricoid cartilage, which may be difficult to identify in female and obese patients.

To perform cricoid pressure, apply firm downward pressure to the anterolateral aspect of the cartilage, using the thumb, index, and middle finger of one hand. If a lesser-trained provider is performing the maneuver, you should confirm that they are in the correct position.

Use caution not to apply so much pressure as to deform and possibly obstruct the trachea; this is a particular danger in infants. The necessary pressure has been estimated as the amount of force that will compress a capped 50-cc syringe from 50 cc to the 30-cc marking. In the event that the patient actively vomits, it is imperative to release the pressure to avoid esophageal rupture. Similarly, if cricoid pressure is being performed during intubation, reduce or release the pressure if the intubator is having difficulty visualizing the vocal cords.

e. demand valve device   **p. 329**

The demand-valve device, also called the manually triggered, oxygen-powered ventilation device or flow-restricted, oxygen-powered ventilation device, will deliver 100 percent oxygen to a patient at its highest flow rates (40 liters per minute maximum). Flow is restricted to 30 cm H_2O or less to diminish gastric distension that can occur with its use.

f. transport ventilator   **pp. 377–380**

In a patient who is not breathing spontaneously, the mechanical ventilator provides "controlled" ventilations. Some mechanical ventilators are designed to provide intermittent "mandatory" ventilation; that is, the ventilator will assist a patient's own spontaneous breaths but will revert to controlled ventilations if the patient stops breathing.

There are two general varieties of ventilators for prehospital use: simple compact devices with a minimum of options for general use and more complicated devices for critical care transport. The simple out-of-hospital ventilator devices are designed for convenience and ease of use during short transports of relatively uncomplicated adult and older pediatric patients. These devices generally allow for control of ventilatory rate and tidal volume only. The inspired oxygen concentration is usually fixed at 100 percent, but it may be adjustable.

Critical care transport ventilators, in contrast to the simple units just described, offer a host of features such as different ventilator modes, enhanced monitoring, alarms, and more. The increased adjustability allows for keeping the patient more comfortable with less sedation, analgesia, and paralysis. These critical transport devices can be used on most pediatric patients and some neonates.

20. Demonstrate modifications of ventilation techniques for pediatric patients.   **p. 329**

The differences in the pediatric patient's anatomy require some variation in ventilation technique. First, the child's relatively flat nasal bridge makes achieving a mask seal more difficult. Pressing the mask against the child's face to improve the seal can actually obstruct the airway, which is more compressible than an adult's. For BVM ventilation, the bag size depends on the child's age. Full-term neonates and infants will require a pediatric BVM with a capacity of at least 450 mL. For children up to 8 years of age, the pediatric BVM is preferred, although for patients in the upper portion of that age range you can use an adult BVM with a capacity of 1,500 mL if you do not maximally inflate it. Children older than 8 years require an adult BVM to achieve adequate tidal volumes. Additionally, be certain that the mask fits properly, from the bridge of the nose to the cleft of the chin. If a length-based resuscitation tape (Broselow tape) is available, you can use it to help determine the proper mask size.

Ventilate according to current standards, obtaining chest rise with each breath. Begin the ventilation and say, "squeeze," providing just enough volume to initiate chest rise, but being very careful not to overinflate the child's lungs. Allow adequate time for exhalation, saying, "release, release."

Content Self-Evaluation

MULTIPLE CHOICE

_____ **1.** In the ear-to-sternal-notch position, the supine patient's head is elevated to the point where the ear and the sternal notch are horizontally aligned.
   A. True
   B. False

2. The strategy for positioning the airway in an unconscious obese patient is the
   A. sniffing position.
   B. decline position.
   C. incline position.
   D. ramped position.
   E. perpendicular ear position.

3. Though oxygen should be administered cautiously in patients with COPD, never withhold oxygen from any patient for whom it is indicated.
   A. True
   B. False

4. Which of the following oxygen delivery devices deliver 40–60 percent oxygen at 6–10 L/min?
   A. Nasal cannula
   B. Venturi mask
   C. Simple face mask
   D. Partial rebreather mask
   E. Nonrebreather mask

5. Bilevel positive airway pressure (BiPAP) maintains a steady level of pressure during both inhalation and exhalation.
   A. True
   B. False

6. Which of the following is an advantage of the nasopharyngeal airway?
   A. It may cause severe nosebleeds if inserted too forcefully.
   B. It is difficult to suction through.
   C. It is smaller than the oropharyngeal airway.
   D. You may not use it if the patient has or is suspected to have a basilar skull fracture.
   E. It bypasses the tongue, providing a patent airway.

7. Insertion of the nasopharyngeal airway directs the soft rubber tube
   A. directly up and into the nostril.
   B. directly along the floor of the nasal cavity.
   C. into the left nostril, most frequently.
   D. laterally along the side of the nasal cavity.
   E. directly into the vallecula space.

8. Which of the following is a disadvantage of the oropharyngeal airway?
   A. It helps manage profoundly unconscious patients who are breathing spontaneously or need mechanical ventilation.
   B. It helps prevent obstruction by the teeth and lips.
   C. It serves as an effective bite block in case of seizures or to protect the endotracheal tube.
   D. It does not isolate the trachea or prevent aspiration.
   E. It is easy to place using proper technique.

9. To insert the oropharyngeal airway
   A. place it directly straight back along the oral cavity floor, parallel to the nasal cavity until fully inserted.
   B. insert with the tip pointing toward the roof of the mouth, advance to the level of the soft palate, and gently rotate $180°$ until it comes to rest over the tongue.
   C. press the tongue upward and forward with a tongue blade. Then, the airway can be advanced until the flange is seated at the teeth.
   D. either B or D.
   E. none of the above.

10. Effective ventilatory support requires a
    A. tidal volume of 6 to 8 mL/kg of ideal body weight at a rate of 12 breaths per minute.
    B. tidal volume of 6 to 8 mL/kg of ideal body weight at a rate of 12–20 breaths per minute.
    C. tidal volume of 10 to 15 mL/kg of ideal body weight at a rate of 12–20 breaths per minute.
    D. tidal volume of 10 to 15 mL/kg of ideal body weight at a rate of 12 breaths per minute.
    E. tidal volume of 12 to 20 mL/kg of ideal body weight at a rate of 6–8 breaths per minute.

11. Mouth-to-mouth and mouth-to-nose ventilation are the most basic methods of rescue ventilation, but their use is limited by exposure to body fluids and by limited oxygen delivery, as expired air contains only
    A. 13 percent oxygen.
    B. 15 percent oxygen.
    C. 17 percent oxygen.
    D. 19 percent oxygen.
    E. 21 percent oxygen.

12. The bag-valve-mask (BVM) consists of
    A. one-way valve.
    B. an oblong, self-inflating bag.
    C. detachable face mask.
    D. oxygen reservoir.
    E. all of the above.

13. Complications of BVM ventilation include all of the following EXCEPT
    A. gastric distension.
    B. adequate tidal volume.
    C. poor mask seal.
    D. barotrauma.
    E. poor compliance.

14. In the event that the patient actively vomits, it is imperative to release the pressure to avoid esophageal rupture.
    A. True
    B. False

15. Which of the following is NOT one of the BVN *Rule of Threes*?
    A. Three providers
    B. Three fingers
    C. Three PSI
    D. Three minutes
    E. Three inches

Special Project

Exhaled carbon dioxide (CO_2) monitoring, also called end-tidal carbon dioxide ($ETCO_2$) monitoring, or capnometry, is a noninvasive method of measuring the levels of carbon dioxide (CO_2) in the exhaled breath.

©2013 Pearson Education, Inc.
Paramedic Care: Principles & Practice, Vol. 2, 4th Ed.

In the table below, list two possible causes of the listed changes in $ETCO_2$.

Sudden drop of $ETCO_2$ to zero	1.
	2.
Sudden decrease of $ETCO_2$ (not to zero)	1.
	2.
Exponential decrease of $ETCO_2$	1.
	2.
Changes in CO_2 baseline	1.
	2.
Sudden increase in $ETCO_2$	1.
	2.
Gradual lowering of $ETCO_2$	1.
	2.
Gradual increase in $ETCO_2$	1.
	2.

Part 3: Advanced Airway Management and Ventilation, p. 330

Review of Chapter Objectives

After reading this part of the chapter, you should be able to:

21. **Describe the indications, contraindications, advantages, disadvantages, complications, equipment, and techniques for the use of advanced airway devices and techniques, including various extraglottic airways, endotracheal intubation, and cricothyrotomy.**   pp. 330–332, 336, 359–360

Esophageal Tracheal Combitube (ETC)
The Esophageal Tracheal Combitube (ETC), also called simply the Combitube, is a dual-lumen retroglottic airway available in two sizes for patients over 4 feet tall. The ETC is inserted blindly through the mouth into the posterior oropharynx and then gently advanced.

Advantages of the ETC
- Insertion is rapid and highly successful.
- It is time tested.
- Insertion does not require visualization.
- It will provide ventilation with either esophageal or tracheal placement.
- The large pharyngeal balloon may tamponade oral bleeding.
- It will generate high airway pressures for ventilation when necessary.
- It offers reasonable aspiration protection in either the esophageal or tracheal position.

- In the esophageal position, gastric decompression is possible through the #2 port.
- When intubating around the ETC, the proximal balloon may be deflated and the distal balloon left inflated to seal off the esophagus.

Disadvantages of the ETC

- Trauma, including esophageal perforation, has been reported.
- It cannot be placed with an intact gag reflex.
- High cuff volumes may result in tissue ischemia.
- It cannot be placed in patients under 4 feet tall.
- Clinical assessment is necessary to ensure ventilation through the correct port.
- It does not completely isolate the trachea in the esophageal position.
- Placement is not 100 percent foolproof.

Pharyngeo-Tracheal Lumen Airway (PtL)

The pharyngeo-tracheal lumen airway (PtL) is a two-tube system. The first tube is short, with a large diameter; its proximal end is green. A large cuff encircles the tube's lower third. When inflated, the cuff seals the entire oropharynx. Air introduced at this tube's proximal end will enter the hypopharynx. The second tube is long, with a small diameter, and clear. It passes through and extends approximately 10 cm beyond the first tube. This second tube may be inserted blindly into either the trachea or the esophagus. A distal cuff, when inflated, seals off whichever anatomical structure the tube has entered. When the second tube enters the trachea, you will ventilate the patient through it.

Advantages of the PtL

- It can function in either the tracheal or esophageal position.
- It has no face mask to seal.
- It does not require direct visualization of the larynx and thus does not require the use of a laryngoscope or additional specialized equipment.
- It can be used in trauma patients, since the neck can remain in neutral position during insertion and use.
- It helps protect the trachea from upper airway bleeding and secretions.

Disadvantages of the PtL

- It does not isolate and completely protect the trachea from aspiration.
- The oropharyngeal balloon can migrate out of the mouth anteriorly, partially dislodging the airway.
- Intubation around the PtL is extremely difficult, even with the oropharyngeal balloon deflated.
- It cannot be used in conscious patients or those with a gag reflex.
- It cannot be used in pediatric patients.
- It can only be passed orally.

Complications of PtL placement include:

- Pharyngeal or esophageal trauma from poor technique.
- Unrecognized displacement of the long tube from the trachea into the esophagus.
- Displacement of the pharyngeal balloon.

Endotracheal Intubation

Endotracheal intubation involves inserting an endotracheal tube into the trachea, usually with direct visualization of the vocal cords, typically via direct laryngoscopy.

Advantages of Endotracheal Intubation

- It isolates the trachea and permits complete control of the airway.
- It impedes gastric distension by channeling air directly into the trachea.
- It eliminates the need to maintain a mask seal.
- It offers a direct route for suctioning of the respiratory passages.
- It permits administration of the medications lidocaine, epinephrine, atropine, and naloxone via the endotracheal tube. (Use the mnemonic LEAN or NAVEL [if vasopressin is added] to remember these medications.)

©2013 Pearson Education, Inc.
Paramedic Care: Principles & Practice, Vol. 2, 4th Ed.

Disadvantages of Endotracheal Intubation

- The technique requires considerable training and experience.
- It requires specialized equipment.
- It requires direct visualization of the vocal cords.
- It bypasses the upper airway's function of warming, filtering, and humidifying the inhaled air.
- It is time consuming.
- It is associated with many potential complications, including aspiration, hypoxemia, airway trauma, increased intracranial pressure, and others.
- It has not been shown to improve survival.

Needle Cricothyrotomy

Needle cricothyrotomy involves placing a large-bore needle with plastic cannula, such as a 14-gauge intravenous catheter, through the cricothyroid membrane into the trachea. Oxygen must then be forced through this small-caliber device, using a bag-valve device or a high-pressure oxygen source.

The potential complications of needle cricothyrotomy include:

- Barotrauma from overinflation if using transtracheal jet insufflation
- Excessive bleeding due to improper catheter placement
- Subcutaneous emphysema from improper placement into the subcutaneous tissue, excessive air leak around the catheter, or laryngeal trauma
- Bleeding
- Hypoventilation and respiratory acidosis
- Aspiration as the airway is unprotected

Open Cricothyrotomy

An open, or surgical, cricothyrotomy involves placing an endotracheal or tracheostomy tube directly into the trachea through a surgical incision at the cricothyroid membrane.

The potential complications of open cricothyrotomy include:

- Incorrect tube placement into a false passage
- Cricoid and/or thyroid cartilage damage
- Thyroid gland damage
- Severe bleeding
- Laryngeal nerve damage
- Subcutaneous emphysema
- Vocal cord damage
- Infection

22. **Under the supervision of a lab instructor or clinical preceptor and as allowed in your scope of practice, demonstrate effective techniques of advanced airway management, including the following:**

    a. **insertion of extraglottic airways**   pp. 331–332

    Esophageal Tracheal Combitube (ETC)
    1. Perform optimal BVM ventilation with high-concentration oxygen.
    2. Place the patient supine in a neutral position if possible.
    3. Prepare and check equipment. Select a Regular size for patients 6 feet tall or taller. Select a Small-Adult size for patients less than 6 feet tall. Note that this sizing instruction is evidence-based but is different from the manufacturer's instructions.
    4. Stabilize the cervical spine if cervical injury is possible.
    5. Perform the Lipp Maneuver (or modified Lipp Maneuver) to preshape the ETC.
    6. Grab and lift the jaw or, if within your scope of practice, use a laryngoscope to create a channel and visualize the esophagus. Insert the ETC gently in midline and advance it past the hypopharynx to the depth indicated by the markings on the tube. The black rings on the tube should be between the patient's teeth.
    7. Inflate the pharyngeal cuff with 100 mL of air and the distal cuff with 10 to 15 mL of air.

8. Ventilate through the longer, blue, #1, proximal port with a bag-valve device connected to 100 percent oxygen, while auscultating over the chest and stomach. If you hear bilateral breath sounds over the chest and none over the stomach (indicating that the device is sitting in and occluding the esophagus while directing oxygen flow into the trachea), secure the tube and continue ventilating.

9. If you hear gastric sounds over the epigastrium and no breath sounds (indicating that the device is sitting in and occluding the trachea while directing oxygen flow into the esophagus), change ports and ventilate through the clear, shorter, #2, distal port to direct oxygen into the trachea. Confirm breath sounds over the chest with absent gastric sounds.

10. Use multiple confirmation techniques. End-tidal CO_2 is reliable with an ETC as long as the patient is producing CO_2. An esophageal detector device (EDD) may be used on an ETC by attaching it to the #2 port that is open on the distal end. Note that failure to inflate indicates appropriate esophageal positioning and you should continue ventilation through the #1 port. This is somewhat backwards compared to using an EDD to confirm endotracheal intubation.

11. Secure the tube and continue ventilating with 100 percent oxygen.

12. Frequently reassess the airway and adequacy of ventilation.

Pharyngeo-Tracheal Lumen Airway (PtL)

1. Complete basic manual and adjunctive maneuvers and provide supplemental oxygen and ventilatory support with a BVM and hyperventilation.

2. Place the patient supine and kneel at the top of his head.

3. Prepare and check the equipment.

4. Place the patient's head in the appropriate position. Hyperextend the neck if there is no risk of cervical spine injury. Maintain neutral position with stabilization of the cervical spine if cervical spine injury is possible.

5. Insert the PtL gently, using the tongue-jaw-lift maneuver.

6. Inflate the distal cuffs on both PtL tubes simultaneously with a sustained breath into the inflation valve.

7. Deliver a breath into the green oropharyngeal tube. If the patient's chest rises and you auscultate bilateral breath sounds, the long clear tube is in the esophagus. Inflate the pharyngeal balloon and continue ventilations via the green tube.

8. If the chest does not rise and you auscultate no breath sounds, the long clear tube is in the trachea. Remove the stylet from the clear tube and ventilate the patient through that tube.

9. Attach the bag-valve device to the 15-mm connector, secure the tube, and continue ventilatory support with 100 percent oxygen.

10. Multiple placement confirmation techniques are again essential, as are good assessment skills. Misidentification of placement has been reported. Frequently reassess the airway and adequacy of ventilation.

b. **orotracheal intubation**   pp. 342–345

1. Use Standard Precautions.

2. Place the patient supine and properly position the patient's head and neck. To visualize the larynx, you must align the three axes of the mouth, the pharynx, and the trachea. To do this, place the patient's head in a "sniffing position" by elevating the head and flexing the neck forward and the head backward. The ear and sternal notch should be on the same horizontal level. In obese patients it is necessary to place padding under the upper back, shoulders, and head to achieve the same position. This is called the "ramped position."

3. Perform BVM ventilation with 100 percent oxygen using the "rule of threes," as discussed earlier in the chapter under the discussion of BVM ventilation. Avoid aggressive hyperventilation, as this is likely to fill the stomach with air and predispose to aspiration.

4. Prepare your intubation equipment.

5. Turn on the suction and attach an appropriate tip.

6. Remove any dentures or partial dental plates.

7. Hold the laryngoscope in your left hand, whether you are right or left-handed. Insert the laryngoscope blade gently into the right side of the patient's mouth. If using a curved blade, gently sweep the tongue to the left and work in the midline. If using a straight blade, remain on the right side of the mouth. Your primary goal at this point is to visualize the epiglottis.

8. Advance the curved blade until the distal end is at the base of the tongue in the vallecula. Advance the straight blade until the distal end is under the epiglottis. Alternatively, with a straight blade, you may fully advance until the distal tip is in the esophagus and then visualize while slowly withdrawing the blade. If you cannot visualize the epiglottis, withdraw the blade, reposition the patient, and repeat.

9. Keeping your left wrist straight, use your left shoulder and arm to continue lifting the mandible and tongue to a 45° angle to the ground (up and toward the feet) until landmarks are exposed. Be careful not to put pressure on the teeth. Consider having an assistant perform the jaw-thrust simultaneously. At this point you may need to suction any large amounts of emesis, blood, or secretions in the posterior pharynx.

10. If you cannot see the landmarks clearly, have your partner release cricoid pressure. If you still cannot visualize the posterior cartilages, perform external laryngeal manipulation. You may not see the entire glottis or even part of it, but you should at least clearly visualize the posterior cartilages and interarytenoid notch.

11. Hold the ETT in your right hand with your fingertips as you would a dart or a pencil. This gives you control to gently maneuver the ETT. Advance the tube through the right corner of the patient's mouth, and direct it toward the midline. Pass the ETT gently through the glottic opening until its distal cuff disappears beyond the vocal cords; then advance it another 1 to 2 cm. Hold the tube in place with your hand to prevent its displacement. Do not let go under any circumstance until it is taped or tied securely in place.

12. Remove the stylet (if used) and attach a bag-valve device to the 15/22-mm connector on the tube.

13. Objectively confirm tube placement with capnography. In addition, check for equal breath sounds to be sure the tube is not too deep.

14. Ventilate the patient with 100 percent oxygen.

15. Gently insert an oropharyngeal airway to serve as a bite block, and secure the ETT with umbilical tape, adhesive tape, or a commercial tube-holding device.

16. Place the patient on the transport ventilator and monitor the continuous capnography waveform.

17. Reconfirm appropriate tube placement periodically, especially after any major patient movement or if there is any deterioration of patient status.

c. blind nasotracheal intubation   pp. 350–351

1. Use Standard Precautions.

2. Using basic manual and adjunctive maneuvers, open the airway and ventilate the patient with 100 percent oxygen.

3. Prepare your equipment.

4. Place the patient in his position of comfort. If the patient is unconscious or if you suspect cervical spine injury, place the patient supine and use manual in-line stabilization as appropriate.

5. Inspect the nose and select the larger nostril as your passageway.

6. Select the correct size endotracheal tube. Normally use a tube one-half to one full size smaller than for oral intubation. For an average adult male, a size 7 mm is appropriate. For an average adult female, a size 6.5 mm is appropriate. Tubes with a directable tip may make the procedure easier, if available. Attach an end-tidal CO_2 detection device to the proximal end of the tube. Alternatively, a device to enhance audible detection of breath sounds, such as the BAAM whistle or the Burden nasoscope, may be used.

7. Lubricate the tube generously. Topical lidocaine may be preferred for long-term comfort but probably does not impact the initial attempt.

8. Insert the ETT into the nostril with the bevel along the floor of the nostril or facing the nasal septum, directed posteriorly. This will help avoid damage to the turbinates. There is some tendency to direct the tube upward, but recall that the nasopharynx runs directly anterior to posterior.

9. As you feel the tube drop into the posterior pharynx, listen closely at its proximal end for the patient's respiratory sounds, and observe for end-tidal CO_2. Sounds are loudest when the ETT is proximal to the epiglottis. When the ETT tip reaches the posterior pharyngeal wall, you must take care to direct it toward the glottic opening. This may be done with an endotracheal tube or by inflating the cuff. At this point, the tip of the ETT may catch in the pyriform sinus. If it does,

you will feel resistance, and the skin on either side of the Adam's apple will tent. To resolve pyriform sinus placement, slightly withdraw the ETT and rotate it to the midline.

10. With the patient's next inhaled breath, advance the ETT gently but quickly into the glottic opening, observing exhaled CO_2.

11. Holding the ETT with one hand to prevent displacement, inflate the distal cuff with enough air to eliminate any audible leak, connect a bag-valve device, ventilate the patient with 100 percent oxygen, and confirm proper placement of the ETT using multiple techniques, including bilateral breath sounds, absent epigastric sounds, and capnography.

12. Secure the ETT and reconfirm proper placement. Continue to observe the patient's condition, maintain ventilatory support, and frequently recheck ETT placement. Use continuous waveform capnography to monitor tube placement and ventilation.

d. digital intubation
pp. 351–352

1. Use Standard Precautions.

2. Continue oxygenation with bag-valve-mask and high-concentration oxygen.

3. Prepare and check your equipment. You will need the following items: an appropriately sized ETT, a malleable stylet, water-soluble lubricant, a 5- to 10-mL syringe, a bite block, and umbilical tape or a commercial anchoring device. Insert the stylet into the endotracheal tube and bend the ETT/stylet into a J shape.

4. Remove the front of the collar and have an assistant stabilize the neck as appropriate.

5. Place a bite block device between the patient's molars to help protect your fingers.

6. Insert your left middle and index fingers into the patient's mouth. By alternating fingers, "walk" your hand down the midline while simultaneously tugging gently forward on the tongue.

7. Advance the tube, pushing it gently with your right hand. Use your left index finger to keep the tip of the ETT against your middle finger. This will direct the tip to the epiglottis.

8. Use your middle and index fingers to direct the tip of the ETT between the epiglottis (in front) and your fingers (behind). Then with your right hand advance the ETT through the cords while simultaneously maneuvering it forward with your left index and middle fingers. This will prevent it from slipping posteriorly into the esophagus.

9. Hold the tube in place with your hand to prevent its displacement, remove stylet, and inflate cuff.

10. Confirm placement with multiple techniques.

11. Ventilate the patient with 100 percent oxygen. Gently insert an oropharyngeal airway to serve as a bite block. Secure the ETT with umbilical tape. Repeat steps to confirm proper ETT placement and maintain ventilatory support. Continue your airway assessment periodically.

e. trauma patient airway management
pp. 352–353

To perform orotracheal intubation on a trauma patient, you need an assistant who will both maintain in-line stabilization and simultaneously perform a jaw-thrust. Maintaining in-line stabilization of the cervical spine is, of course, critical for the trauma patient who may have suffered spinal injury. The jaw-thrust maneuver will not only open the airway but also will assist with direct laryngoscopy, since the patient cannot be placed into the optimal ear-to-sternal notch position.

f. verification of endotracheal tube placement
pp. 345–346

It is absolutely imperative that endotracheal placement of the tube be objectively confirmed immediately after placement and continuously throughout care, particularly if the patient is moved or deteriorates.

Subjective methods of tube placement confirmation include direct visualization, tube misting, and auscultation for breath sounds.

Objective methods of tube confirmation include capnography, esophageal detector device (EDD), endotracheal tube introducer, pulse oximetry, chest rise and fall, and presence or absence of gastric distention. Remember that objective methods such as these must be used, in addition to subjective observations, to confirm proper tube placement.

g. foreign body removal under direct laryngoscopy
p. 355

When confronted with a patient who has apparently choked, you should initially carry out basic maneuvers for airway obstruction that are appropriate to the patient's age and mental status, such as abdominal thrusts or chest thrusts. If these fail to alleviate the obstruction, direct visualization of the airway with a laryngoscope may enable you to remove an obstructing foreign body using Magill forceps or a suction device. The procedure for visualizing the airway is identical to that used for orotracheal intubation

h. pediatric intubation pp. 356–358

1. Use Standard Precautions.
2. Continue BVM ventilation with 100 percent oxygen while using a towel roll under the shoulders of an infant or towels under the head in older children (if not in cervical spine precautions) to achieve a sniffing position.
3. Prepare and check your equipment. As stated earlier, a straight blade is usually preferred in infants and small children, but it is suggested to have an age-appropriate curved blade available as well in case tongue control becomes critical. With children younger than 8 years, you will either use an uncuffed endotracheal tube or a cuffed tube that is a half size smaller than calculated with standard formulas. Because of the short distance between the mouth and the trachea, you rarely need a stylet to position the tube properly. Remember to lubricate the ETT with water-soluble gel.
4. In case of trauma, remove the front of the cervical collar and have an assistant maintain manual in-line stabilization of the cervical spine.
5. Hold the laryngoscope in your left hand and insert it gently into the right side of the patient's mouth. Do not attempt to sweep the tongue with a straight blade.
6. Advance the straight blade on the right side of the tongue with the tip directed toward the midline until the distal end reaches the base of the tongue. Alternatively, you may use the "hub technique" by initially advancing the straight blade gently into the esophagus as far as it will go without resistance, then withdrawing while performing ELM. If using a curved blade, sweep the tongue from right to left and advance in the midline.
7. Look for the tip of the epiglottis and gently lift with the tip of the blade while simultaneously performing ELM with an assistant's hand until the glottis or posterior cartilages are visualized. Keep in mind that a child—particularly an infant—has a shorter airway and a higher glottis than an adult. Because of this, you may see the cords much sooner than you expect.
8. If you cannot see the epiglottis, you are likely too deep. Gently and slowly withdraw while continuing to visualize until the vocal cords fall into view.
9. Grasp the endotracheal tube in your right hand and, under direct visualization of the vocal cords or posterior cartilages, insert it through the right corner of the patient's mouth into the glottic opening.

   Pass it through until the vocal cord marking on the tube is at the level of the cords or until the distal cuff of the ETT just disappears beyond the vocal cords. In some cases, advancing an endotracheal tube will be difficult at the level of the cricoid. Do not force the ETT through this region, as it may cause laryngeal edema and bleeding. Confirm correct placement of the ETT. Hold the tube in place with your left hand, attach an age-appropriate bag-valve device to the 15/22-mm connector, and deliver several breaths with an end-tidal CO_2 detector in-line. For additional confirmation, observe for symmetrical chest rise and fall with each ventilation. Also auscultate for equal, bilateral breath sounds at the lateral chest wall, high in the axilla, and absent breath sounds over the epigastrium. An esophageal detector device may also be used for patients over 10 kg as long as you squeeze the bulb before attaching it to the tube.
10. If the tube has a distal cuff, do not inflate it unless there is a detectable air leak. If a leak is audible, inflate the distal cuff with just enough air to stop the leak.
11. Secure the ETT with tape or a commercial device, being very careful not to compress the tube. Note placement of the distance marker at the teeth/gums, recheck for proper placement, and continue ventilatory support. Periodically reassess ETT placement and watch the patient carefully for any clinical signs of difficulty. Continue ongoing waveform capnography monitoring if possible.
12. Place a gastric tube if allowed by protocol.

i. needle cricothyrotomy pp. 360–361

1. Use Standard Precautions, including face mask and shield.
2. Manage the patient's airway as well as possible with basic maneuvers and supplemental oxygen while you prepare your equipment. Attach a large-bore IV needle with a catheter (adults: 14- or 16-gauge; pediatrics: 18- or 20-gauge) to a 10- or 20-mL syringe. If time permits you may fill the syringe with sterile water or saline to facilitate detection of air when aspirating.

©2013 Pearson Education, Inc.
Paramedic Care: Principles & Practice, Vol. 2, 4th Ed.

CHAPTER 5 *Airway Management and Ventilation* **143**

3. Place the patient supine and hyperextend the head and neck. (Maintain neutral position if you suspect cervical spine injury.) Position yourself at the patient's side.

4. Palpate the inferior portion of the thyroid cartilage and the cricoid cartilage. The indention between the two is the cricothyroid membrane.

5. Prepare the anterior neck with antiseptic solution.

6. Firmly grasp the laryngeal cartilages and reconfirm the site of the cricothyroid membrane.

7. Carefully insert the needle into the cricothyroid membrane at midline, directed 45° caudally (towards the feet). Often you will feel a pop as the needle penetrates the membrane.

8. Advance the needle while aspirating with the syringe. If air returns easily, the catheter is in the trachea. If blood returns or you feel resistance to return, reevaluate needle placement.

9. After you confirm proper placement, hold the needle steady and advance the catheter. Then withdraw the needle.

10. Reconfirm placement by again withdrawing air from the catheter with the syringe. Secure the catheter in place.

11. Attach the jet-ventilation device to the catheter and a 50-psi oxygen supply. If this is unavailable, you may connect a bag-valve device to the catheter using the inner adapter from a 7.5-mm endotracheal tube. The bag-valve device must be connected to oxygen.

12. Open the release valve to introduce an oxygen jet into the trachea. Then adjust the pressure to allow adequate lung expansion (usually about 50 psi, compared with about 1 psi through a regulator).

13. Watch the chest carefully, turning off the release valve as soon as the chest rises. Exhalation then occurs passively through the glottis as a result of elastic recoil of the lungs and chest wall. Deliver at least 20 breaths per minute, keeping the inflation-to-deflation time approximately 1:3. Keep in mind that you may need to adjust this to the patient's needs, particularly in COPD and asthma patients, who often require a longer expiration time.

14. Continue ventilatory support, assessing for adequacy of ventilations and looking for the development of any potential complications.

15. You should be anticipating the need for an alternative means of oxygenation and ventilation within approximately 30 minutes.

j. open cricothyrotomy   **p. 362**

1. Use Standard Precautions, including face mask and shield.

2. Use BVM ventilation and supplemental oxygen to maintain oxygenation and ventilation as well as possible while preparing supplies.

3. Locate the thyroid cartilage and the cricoid cartilage. Identify the cricothyroid membrane between these two cartilages.

4. Clean the area with antiseptic solution.

5. Stabilize the cartilages with one hand, while using a scalpel in the other hand to make a 2- to 4-cm vertical skin incision in the midline over the membrane.

6. Locate the cricothyroid membrane again, using blunt dissection if necessary.

7. Make a 1- to 2-cm incision in the horizontal plane through the membrane.

8. Insert a tracheal hook on the inferior portion of the thyroid cartilage to help maintain the opening. This may also be improvised with an adult or pediatric stylet.

9. Insert curved hemostats into the membrane incision and spread it open.

10. Insert either a cuffed endotracheal tube or a tracheostomy tube into the opening, directing the tube distally into the trachea. Ideally a 6-mm tube will fit, although smaller patients may require a smaller size.

11. Inflate the cuff and ventilate.

12. Confirm placement with multiple methods as available and appropriate.

13. Secure the tube in place.

Variations on the traditional open cricothyrotomy technique include the rapid four-step technique and the bougie-aided technique.

Rapid four-step. In this technique, a single incision is made horizontally through the skin and cricoid membrane, then a tracheal hook is held in the left hand and traction is applied against the cricoid membrane, directed toward the feet, and the tube is inserted with the right hand, mimicking endotracheal intubation. This technique has been associated with more complications in some studies.

©2013 Pearson Education, Inc.
Paramedic Care: Principles & Practice, Vol. 2, 4th Ed.

Bougie-aided. An endotracheal tube introducer (bougie) may be used with either the traditional or the rapid four-step technique to minimize the risk of placement in a false passage, to allow the operator to let go without losing critical landmarks, and to ease threading of the tube. In the simplest version of this technique, an adult bougie is passed into the trachea through the incision in the cricothyroid membrane, directed distally, and intratracheal placement is confirmed with palpation of clicks as the bougie passes over the cartilage rings and/or palpation of hold-up within 20 cm. Note that the distance to hold-up is much shorter than when using the introducer/bougie through the mouth. Once placement is confirmed, the endotracheal or tracheostomy tube is threaded over the bougie into the trachea.

23. **Recognize complications of advanced airway management.** pp. 331–332, 335–336, 341, 351, 358–360, 362, 364–365

Potential complications of using extraglottic airway devices

- Pharyngeal or esophageal trauma
- Tissue ischemia due to excessive cuff volumes
- Improper tube placement
- Aspiration
- Gastric distension

Potential complications of endotracheal intubation

- Bypasses the upper airway's function of warming, filtering, and humidifying
- Time consuming.
- Equipment malfunction
- Tooth breakage and soft-tissue lacerations
- Aspiration
- Elevated intracranial pressure
- Transport delays
- Hypoxemia
- Esophageal intubation
- Endobronchial intubation
- Tension pneumothorax
- Digital intubation may stimulate patient to clamp down and bite provider's fingers

Potential complications of needle cricothyrotomy with jet ventilation

- Barotrauma from overinflation
- Excessive bleeding
- Subcutaneous emphysema
- Excessive air leak around the catheter
- Hypoventilation and respiratory acidosis
- Aspiration as the airway is unprotected

Potential complications of open cricothyrotomy with jet ventilation

- Incorrect tube placement into a false passage
- Cricoid and/or thyroid cartilage damage
- Thyroid gland damage
- Severe bleeding
- Laryngeal nerve damage
- Subcutaneous emphysema
- Vocal cord damage
- Infection

Potential complications of medication-assisted intubation

These procedures come with great risk, as you are employing very powerful medications that may result in severe morbidity and death when the paramedic is unable to intubate and cannot maintain adequate oxygenation through other means. In the setting of cardiac arrest, of course, you cannot realistically make the situation any worse. MAI, however, is employed in patients who are alive and sometimes conscious, when both the potential benefits and the potential harms are greater.

24. Take actions to correct complications of advanced airway management. pp. 331–374

As new and improved airway devices are introduced, the paramedic must remain current on manufacturers' recommendations for use and local protocols for approved devices.

Look for and heed obvious warning signs of difficult intubation or BVM ventilation and prepare accordingly.

Use care in placing the device, including use of appropriate pre-insertion preparation and device lubrication to help avoid trauma to airway tissues and structures.

Assure the device is placed, inflated, confirmed, and secured as directed. This will help to avoid aspiration, trauma, and misplaced device.

To reduce hypoxia, limit the amount of time used for each attempt. Remember, while you are placing the device the patient is not being ventilated.

Monitor assisted ventilation rates and tidal volume to help reduce the risk of gastric distension, aspiration, and subcutaneous emphysema.

Frequently reconfirm appropriate device placement and document your findings.

25. Discuss management of post-intubation agitation and field extubation. pp. 358–359

Occasionally, an intubated patient will awaken and be intolerant of the ETT. This happens most often with patients who undergo rapid sequence intubation and then awaken from the sedative agent and paralytic. This occurrence usually indicates inadequate sedation/analgesia and/or inappropriate ventilator settings. Paralytics alone should never be given to treat agitation.

Only rarely should extubation be considered in the field, because this may be associated with serious complications such as aspiration, laryngospasm, and negative-pressure pulmonary edema. The patient may deteriorate again and be difficult to reintubate. If the patient is clearly able to maintain and protect his airway, is intolerant of the tube and ventilator, no medications are available to make him comfortable, and reassessment indicates that the problem that led to endotracheal intubation is resolved (such as a narcotic overdose), extubation may be indicated.

To perform field extubation:
1. Use Standard Precautions.
2. Ensure adequate oxygenation. A crude method for accomplishing this in the field is to be certain that the patient's mental status, skin color, and pulse oximetry are optimal on room air with the ETT in place.
3. Prepare intubation equipment and suction.
4. Confirm patient responsiveness.
5. Position patient on his side if possible.
6. Suction the patient's oropharynx.
7. Deflate the ETT cuff.
8. Remove the ETT upon cough or expiration.
9. Provide supplemental oxygen as indicated.
10. Reassess the adequacy of the patient's ventilation and oxygenation.

26. Explain the considerations in medication-assisted intubation. pp. 365, 369

Rapid sequence intubation (RSI) involves a series of steps that includes administration of a neuromuscular blocking drug to a critically ill or injured patient, who is presumed to have a full stomach, in order to facilitate oral intubation without aspiration or other complications.

Indications for RSI include: impending or actual respiratory failure from any cause, impending or actual inability to protect the airway from any cause, combativeness secondary to presumed head trauma, and hypoxemia despite maximal therapy.

Relative contraindications for RSI include: predicted difficult airway, short eta to hospital or more experienced providers, only one paramedic on scene, ability to manage the patient with less risky procedures, and when the only indication is airway protection.

Absolute contraindications for RSI include: respiratory arrest and cardiac arrest.

Rapid sequence airway (RSA) is a new airway management technique in which the preparation and pharmacology of rapid sequence intubation (RSI) is paired with intentional placement of an extraglottic airway device, without prior attempt at direct laryngoscopy, in selected patients.

Indications for RSA include: impending or actual respiratory failure from any cause, impending or actual inability to protect the airway from any cause, combativeness secondary to presumed head trauma, and hypoxemia despite maximal therapy.

Relative contraindications for RSA include: patient's airway may be managed by other means, anticipated inability to ventilate by BVM, anticipated need for very high airway pressures, very high aspiration risk, short eta to hospital or arrival of help with more resources, and only one paramedic on scene.

Absolute contraindications for RSA include: upper airway pathology known or suspected, blunt or penetrating anterior neck trauma, inhalation injury, angioedema, anaphylaxis, upper airway tumor, obstructing upper airway infection (croup, epiglottitis), parapharyngeal abscess, and caustic ingestion.

27. **Describe procedures for medication-assisted intubation.** p. 369

1. Preoxygenate to achieve nitrogen washout and create an oxygen reserve (as discussed earlier). Use a nonrebreather mask with high-concentration oxygen for at least 3 minutes if possible. Consider CPAP, assisted respiration, and BVM ventilation as indicated. Avoid positive pressure if the patient is not hypoxemic.
2. Protect the C-spine if indicated. The front of the cervical collar should be removed and manual in-line stabilization performed by an assistant who is also ready to perform a jaw-thrust maneuver.
3. Position optimally if possible. Patients not in cervical precautions should be placed in sniffing or ramped position.
4. Apply pressure to the cricoid if there is sufficient assistance available. The individual providing pressure should be prepared to release pressure and assist with external laryngeal manipulation (ELM) as directed by the intubator.
5. Ponder if intubation is really necessary. Are there other management options, if this is likely to be a difficult airway? Use a checklist if possible.
6. Premedicate if time permits and allowed by protocol and scope of practice. Consider regular-dose fentanyl for most patients, high-dose fentanyl for suspected critical ICP, and lidocaine for severe asthmatics.
7. Prepare equipment, using a checklist to ensure that all supplies are ready. This includes intubation, BVM ventilation, rescue, and post-intubation supplies.
8. Sedate and paralyze, using appropriate medications and doses. Most patients should receive both an induction agent and paralytic. The induction agent should routinely be given before the paralytic.
9. Pass the tube with direct or indirect visualization or an endotracheal tube introducer. Use all available adjunctive techniques including external laryngeal manipulation (ELM). Monitor oxygenation and be ready to abort the attempt before the oxygen level reaches a critical point. In most cases, where the patient is adequately preoxygenated and has a saturation of 100 percent beforehand, the attempt should be stopped when the saturation reaches about 93 percent.
10. Post-intubation management begins with objective tube confirmation, using capnography. Lung sounds should be used to help guide tube depth. A bite block should be inserted, and the tube should be secured in place and the cervical collar replaced if indicated. The patient should be placed on the transport ventilator including in-line continuous capnography. The patient should then receive analgesia and sedation. Ongoing paralytics should be administered only if absolutely necessary to manage the patient on the ventilator and never without analgesia and sedation. Monitor oxygen saturation (SpO_2), end-tidal CO_2, blood pressure, clinical exam, and ventilator parameters.

28. **Describe the pharmacology of agents commonly used in medication-assisted intubation.** pp. 366–369

Premedications are drugs given early in the course of RSI to mitigate anticipated complications:

Fentanyl. At routine doses, fentanyl is an excellent analgesic (pain reliever) that may keep a patient more comfortable during a painful procedure such as intubation. At higher doses, fentanyl is a sympatholytic agent that blunts the hypertension, tachycardia, and ICP elevation associated with laryngoscopy. It is reasonable to consider giving all patients analgesic doses of fentanyl at least 3 minutes before the procedure and higher doses to patients at risk for life-threatening elevations of ICP. While fentanyl is highly regarded for its hemodynamic (blood flow/blood pressure) stability, it may occasionally cause hypotension (a drop in blood pressure) in patients who are dependent on their sympathetic drive for blood pressure maintenance, especially at higher doses.

Atropine. Succinylcholine is associated with bradycardia (slow heartbeat) in younger children and in any patient receiving a second dose. Historically, atropine was recommended routinely 2 to 3 minutes before administration of succinylcholine to children less than 6 to 8 years of age to reduce the risk of bradycardia. Evidence now shows that this is optional, although atropine must always be at the bedside.

Lidocaine. While commonly used in head injury patients to blunt an increase in ICP, there has been a movement away from this practice in some circles because of limited evidence for benefit and the potential risk of hypotension as well as time delays. There is evidence that lidocaine is useful in asthmatic patients to avoid or lessen bronchospasm triggered by airway manipulation.

Induction agents render the patient unaware during the procedure:

Etomidate. Etomidate is a great agent for induction since it rarely causes any rise or drop in blood pressure or pulse. It also works extremely fast with a relatively consistent dose response. There has been concern about suppression of adrenal gland function in septic patients, but thus far there is no evidence that this is a significant enough safety concern to cause EMS to avoid it.

Midazolam. Midazolam is a benzodiazepine sedative/hypnotic. The major advantage of midazolam is amnesia. That is, the patient is unlikely to recall the procedure. The major disadvantage is that the dose required for induction is commonly associated with hypotension. It is also hard to predict the dose that will make any particular patient unaware.

Ketamine. Ketamine is a dissociative agent that is being used more in emergency medicine and critical care transport with some use in EMS as well. The advantages of ketamine are that it has a predictable dose response, does not cause hypotension, and provides analgesia as well as sedation. The major disadvantage is hypertension and tachycardia in some patients. There used to be concern about using ketamine in patients with head trauma and stroke, but that has largely been disproved as long as the patient is not hypertensive.

Propofol. Propofol is commonly used in the hospital for induction, but its use is limited in EMS by potentially profound hypotension.

Paralytics, or neuromuscular blocking agents, are drugs that temporarily stop skeletal muscle function without affecting cardiac or smooth muscle:

Succinylcholine. Succinylcholine is the prototype noncompetitive depolarizing neuromuscular blocker. Because of its fast onset (about 45 seconds) and short duration (about 8 minutes) this is the preferred agent for most EMS services. Unfortunately, succinylcholine has a host of potential adverse effects that result in a number of contraindications that must be considered in all patients. Succinylcholine is not routinely recommended for maintaining paralysis, so a second competitive agent must usually be carried as well.

Rocuronium. Rocuronium is now the most commonly used competitive agent in emergency medicine and EMS. The onset time with rocuronium is only slightly longer than with succinylcholine (60 seconds) as long as higher doses are used. At the recommended intubation doses, rocuronium may last 30 minutes or longer. While this is often used as an argument against rocuronium for EMS use, it is used successfully by many services that argue that even 8 minutes is too long with succinylcholine before moving on to a rescue airway. Rocuronium has few adverse effects and may be used for initial and ongoing paralysis.

Vecuronium. Vecuronium is a competitive agent that is commonly used to maintain paralysis after succinylcholine. Vecuronium is a second- or third-line agent for RSI because of its long onset time. While there are tricks that may be used to shorten the onset time, they add complexity and a very long duration of action.

©2013 Pearson Education, Inc.
Paramedic Care: Principles & Practice, Vol. 2, 4th Ed.

Sedatives and analgesics are essential for keeping a patient comfortable after intubation:

Narcotics. Narcotics are critical to provide analgesia. Fentanyl is used most commonly because it has a rapid onset and minimal effects on blood pressure unless the patient is sympathetic dependent. Other narcotics such as morphine may also be used cautiously.

Benzodiazepines. Benzodiazepines are optimal for keeping patients sedated while intubated. Midazolam is a favorite among critical care transport crews because of its rapid onset and short duration. Lorazepam and diazepam may also be used. All benzodiazepines must be used cautiously in volume-depleted and hypotensive patients.

Propofol. Propofol infusions are commonly used in the intensive care unit and during critical care transport to maintain sedation. The very short duration of action facilitates neurologic examination when the infusion is stopped. Propofol is even more prone to cause hypotension than the benzodiazepines and must be used cautiously.

29. **Given a variety of scenarios of patients requiring airway management, including patients with a difficult airway, intervene to establish an effective airway and ventilation without delay.** pp. 309–311, 313–329, 330–369, 374–380

Perform a primary assessment to identify any immediate threats to the patient's life, specifically, airway, breathing, and circulation problems. Feel for air movement with your hand or cheek. Look for the chest to rise and fall normally with each respiratory cycle. Listen for air movement and equal bilateral breath sounds.

If the patient is not breathing or if you suspect airway problems, open the airway using the head-tilt/chin-lift or jaw-thrust maneuver, as appropriate. Once the airway is open, reevaluate the breathing status. If breathing is adequate, provide supplemental oxygen and assess circulation. Consider the use of airway adjuncts. If breathing is inadequate or absent, begin artificial ventilation.

After you complete the primary assessment and correct any immediate life threats, conduct the secondary assessment while continuously monitoring the patient's airway, breathing, and circulation. The patient's past medical history will put his present complaints into perspective and help to identify the risk factors for a variety of likely diagnoses. Your physical examination of a patient with respiratory problems should continue the evaluation of his airway, breathing, and circulation begun during your primary assessment. Now you will use the physical examination techniques of inspection, auscultation, and palpation to evaluate his injury or illness in more detail and determine your plan of action.

Several available noninvasive respiratory monitoring devices will help you measure the effectiveness of oxygenation and ventilation and maintain parameters at the appropriate levels. Those measurements used most commonly in prehospital care are pulse oximetry, CO-oximetry, and capnography. Peak expiratory flow testing can also be useful in the prehospital setting for some respiratory diseases, although it is not widely employed. These measurements use various devices and methodologies that, when used alone, have their imitations. However, when used together they can provide a fairly comprehensive and reliable picture of the patient's respiratory status.

Basic airway management and ventilation includes most airway maneuvers that have been shown to be lifesaving, including proper positioning, suctioning, oxygen administration, and bag-valve-mask (BVM) ventilation. Providing supplemental oxygen to patients who are frankly hypoxemic will diminish the hypoxia's secondary effects on organs such as the brain and the heart and lessen subjective respiratory distress.

Advanced airway management includes the proper placement of extraglottic airway devices, orotracheal intubation, blind nasotracheal intubation, digital intubation, cricothyrotomy, and medication-assisted intubation, Additional airway and ventilation issues included patients with stoma sites, tracheobronchial suctioning, gastric distension decompression, and transport ventilators.

It is important, however, to think globally in terms of the difficult airway rather than considering only difficult intubation. The concept of the difficult airway includes difficult BVM ventilation, difficult extraglottic airway placement and ventilation, difficult intubation, and difficult cricothyrotomy.

Accurate and thorough documentation of airway management is critical for clinical care after the patient is transported, for quality assurance, and for medical/legal defense.

30. Recognize predictors of a difficult airway.   p. 370

Predictors of difficult BVM ventilation include: facial trauma, facial hair, obesity, lack of teeth or lack of dentures, history of snoring, Mallampati grade 3 or 4, severely limited jaw protrusion, and thyromental distance less than 6 cm.

Predictors of difficult extraglottic airway insertion or ventilation include: limited mouth opening, massive secretions, morbid obesity, severe pulmonary disease, and pathology below the device (e.g., inhalation burns, laryngeal trauma, angioedema)

Predictors of difficult laryngoscopy and orotracheal intubation include: facial trauma or anomalies, increasing Mallampati grade, short thyromental distance, short sternomental distance, limited mouth opening, limited neck mobility, obesity, and buckteeth.

Predictors of difficult surgical airway (cricothyrotomy) placement include: morbid obesity, anterior neck trauma, prior radiation therapy, Ludwig's angina (skin infection to anterior neck), tumor, infection, swelling, and foreign body.

31. Defend your decision-making processes in scenarios involving airway management and ventilation.   pp. 298, 380

Airway management and ventilation are the first and most critical steps in the primary assessment of every patient you will encounter (unless the patient is in cardiac arrest, when chest compressions will come first). Airway management and ventilation go hand in hand. You must immediately establish and maintain an open airway while providing adequate oxygen delivery and carbon dioxide elimination for all patients. Without adequate airway maintenance and ventilation, the patient will succumb to brain injury or even death in as little as 4 minutes. Early detection and intervention of airway and breathing problems, including dispatcher-guided interventions by bystanders, are vital to patient survival.

With regard to airway and/or ventilation problems, paramedics should approach the patient more globally and consider the whole picture, rather than blindly following predetermined steps. You cannot assess an airway if the patient is not breathing. You cannot assess breathing if there is no airway. Therefore, airway and ventilation need to be considered and managed together. Ultimately, circulation also will depend on an intact airway and adequate ventilation and respiration. The respiratory, cardiovascular, and neurologic systems all play an important role in airway management and ventilation. Stated another way, airway and ventilation problems must be approached in a nonlinear fashion with a number of factors considered simultaneously.

Your deliberate and precise use of simple, basic airway skills is the key to successful airway management and good patient outcome. Once you have applied the basic airway techniques to properly provide oxygenation and ventilation for your patient, you can then use more sophisticated airway maneuvers and skills, if necessary, to further stabilize his airway. You must continually monitor and reassess the airway, being careful to watch for displacement of any placed airway devices, mucous plugging, equipment failure, or the development of a pneumothorax.

Accurate and thorough documentation of airway management is critical for clinical care after the patient is transported, for quality assurance, and for medical/legal defense. Documentation should include not only what was done but also the thought process of why it was done and any complications that occurred. A significant percentage of claims and lawsuits that are filed against prehospital providers involve airway issues, and often these cases are won or lost based on the field documentation. Therefore, it is crucial that the provider learn to document in medically correct and legally sufficient terms exactly what was done in managing the airway.

Content Self-Evaluation

MULTIPLE CHOICE

_____ 1. Which of the following are considered retroglottic airway devices?
   A. Esophageal Obturator Airway and Esophageal Gastric Tube Airway
   B. Esophageal Tracheal Combitube Airway and Laryngeal Mask Airway
   C. Supraglottic Airway Laryngopharyngeal Tube and Laryngeal Mask Airway

D. Esophageal Tracheal Combitube and Pharyngeal Tracheal Lumen Airway
E. CookGas AirQ and Pharyngeal Tracheal Lumen Airway

_____ **2.** All of the following are advantages of the Esophageal Tracheal Combitube (ETC) EXCEPT
A. insertion does not require visualization.
B. it does not completely isolate the trachea in the esophageal position.
C. it offers reasonable aspiration protection in either the esophageal or tracheal position.
D. when intubating around the ETC, the proximal balloon may be deflated and the distal balloon left inflated to seal off the esophagus.
E. the large pharyngeal balloon may tamponade oral bleeding.

_____ **3.** When inserting the ETC, inflate the:
A. pharyngeal cuff with 10 to 15 mL of air and the distal cuff with 100 mL of air.
B. pharyngeal cuff with 50 mL of air and the distal cuff with 10 to 15 mL of air.
C. pharyngeal cuff with 100 mL of air and the distal cuff with 10 to 15 mL of air.
D. pharyngeal cuff with 100 mL of air and the distal cuff with 15 to 20 mL of air.
E. pharyngeal cuff with 120 mL of air and the distal cuff with 10 to 15 mL of air.

_____ **4.** Complications of PtL placement include
A. displacement of the pharyngeal balloon.
B. pharyngeal or esophageal trauma from poor technique.
C. unrecognized displacement of the long tube from the trachea into the esophagus.
D. pharyngeal or esophageal trauma from poor technique.
E. all of the above.

_____ **5.** The supraglottic airway laryngopharyngeal tube (S.A.L.T.) airway can be used as a simple mechanical airway adjunct, much like an oropharyngeal airway, or as a blind endotracheal tube introducer in situations where laryngoscopy is difficult or impossible.
A. True
B. False

_____ **6.** All of the following are laryngeal airways EXCEPT
A. LMA-Fastrach.
B. LMA-Supreme.
C. CookGas AirQ.
D. S.A.L.T.
E. Ambu Laryngeal Mask.

_____ **7.** While endotracheal intubation provides optimal aspiration protection and ventilation, it comes at a high cost, including
A. prolonged scene times.
B. potential airway trauma.
C. potential hypoxemia.
D. potential aspiration.
E. all of the above.

_____ **8.** The light of the laryngoscope should be a bright yellow and flicker slightly when pressure is placed on the blade.
A. True
B. False

_____ **9.** The tip of the curve of the Macintosh laryngoscope blade is designed to fit into the
A. nasopharynx.   **D.** arytenoid fossa.
B. glottic opening.   **E.** epiglottis.
C. vallecula.

_____ **10.** The laryngoscope blade considered to be best designed for intubation of the infant is
A. the Macintosh blade.   **D.** B or C.
B. the curved blade.   **E.** none of the above.
C. the straight blade.

11. The purpose of the cuff on the end of the endotracheal tube is to
    A. help guide the tube to its proper location.
    B. prevent dislodging of the tube after it is correctly placed.
    C. provide a seal between the tube and the trachea.
    D. center the tube in the trachea.
    E. widen the opening of the vocal cords.

12. In the intubation of a neonate, it is recommended that the paramedic use a(n)
    A. cuffed endotracheal tube and a straight laryngoscope blade.
    B. uncuffed endotracheal tube and a straight laryngoscope blade.
    C. cuffed endotracheal tube and a curved laryngoscope blade.
    D. uncuffed endotracheal tube and a curved laryngoscope blade.
    E. uncuffed endotracheal tube and digital technique.

13. Because overinflation of the pilot balloon may lead to tracheal mucosal damage, it is suggested that a manometer be used to ensure proper pressures, especially during longer transports.
    A. True
    B. False

14. Paramedics should learn to listen for air leakage and place only enough air in the cuff to inflate it without causing a leak.
    A. True
    B. False

15. The major purpose for using a malleable stylet during endotracheal intubation is to
    A. maintain optimal shape of the tube.
    B. keep the tube's lumen open.
    C. stiffen the tube so it can be pushed through the glottis.
    D. prevent foreign matter from entering the tube.
    E. all of the above.

16. Because of the anterior location of the glottic opening, it is essential to use a stylet with the endotracheal tube during pediatric intubation.
    A. True
    B. False

17. Complications of endotracheal intubation include all of the following EXCEPT
    A. equipment malfunction.
    B. tooth breakage.
    C. transport delays.
    D. endobronchial intubation.
    E. decreased intracranial pressure.

18. When using the laryngoscope to visualize the glottis, it is best to use the teeth as a fulcrum to increase your ability to lift the tissue.
    A. True
    B. False

19. To reduce the risk for hypoxia, limit attempts at intubation to no more than
    A. 15 seconds.   D. 45 seconds.
    B. 20 seconds.   E. 60 seconds.
    C. 30 seconds.

20. Which of the following is NOT an indication of esophageal intubation?
    A. Absence of chest rise with ventilation   C. A falling pulse oximetry reading
    B. Gurgling sound over the epigastrium   D. Skin color turning pink

©2013 Pearson Education, Inc.
Paramedic Care: Principles & Practice, Vol. 2, 4th Ed.

_____ **21.** Upon placing the endotracheal tube in a patient, you determine that you can only auscultate breath sounds on the right side. You should next
  A. withdraw the tube until breath sounds are equal.
  B. withdraw the tube completely.
  C. pass the tube a few centimeters further.
  D. secure the tube and ventilate more aggressively.
  E. check the mask seal.

_____ **22.** All of the following are objective techniques for confirming proper tube placement EXCEPT
  A. capnography.
  B. auscultation.
  C. esophageal detector device.
  D. pulse oximetry.
  E. endotracheal tube introducer.

_____ **23.** All of the following are relative contraindications of blind nasotracheal intubation EXCEPT
  A. suspected elevation of intracranial pressure.
  B. cardiac or respiratory arrest.
  C. coagulopathy, including therapeutic warfarin or heparin.
  D. combative/uncooperative patient.
  E. suspected basilar skull fractures.

_____ **24.** Digital intubation may be indicated in all of the following EXCEPT a(n)
  A. unconscious trauma patient with suspected C-spine injury.
  B. patient with facial injuries that distort the anatomy.
  C. unconscious patient with a gag reflex.
  D. entrapped patient who cannot be properly positioned.
  E. patient with copious amounts of blood or other fluids remaining in the airway.

_____ **25.** The primary danger associated with extubation is
  A. fasciculations.   **D.** tracheal damage.
  B. vomiting.   **E.** none of the above.
  C. laryngospasm.

_____ **26.** The only indication for a surgical airway is the inability to establish an airway by any other means.
  A. True
  B. False

_____ **27.** The open cricothyrotomy should not be performed on the patient under 10 years of age because the cricothyroid membrane is small and underdeveloped.
  A. True
  B. False

_____ **28.** Medication-assisted intubation (MAI) may take several forms, including rapid sequence intubation (RSI) and sedation-facilitated intubation.
  A. True.
  B. False.

_____ **29.** The current evidence has not found a survival benefit to prehospital RSI outside the air-medical setting, and in some cases survival rates are notably worse with RSI.
  A. True
  B. False

_____ **30.** Indications for rapid sequence intubation include which of the following?
  A. Impending or actual respiratory failure
  B. Impending or actual inability to protect the airway
  C. Combativeness secondary to presumed head trauma
  D. Hypoxemia despite maximal therapy
  E. All of the above

_____ 31. Which of the following is NOT an induction agent used for rapid sequence intubation?
- A. Propofol
- B. Succinylcholine
- C. Midazolam
- D. Ketamine
- E. Etomidate

_____ 32. The duration of action of succinylcholine is approximately
- A. 2 minutes.
- B. 4 minutes.
- C. 6 minutes.
- D. 8 minutes.
- E. 10 minutes.

_____ 33. The reason the succinylcholine is used in prehospital care is that it
- A. is fast acting and of short duration.
- B. is the easiest to administer.
- C. does not cause muscle fasciculations.
- D. can be used with massive crush injuries.
- E. has a half-life of 30 minutes.

_____ 34. All of the following are predictors of difficult BVM ventilation EXCEPT
- A. facial hair.
- B. short sternomental distance.
- C. facial trauma
- D. Mallampati grade 3 or 4.
- E. history of snoring.

_____ 35. The most frequently used system of pre-intubation airway assessment is the
- A. POGO scoring system.
- B. Cormack and LeHane grading system.
- C. LEMON grading scale.
- D. Mallampati classification system.
- E. none of the above.

Special Project

Problem Solving: Airway Maintenance

You have been called to a report of a man down and arrive with one EMT and another paramedic. You find bystanders doing CPR on a male in his mid-50s in a parking lot. You take position at the patient's head and determine that the bystanders are doing a fine job of ventilating the patient. You get out your airway bag and prepare to place an endotracheal tube.

1. What equipment would you prepare?

_____

_____

_____

2. How would you check your equipment?

_____

_____

_____

_____

©2013 Pearson Education, Inc.
Paramedic Care: Principles & Practice, Vol. 2, 4th Ed.

3. What would you ask the ventilator to do before your attempt?

_____

_____

4. Identify the ten steps of the procedure you are about to attempt.

_____

_____

_____

_____

_____

_____

_____

_____

_____

_____

5. You place the endotracheal tube. What actions would you take to ensure it is properly placed?

_____

_____

_____

_____

_____

_____

_____

6. You place the endotracheal tube and notice no chest rise with the first breath. Auscultation reveals diminished breath sounds and gurgling over the epigastric area. What actions would you take?

_____

_____

_____

_____

_____

Drugs Used in the Care of Patients with Airway Problems

Emergency management for patients with airway problems utilizes many of the pharmacological agents that are available to the paramedic. Please review and memorize the various names, indications, therapeutic effects, contraindications, side effects, routes of administration, and recommended dosages for the following medications. You can use the drug cards found at the back of this workbook for review.

Atropine
Diazepam
Etomidate
Fentanyl

Ketamine
Lidocaine
Midazolam
Oxygen
Propofol
Rocuronium
Sodium thiopental
Succinylcholine
Vecuronium

Part 4: Additional Airway and Ventilation Issues, p. 374

Review of Chapter Objectives

After reading this part of the chapter, you should be able to:

32. Manage airway and ventilation in patients with stomas.   p. 374

Tube clogging is a common problem because a laryngectomy produces a less-effective cough, making it more difficult to clear secretions. If these secretions organize, they form a mucous plug that can occlude the stoma. A clogged tube can usually be managed easily by removing the inner cannula from the fixed external cannula and cleaning it.

If a tracheostomy tube becomes completely dislodged, it should be replaced as soon as possible. This is particularly critical if the tracheostomy is less than a few weeks old. If another tube is not available, an endotracheal tube may be used temporarily.

Bleeding may come from irritation of the skin externally around the stoma site or internally. External bleeding is usually minor, although it may scare the patient, especially if the tracheostomy is new or bleeding has not occurred previously. Internal bleeding, on the other hand, may be catastrophic. This warrants very expeditious transport and contact with medical direction.

Other stoma-related problems to consider are excessive secretions that are not obstructing the lumen of the tube but are nevertheless causing respiratory problems. You may suction the airway through the stoma, but you must use extreme caution as this process can, itself, cause soft-tissue swelling.

33. Demonstrate effective suctioning of the oropharynx and trachea (in an intubated patient).   pp. 376–377

Oropharyngeal Suctioning
1. Use Standard Precautions, including protective eyewear, gloves, and face mask.
2. Preoxygenate the patient; this may require brief hyperventilation.
3. Determine the depth of catheter insertion by measuring from the patient's earlobe to his lips.
4. With the suction turned off, insert the catheter into your patient's pharynx to the predetermined depth.
5. Turn on the suction unit and place your thumb over the suction control orifice; limit suction to 10 seconds.
6. Continue to suction while withdrawing the catheter. When using a whistle-tip catheter, rotate it between your fingertips.
7. While maintaining ventilatory support, hyperventilate the patient with 100 percent oxygen.

Tracheobronchial Suctioning
1. Preoxygenate the patient with 100 percent oxygen.

2. You may need to inject 3 to 5 cc of sterile water or saline down the endotracheal tube before suctioning to help loosen thick secretions.
3. Gently insert the lubricated tube, using sterile gloves, until you feel resistance.
4. Apply suction for only about 10 seconds while withdrawing the catheter.

34. Take steps to minimize and manage gastric distension. p. 377

Ideally, gastric insufflation should be prevented rather than treated, as it is much less likely to occur with optimal BVM ventilation technique. Gastric insufflation is even less likely to occur with an extraglottic airway (EGA) device. Gastric insufflation increases the risk of vomiting and regurgitation with subsequent aspiration. The enlarged stomach also pushes against the diaphragm, inhibiting the lungs' expansion and increasing resistance to ventilation. Pediatric patients are prone to bradycardia from vagal stimulation that may result.

Nasogastric tube placement is generally preferred in awake patients, as it is more comfortable than orogastric placement and does not interfere with speech. However, placement in an awake patient is rarely necessary in prehospital care.

To place an orogastric tube in the unconscious patient:
1. Take Standard Precautions.
2. Place the patient's head in a neutral position while ventilating via the endotracheal tube or EGA.
3. Select the correct-size gastric tube. Most adults take a 16 Fr when placed orally. Some EGAs will accommodate only larger or only smaller sizes, and this should be checked in advance.
4. Determine the approximate length of tube insertion by measuring from the epigastrium to the angle of the jaw, then to the mouth opening or to the proximal end of the EGA.
5. Generously lubricate the distal tip of the gastric tube and gently insert it into the oral cavity at midline.
6. Advance the tube gently to the length you determined prior to insertion.
7. Check that the tube has not curled in the mouth.
8. Confirm placement by injecting 30 to 50 mL of air while listening to the epigastric region for air entry into the stomach. In addition, end-tidal CO_2 detectors are now available that will attach to a gastric tube. In this case the detection of CO_2 indicates incorrect placement in the lungs, rather than correct placement in the stomach. Coughing also suggests malposition in the lungs, although this is unreliable in unconscious patients.
9. Apply gentle suction to the tube to evacuate gastric fluids and gas.
10. Secure the tube in place.
11. Document the indication for gastric decompression, the size of tube placed, the technique, means of confirmation, any complications incurred, the type and volume of gastric contents evacuated, and the clinical response.

35. Accurately and completely document relevant information about assessment and management of the airway, ventilation, and oxygenation in patient-care reports. p. 380

Accurate and thorough documentation of airway management is critical for clinical care after the patient is transported, for quality assurance, and for medical/legal defense. Documentation should include not only what was done but also the thought process of why it was done and any complications that occurred. A significant percentage of claims and lawsuits that are filed against prehospital providers involve airway issues, and often these cases are won or lost based on the field documentation. Therefore, it is crucial that the provider learn to document in medically correct and legally sufficient terms exactly what was done in managing the airway.

Because patients who require prehospital airway management are at high risk for a bad outcome from the outset, and because airway management literally determines whether the patient lives or dies, it stands to reason that the greatest emphasis should be placed on detailed documentation of these issues.

Content Self-Evaluation

MULTIPLE CHOICE

_____ 1. An opening in the anterior neck that connects the trachea with the ambient air is called a
A. laryngectomy.
B. larynx tube.
C. tracheostomy.
D. stoma larynx tube.
E. tracheostomy tube.

_____ 2. Which of the following is a part of suctioning the stoma patient?
A. Preoxygenating with 100 percent oxygen
B. Injecting 3 mL of saline
C. Inserting the catheter until resistance is met
D. Withdrawing the catheter while the patient exhales or coughs
E. All of the above

_____ 3. You should limit each suctioning attempt to
A. 5 seconds.
B. 10 seconds.
C. 15 seconds.
D. 20 seconds.
E. 25 seconds.

_____ 4. You should apply suction
A. only while inserting the catheter.
B. both while inserting and while withdrawing the catheter.
C. either while inserting or while withdrawing the catheter.
D. only while withdrawing the catheter.
E. only while holding the catheter in place.

_____ 5. Which of the following is NOT indicated when suctioning through the endotracheal tube?
A. Suction only during insertion.
B. Insert the tube until you meet resistance.
C. Preoxygenate the patient.
D. Lubricate the tube.
E. Suction no longer than 10 seconds.

_____ 6. Pediatric patients are prone to tachycardia from vagal stimulation that may result from gastric distension.
A. True.
B. False.

_____ 7. Nasogastric tube placement is indicated in a patient
A. with facial fractures.
B. with a possible basilar skull fracture.
C. who is awake.
D. for whom a relatively large gastric tube is indicated.
E. all of the above

_____ 8. How much air do you inject down the orogastric tube to confirm placement?
A. 10–20 mL
B. 20–40 mL
C. 30–50 mL
D. 40–60 mL
E. 50–100 mL

_____ **9.** Transport ventilator pop-off valves may hinder ventilation in patients who require greater positive pressure, including patients with
   A. adult respiratory distress syndrome.
   B. cardiogenic pulmonary edema.
   C. pulmonary contrusion.
   D. bronchospasm.
   E. all of the above.

_____ **10.** A significant percentage of claims and lawsuits that are filed against prehospital providers involve airway issues, and often these cases are won or lost based on the field documentation.
   A. True
   B. False

Special Project

Complete the following chart by listing two advantages and two disadvantages of various types of suction units.

TYPE OF SUCTION UNIT	ADVANTAGES	DISADVANTAGES
Hand-powered	1.	1.
	2.	2.
Oxygen-powered	1.	1.
	2.	2.
Battery-powered	1.	1.
	2.	2.
Mounted	1.	1.
	2.	2.

PARAMEDICINE FUNDAMENTALS
Content Review
Content Self-Evaluation

Chapter 1: Pathophysiology, Part 1

____ 1. The study of disease is called
   A. pathophysiology.
   B. etiology.
   C. physiology.
   D. immunology.
   E. biology.

____ 2. All of the following are levels of life beyond the individual organism EXCEPT
   A. population.
   B. community.
   C. ecosystem.
   D. biosphere.
   E. ionosphere.

____ 3. A defined sequence of events that leads to development of an abnormal structural or functional change within the body is called
   A. pathophysiology.
   B. etiology.
   C. immunology.
   D. pathogenesis.
   E. clinical presentation.

____ 4. Nutritional diseases primarily result from a deficiency in
   A. proteins.
   B. carbohydrates.
   C. fats.
   D. vitamins.
   E. any of the above.

____ 5. In many instances the specific cause of a disease is unknown. In this case, the disease is classified as idiopathic.
   A. True.
   B. False.

Chapter 1: Pathophysiology, Part 2

____ 6. Which of the following is the weakest bond?
   A. Covalent bond
   B. Metallic bond
   C. Ionic bond
   D. Hydrogen bond
   E. Valence bond

____ 7. An unsaturated fatty acid has a single bond between each carbon atom, leaving room on the atom for two hydrogen atoms.
   A. True
   B. False

____ 8. The term that applies to the building up of biochemical substances to produce energy is
   A. anatomy.
   B. physiology.
   C. catabolism.
   D. anabolism.
   E. metabolism.

____ **9.** The lower the pH value, the lower the concentration of hydrogen ions.
  A. True
  B. False

____ **10.** A drop in the pH scale of 1 unit indicates a
  A. 10-fold decrease in H^+.
  B. 100-fold decrease in H^+.
  C. 10-fold increase in H^+.
  D. 100-fold increase in H^+.
  E. none of the above.

____ **11.** A pH value that would be considered acidosis in the human is
  A. 6.9 to 7.35.
  B. 7.35 to 7.45.
  C. 7.45 to 7.5.
  D. 7.6 to 7.75.
  E. 7.75 and greater.

____ **12.** The mechanism that responds most slowly to a change in the pH of the body is
  A. endocrine function.
  B. kidney function.
  C. the digestive system.
  D. the buffer system.
  E. none of the above.

____ **13.** Respiratory acidosis is caused by retention of carbon dioxide in the lungs.
  A. True
  B. False

____ **14.** The addition of carbon dioxide to the bloodstream will result in an increase in hydrogen ions.
  A. True
  B. False

____ **15.** The acid-base disorder resulting from an increase in bicarbonate or a decrease in circulating acids is:
  A. respiratory alkalosis.
  B. respiratory acidosis
  C. metabolic alkalosis.
  D. metabolic acidosis.
  E. hypocapnia.

Chapter 1: Pathophysiology, Part 3

____ **16.** The main elements of a typical cell include all of the following EXCEPT the
  A. cilia.
  B. cell membrane.
  C. organelles.
  D. cytoplasm.
  E. all except B and D.

____ **17.** The process of moving substances from an area of lower solute concentration to higher solute concentration is called
  A. simple diffusion.
  B. facilitated diffusion.
  C. osmosis.
  D. complex diffusion.
  E. active transport.

____ **18.** Water accounts for approximately what percent of total body weight?
  A. 25 percent
  B. 35 percent
  C. 50 percent
  D. 60 percent
  E. 75 percent

____ **19.** The interstitial compartment contains all the fluids found outside the cellular compartment.
  A. True
  B. False

____ **20.** The percentage of total body water made up of intravascular fluid is
  A. 75 percent.
  B. 60 percent.
  C. 25 percent.
  D. 15 percent.
  E. 5 percent.

©2013 Pearson Education, Inc.
Paramedic Care: Principles & Practice, Vol. 2, 4th Ed.

_____ 21. The universal solvent is
A. water.
B. sodium.
C. plasma.
D. calcium.
E. hydrogen.

_____ 22. Dehydration from plasma loss can result from
A. hyperventilation.
B. poor nutritional states.
C. pancreatitis.
D. burns.
E. all of the above.

_____ 23. A negatively charged ion is called a(n)
A. anion.
B. cation.
C. electrolyte.
D. dissociated element.
E. none of the above.

_____ 24. Which of the following is NOT an electrolyte?
A. Bicarbonate
B. Chloride
C. Glucose
D. Magnesium
E. Potassium

_____ 25. The most frequently occurring anion in the human body is
A. magnesium.
B. chloride.
C. potassium.
D. calcium.
E. sodium.

_____ 26. The movement of a solute from an area of higher concentration to an area of lower concentration is:
A. diffusion.
B. osmosis.
C. active transport.
D. facilitated transport.
E. oncosis.

_____ 27. The mechanism by which glucose is transported across a cell membrane using helper proteins is
A. diffusion.
B. osmosis.
C. active transport.
D. facilitated transport.
E. oncosis.

_____ 28. The pressure pushing water out of plasma and across the capillary wall into the interstitial space is
A. osmolarity.
B. osmotic pressure.
C. hydrostatic pressure.
D. oncotic force.
E. filtration.

_____ 29. Which of the following is NOT a mechanism that commonly produces edema?
A. A decrease in plasma osmotic force
B. An increase in hydrostatic pressure
C. Increased capillary permeability
D. Venous dilation
E. Lymphatic channel obstruction

_____ 30. The blood component that comprises 99 percent of the formed elements is
A. plasma.
B. platelets.
C. erythrocytes.
D. leukocytes.
E. hemoglobin.

_____ 31. The blood component that contains hemoglobin and is responsible for transporting most of the oxygen from the lungs to the body cells is
A. plasma.
B. platelets.
C. erythrocytes.
D. leukocytes.
E. hemoglobin.

____ 32. The blood component that helps the body fight infection is
  A. plasma.
  B. platelets.
  C. erythrocytes.
  D. leukocytes.
  E. hemoglobin.

____ 33. Common signs of a transfusion reaction include
  A. hypotension.
  B. tachycardia.
  C. headache.
  D. vomiting.
  E. all of the above.

____ 34. A small volume of colloid solution can be administered to a patient with a greater-than-expected increase in the intravascular volume.
  A. True
  B. False

____ 35. The solution that will cause a net movement of water into the intravascular space is
  A. a colloid solution.
  B. a hypertonic solution.
  C. a hypotonic solution.
  D. an isotonic solution.
  E. A and B.

____ 36. The solution that will cause a net movement of water out of the erythrocytes is
  A. a colloid solution.
  B. a hypertonic solution.
  C. a hypotonic solution.
  D. an isotonic solution.
  E. A and B.

____ 37. A solution that contains a lesser concentration of solute molecules than another is referred to as
  A. hypertonic.
  B. isotonic.
  C. hypotonic.
  D. osmotic.
  E. hyperbaric.

____ 38. When a hypotonic solution is placed in the human bloodstream, water moves in what manner?
  A. Into the vascular space
  B. It does not move
  C. Out of the vascular space
  D. Both into and out of the vascular space
  E. None of the above

____ 39. An example of a hypotonic solution is
  A. lactated Ringer's solution.
  B. normal saline.
  C. dextran.
  D. D_5W.
  E. plasmanate.

____ 40. Which of the following is NOT an organelle?
  A. Golgi apparatus
  B. Mitochondria
  C. Endoplasmic reticulum
  D. Lysosome
  E. Cytoplasm

____ 41. The component of the cell that converts carbohydrates into energy sources is the
  A. mitochondria.
  B. lysosome.
  C. nucleus.
  D. Golgi apparatus.
  E. cytoplasm.

____ 42. The form of cellular adaptation in which there is an increase in the number of cells due to an increase in workload is
  A. atrophy.
  B. hypertrophy.
  C. hyperplasia.
  D. metaplasia.
  E. dysplasia.

____ 43. An increase in the size of cells in a tissue or organ is referred to as
  A. hyperplasia.
  B. atrophy.
  C. hypertrophy.
  D. metaplasia.
  E. ischemia.

©2013 Pearson Education, Inc.
Paramedic Care: Principles & Practice, Vol. 2, 4th Ed.

_____ **44.** The form of cellular adaptation in which cell size decreases due to a decrease in workload is
A. atrophy.
B. hypertrophy.
C. hyperplasia.
D. metaplasia.
E. dysplasia.

_____ **45.** The body's natural process for removal of the body's dead and nonfunctioning cells is
A. apoptosis.
B. fatty change.
C. necrosis.
D. gangrene.
E. none of the above.

Chapter 1: Pathophysiology, Part 4

_____ **46.** Ductless or endocrine glands secrete directly onto the surface of the body.
A. True
B. False

_____ **47.** The type of tissue that includes squamous, cuboidal, and columnar shapes is
A. connective tissue.
B. epithelial tissue.
C. muscle tissue.
D. nerve tissue.
E. none of the above.

_____ **48.** All of the following are types of connective tissue EXCEPT
A. cartilage.
B. bone.
C. adipose.
D. striated.
E. blood.

_____ **49.** The tissue type that can spontaneously contract is
A. epithelial.
B. cardiac muscle.
C. nerve.
D. connective.
E. skeletal muscle.

_____ **50.** The tissue type that transmits electrical impulses throughout the body is
A. epithelial.
B. cardiac muscle.
C. nerve.
D. connective.
E. skeletal muscle.

Chapter 1: Pathophysiology, Part 5

_____ **51.** The proportion of the population affected by a disease at a given point in time is that disease's
A. prevalence.
B. morbidity.
C. mortality.
D. incidence.
E. average.

_____ **52.** Few diseases with a genetic disposition have risk factors that are modifiable.
A. True
B. False

_____ **53.** The percentage of lung cancer in men associated with smoking is
A. 40 percent.
B. 60 percent.
C. 70 percent.
D. 75 percent.
E. 90 percent.

_____ **54.** Which of the following are associated with ulcer development?
A. Stress
B. Nonsteroidal anti-inflammatory drugs
C. Diet
D. Alcohol consumption
E. All of the above

_____ 55. Which of the following may cause hypoperfusion?
  A. Blood loss
  B. Spinal cord injury
  C. Myocardial infarction
  D. Allergic reaction
  E. All of the above

_____ 56. The portion of the cardiovascular system that is known as the capacitance system is the
  A. venous system.
  B. heart.
  C. arterial system.
  D. capillary beds.
  E. lymphatic system.

_____ 57. Cardiac afterload is determined by
  A. peripheral vascular resistance.
  B. cardiac output.
  C. blood pressure.
  D. the Frank-Starling mechanism.
  E. all of the above.

_____ 58. Which of the following is NOT one of the conditions of oxygen movement and utilization that make up the Fick principle?
  A. Adequate exhaled carbon dioxide
  B. Adequate oxygen diffusion in lungs
  C. Proper tissue perfusion
  D. Efficient oxygen off-loading
  E. Adequate red blood cells

_____ 59. Ultimately, all types of shock result in impairment of cellular metabolism.
  A. True
  B. False

_____ 60. Anaerobic metabolism occurs in the absence of
  A. carbon dioxide.
  B. tissue perfusion.
  C. oxygen.
  D. pyruvic acid.
  E. nitrogen.

_____ 61. When baroreceptors detect a fall in blood pressure, they cause
  A. an increase in heart rate.
  B. an increase in the strength of myocardial contraction.
  C. venous constriction.
  D. arteriolar constriction.
  E. all of the above.

_____ 62. During hypoperfusion, the catecholamines epinephrine and norepinephrine are responsible for
  A. increasing heart rate.
  B. increasing cardiac contractile strength.
  C. arteriolar constriction.
  D. increasing blood pressure.
  E. all of the above.

_____ 63. During hypoperfusion, the hormone ADH is responsible for
  A. increasing red blood cell production.
  B. causing the spleen to release blood.
  C. producing a potent vasoconstrictor.
  D. increasing re-absorption of water by the kidneys.
  E. increasing the heart rate.

_____ 64. During decompensated shock, which of the following is likely to occur?
  A. Myocardial hypoxia and reduced output
  B. A speeding up of sympathetic activity
  C. Dilution of the blood
  D. Decreased capillary permeability
  E. Release of $beta_2$

_____ 65. The type of shock resulting from severe heart damage from an MI is
  A. cardiogenic.
  B. hypovolemic.
  C. neurogenic.
  D. septic.
  E. anaphylactic.

©2013 Pearson Education, Inc.
Paramedic Care: Principles & Practice, Vol. 2, 4th Ed.

_____ 66. The type of shock resulting from dehydration from prolonged vomiting is
A. cardiogenic.
B. hypovolemic.
C. neurogenic.
D. septic.
E. anaphylactic.

_____ 67. The type of shock resulting from a severe spinal cord injury is
A. cardiogenic.
B. hypovolemic.
C. neurogenic.
D. septic.
E. anaphylactic.

_____ 68. Pharmacological treatment for anaphylaxis may include all of the following EXCEPT
A. beta agonists.
B. vasopressors.
C. corticosteroids.
D. vasodilators.
E. antihistamines.

_____ 69. Multiple organ dysfunction syndrome is a massive inflammatory response triggered by a severe disease or injury.
A. True
B. False

_____ 70. In a patient with MODS, renal failure usually begins
A. within 24 hours.
B. within 24 to 72 hours.
C. within 7 to 10 days.
D. within 14 to 21 days.
E. after 21 days.

Chapter 1: Pathophysiology, Part 6

_____ 71. Which of the following are released by bacteria during their destruction?
A. Antibiotics
B. Gram-negative material
C. Exotoxins
D. Endotoxins
E. Histamines

_____ 72. The infectious agents that are made almost entirely of protein and do not have protective capsids are
A. viruses.
B. bacteria.
C. fungi.
D. parasites.
E. prions.

_____ 73. When the body is infected, the skin provides an
A. external, specific response to infection.
B. external, nonspecific response to infection.
C. internal, specific response to infection.
D. internal, nonspecific response to infection.
E. A and B.

_____ 74. The inflammatory response to infection is more rapid than the immune response and is not specific to the invading organism.
A. True
B. False

_____ 75. The principal agent of the immune response that identifies "non-self" proteins located on the surface of many cells is called a(n)
A. antigen.
B. antibody.
C. B cell.
D. T cell.
E. lymphocyte.

_____ 76. The type of immunity that is an outcome of an immune response is
A. primary.
B. acquired.
C. natural.
D. secondary.
E. B and D.

____ 77. Infants are given some immunity from antibodies that cross the placental barrier.
  A. True
  B. False

____ 78. The type of immunity that does not produce antibodies but attacks the invading agent directly is
  A. cell-mediated.
  B. humoral.
  C. natural.
  D. primary.
  E. A and C.

____ 79. Which of the following is NOT one of the essential characteristics of an immunogen?
  A. Sufficient foreignness
  B. Sufficient size
  C. Sufficient complexity
  D. Sufficient density
  E. Sufficient quantity

____ 80. The erythrocytes (red blood cells) have HLA antigens on their surface like all other body cells.
  A. True
  B. False

____ 81. Under the ABO classification of blood antigens, the universal blood recipient is blood type
  A. A.
  B. B.
  C. O.
  D. AB.
  E. both C and D.

____ 82. With which of the following blood types would an individual have only the anti-A antibody?
  A. A
  B. B
  C. O
  D. AB
  E. both B and D

____ 83. Which of the following is NOT a function of the inflammatory response?
  A. Destroying and removing unwanted substances
  B. Recognizing "non-self" antigens
  C. Stimulating the immune response
  D. Promoting healing
  E. Walling off the infected and inflamed area

____ 84. When cells are injured, the inflammatory response begins within seconds.
  A. True
  B. False

____ 85. The cell that is the chief activator of the inflammatory response is the
  A. mast cell.
  B. T cell.
  C. B cell.
  D. C cell.
  E. phagocyte.

____ 86. The agent released by mast cells during the inflammatory response that increases blood flow to the injury site is
  A. the chemotaxic factor.
  B. IgE.
  C. histamine.
  D. serotonin.
  E. cortisol.

____ 87. To help corral an invading organism, the coagulation system produces a protein fiber called
  A. bradykinin.
  B. fibrin.
  C. fibrous enzyme.
  D. fibrinogen.
  E. serotonin.

____ 88. The collection of white cells along blood vessel walls during the early stages of inflammation is
  A. margination.
  B. diapedesis.
  C. granulocytosis.
  D. active transport.
  E. exudation.

©2013 Pearson Education, Inc.
Paramedic Care: Principles & Practice, Vol. 2, 4th Ed.

_____ 89. Which of the following cells are involved in the immune response?
  A. Monocytes   D. Eosinophils
  B. Neutrophils   E. All of the above
  C. Basophils

_____ 90. A growth that forms to wall off infection from the rest of the body is
  A. pus.   D. a granulocyte.
  B. a fibroblast.   E. a phagocyte.
  C. a granuloma.

_____ 91. Scab generation occurs during which stage of the wound healing process?
  A. Initial response   D. Contraction
  B. Granulation   E. None of the above
  C. Epithelialization

_____ 92. The impaired wound healing experienced by the elderly is most commonly due to the incidence of chronic disease.
  A. True
  B. False

_____ 93. The hypersensitivity associated with disturbance in tolerance for one's own "self" antigens is
  A. allergy.   D. isoimmunity.
  B. anaphylaxis.   E. monoimmunity.
  C. autoimmunity.

_____ 94. Rheumatoid arthritis is a disease involving
  A. allergy.   D. isoimmunity.
  B. anaphylaxis.   E. none of the above.
  C. autoimmunity.

_____ 95. The type of immune deficiency related to medical treatment is
  A. nutritional.   D. trauma induced.
  B. iatrogenic.   E. all of the above.
  C. stress induced.

_____ 96. The second stage of the general adaptation syndrome in response to stress involves
  A. exhaustion.   D. alarm.
  B. resistance.   E. B and C.
  C. adaptation.

_____ 97. The category of hormones called catecholamines includes
  A. epinephrine.   D. norepinephrine.
  B. endorphins.   E. A and D.
  C. cortisol.

_____ 98. Stimulation of the alpha$_2$ receptors will cause
  A. increased heart rate.   D. bronchodilation.
  B. inhibition of norepinephrine release.   E. all of the above.
  C. vasoconstriction.

_____ 99. Stimulation of the beta$_1$ receptors will cause
  A. increased heart rate.   D. bronchodilation.
  B. inhibition of the effects of norepinephrine.   E. lacrimation.
  C. vasoconstriction.

_____ 100. Cortisol has a harmful immunosuppressive action that may, however, be beneficial in protecting against stress.
  A. True
  B. False

Chapter 2: Human Life Span Development

____101. The preschooler represents a child between the ages of
    A. birth and 1 year.
    B. 1 and 3 years.
    C. 3 and 5 years.
    D. 6 and 12 years.
    E. 13 and 18 years.

____102. The infant represents a child between the ages of
    A. birth and 1 year.
    B. 1 and 3 years.
    C. 3 and 5 years.
    D. 6 and 12 years.
    E. 13 and 18 years.

____103. The respiratory rate generally falls with age.
    A. True
    B. False

____104. The pulse rate generally increases with age.
    A. True
    B. False

____105. During the first 6 months of life, the infant's birth weight is expected to
    A. increase by 2 kg per week.
    B. decrease by 5 to 10 percent.
    C. double.
    D. triple.
    E. none of the above.

____106. The reflex that causes the infant to turn his head toward a touch to the cheek is the
    A. Moro reflex.
    B. palmar reflex.
    C. rooting reflex.
    D. sucking reflex.
    E. vagal reflex.

____107. The formation of a close personal relationship through frequent or constant association is called
    A. bonding.
    B. secure attachment.
    C. scaffolding.
    D. benchmarking.
    E. modeling.

____108. By the time an infant becomes a toddler, the respiratory system has matured and is able to maintain an excessive respiratory rate.
    A. True
    B. False

____109. The age at which children begin to understand the concept of cause and effect is
    A. 1 to 2 years.
    B. 2 to 3 years.
    C. 3 to 4 years.
    D. 4 to 5 years.
    E. 5 to 6 years.

____110. The school-age child grows by about what amount per year?
    A. 2 cm
    B. 3 cm
    C. 4 cm
    D. 5 cm
    E. 6 cm

____111. Female children generally finish growing at the age of
    A. 12.
    B. 14.
    C. 16.
    D. 18.
    E. 20.

____112. The development stage at which smoking and alcohol and illicit drug use is most likely is
    A. preschool.
    B. school age.
    C. adolescent.
    D. early adult.
    E. middle adult.

©2013 Pearson Education, Inc.
Paramedic Care: Principles & Practice, Vol. 2, 4th Ed.

_____113. The stage of development in which lifelong habits and routines are established is
A. late adult.
B. school age.
C. adolescent.
D. early adult.
E. middle adult.

_____114. Cardiovascular changes associated with late adulthood include
A. cardiac valve disease.
B. diminishing of pacemaker cells.
C. decreased tolerance of tachycardia.
D. heart enlargement.
E. all of the above.

_____115. The stage of development in which individuals are more concerned with the "social clock" and become more task oriented as they see the time for accomplishing their lifetime goals recede is
A. late adult.
B. school age.
C. adolescent.
D. early adult.
E. middle adult.

Chapter 3: Emergency Pharmacology, Part 1

_____116. "Valium" is an example of what type of drug name?
A. Chemical
B. Generic
C. Official
D. Brand
E. Common

_____117. "Diazepam, USP" is an example of what type of drug name?
A. Chemical name
B. Generic name
C. Official name
D. Brand name
E. Common name

_____118. Which of the following is a common source of drugs?
A. Plant
B. Animal
C. Mineral
D. Synthetic
E. All of the above

_____119. Calcium chloride is an example of a drug from
A. plant sources.
B. animal sources.
C. mineral sources.
D. synthetic sources.
E. all of the above.

_____120. The current oversight of narcotics and addictive substances is regulated under the
A. Pure Food and Drug Act of 1906.
B. Harrison Narcotic Act of 1914.
C. Federal Food and Cosmetic Act of 1938.
D. Controlled Substances Act of 1970.
E. Prescription Drug Amendments.

_____121. The bioassay of a drug in a preparation is a test to determine the drug's
A. potency.
B. amount and purity.
C. effectiveness.
D. availability in a biological model.
E. effectiveness compared to other like drugs.

_____122. Drugs that are classified as Schedule I controlled substances include
A. heroin.
B. morphine.
C. codeine.
D. diazepam.
E. B and C.

_____123. You should inspect the label of a drug you are about to administer
A. when you remove the medication from the drug box.
B. as you draw up the medication.
C. immediately before administering to the patient.
D. A and C.
E. A, B, and C.

____124. During the last trimester of pregnancy, medication administration does not present as great a risk as earlier in the pregnancy because most drugs will not cross the placenta to the fetus.
A. True
B. False

____125. Drugs confer new properties on cells or tissues through complicated biochemical reactions.
A. True
B. False

____126. Which of the following is NOT one of the processes of pharmacokinetics?
A. Absorption
B. Distribution
C. Biotransformation
D. Antagonism
E. Elimination

____127. The movement of large molecules through the cell membrane using special carrier proteins is
A. diffusion.
B. active transport.
C. osmosis.
D. filtration.
E. facilitated diffusion.

____128. The movement of solvent in solution from an area of lower concentration to an area of higher concentration is
A. diffusion.
B. active transport.
C. osmosis.
D. filtration.
E. facilitated transport.

____129. The breaking down of a drug by the body that facilitates the drug's activity or elimination is its
A. bioavailability.
B. biotransformation.
C. metabolism.
D. prodrug effect.
E. none of the above.

____130. Which of the following is a medium for elimination of a drug from the body?
A. Urine
B. Respiratory air
C. Feces
D. Sweat
E. All of the above

____131. Which of the following is NOT an enteral route of drug administration?
A. Oral
B. Intraosseous
C. Umbilical
D. Sublingual
E. Rectal

____132. The administration route that delivers medication most quickly and specifically to the lungs is
A. intramuscular.
B. nebulization.
C. topical.
D. intravenous.
E. endotracheal.

____133. Drugs that are mixed with a wax-like base that dissolves at body temperature are
A. pills.
B. suppositories.
C. tablets.
D. capsules.
E. suspensions.

____134. Drugs that are powders or small pills placed in gelatin containers are
A. pills.
B. suppositories.
C. tablets.
D. capsules.
E. suspensions.

____135. Preparations made using an alcohol extraction process are
A. solutions.
B. tinctures.
C. suspensions.
D. spirits.
E. elixirs.

©2013 Pearson Education, Inc.
Paramedic Care: Principles & Practice, Vol. 2, 4th Ed.

_____136. Preparations of volatile drugs in alcohol are called
  A. solutions.   D. spirits.
  B. tinctures.   E. elixirs.
  C. suspensions.

_____137. Variables that must be considered when determining the proper method for storing drugs include
  A. temperature.   D. shelf life.
  B. light.   E. all of the above.
  C. moisture.

_____138. The force of attraction between a drug and its receptor site is referred to as its
  A. affinity.   D. antagonism.
  B. efficacy.   E. none of the above.
  C. agonism.

_____139. A chemical that binds to a receptor site and causes the expected effect is called a(n)
  A. partial antagonist.   D. antagonist.
  B. competitive antagonist.   E. noncompetitive antagonist.
  C. agonist.

_____140. Nalbuphine (Nubain) is a(n)
  A. agonist-antagonist.   D. pseudoantagonist.
  B. competitive antagonist.   E. noncompetitive antagonist.
  C. agonist.

_____141. A chemical that binds to a receptor site, causes the expected effect, changes the receptor site, and prevents other drugs from triggering it is called a(n)
  A. partial antagonist.   D. antagonist.
  B. competitive antagonist.   E. noncompetitive antagonist.
  C. agonist.

_____142. A rapidly occurring tolerance to a drug is called
  A. idiosyncrasy.   D. synergism.
  B. tachyphylaxis.   E. potentiation.
  C. antagonism.

_____143. The response in which a drug enhances the actions of another is called
  A. idiosyncrasy.   D. synergism.
  B. tachyphylaxis.   E. potentiation.
  C. antagonism.

_____144. The time from administration until the drug reaches the minimum effective dose is its
  A. onset of action.   D. biological half-life.
  B. duration of action.   E. termination of action.
  C. therapeutic index.

_____145. The time it takes to reduce the concentration of a drug in the body by 50 percent is its
  A. onset of action.   D. biological half-life.
  B. duration of action.   E. termination of action.
  C. therapeutic index.

Chapter 3: Emergency Pharmacology, Part 2

_____146. Control of the body's voluntary functions is provided by the
  A. somatic nervous system.   D. central nervous system.
  B. autonomic nervous system.   E. voluntary nervous system.
  C. peripheral nervous system.

____147. Control of the body's automatic functions is provided by the
    A. somatic nervous system.
    B. autonomic nervous system.
    C. peripheral nervous system.
    D. central nervous system.
    E. voluntary nervous system.

____148. The "fight-or-flight" response is controlled by the
    A. somatic nervous system.
    B. autonomic nervous system.
    C. sympathetic nervous system.
    D. parasympathetic nervous system.
    E. voluntary nervous system.

____149. Anesthetics, as a group, tend to cause
    A. reduced sensation.
    B. respiratory stimulation.
    C. central nervous system elevation.
    D. cardiovascular stimulation.
    E. all of the above.

____150. Sedation is a term that describes
    A. decreased anxiety.
    B. induction of sleep.
    C. reduced sensation.
    D. decreased pain sensation.
    E. opioid antagonism.

____151. The class of drugs called amphetamines cause
    A. the release of norepinephrine.
    B. the release of dopamine.
    C. an increased wakefulness.
    D. decreased appetite.
    E. all of the above.

____152. Extrapyramidal symptoms associated with psychotherapeutic medication administration include
    A. muscle tremors.
    B. fatigue.
    C. tachycardia.
    D. anxiety.
    E. all of the above.

____153. The side effects of the antipsychotic drugs include
    A. extrapyramidal symptoms.
    B. orthostatic hypotension.
    C. sedation.
    D. sexual dysfunction.
    E. all of the above.

____154. Which of the following is NOT a sign or symptom of depression?
    A. Weight loss or gain
    B. Loss of energy
    C. Enhanced concentration
    D. Suicide attempts
    E. Feelings of hopelessness

____155. Tricyclic antidepressants (TCAs) act by blocking the uptake of serotonin and dopamine, thereby extending their duration of action.
    A. True
    B. False

____156. When taken in overdose, tricyclic antidepressants can cause
    A. CNS depression.
    B. respiratory depression.
    C. cardiotoxic effects.
    D. neurotoxic sedation.
    E. none of the above.

____157. Parkinson's disease is a nervous disorder caused by the destruction of dopamine-releasing neurons in the substantia nigra, a part of the basal ganglia, which is a specialized area of the brain involved in controlling fine movements.
    A. True
    B. False

____158. The system that works in opposition to the sympathetic nervous system is the
    A. somatic nervous system.
    B. autonomic nervous system.
    C. central nervous system.
    D. peripheral nervous system.
    E. none of the above.

____159. The adrenergic neurotransmitter is
  A. acetylcholine.
  B. epinephrine.
  C. norepinephrine.
  D. muscarinic antagonist.
  E. muscarinic agonist.

____160. The parasympathetic nervous system originates from which nerve root regions?
  A. Cranial and sacral
  B. Cranial and lumbar
  C. Cranial and thoracic
  D. Thoracic and lumbar
  E. Thoracic and sacral

____161. A drug that stimulates the parasympathetic nervous system is a
  A. sympatholytic.
  B. sympathomimetic.
  C. parasympatholytic.
  D. parasympathomimetic.
  E. none of the above.

____162. A drug that blocks or inhibits the actions of the parasympathetic nervous system is a
  A. sympatholytic.
  B. sympathomimetic.
  C. parasympatholytic.
  D. parasympathomimetic.
  E. none of the above.

____163. The effects of cholinergic stimulation include all of the following EXCEPT
  A. salivation.
  B. lacrimation.
  C. defecation.
  D. blurred vision.
  E. emesis.

____164. Side effects of atropine include
  A. blurred vision.
  B. dry mouth.
  C. photophobia.
  D. anhidrosis.
  E. all of the above.

____165. Epinephrine accounts for what percentage of the neurotransmitters released by the adrenal gland when it is stimulated?
  A. 20 percent
  B. 40 percent
  C. 60 percent
  D. 80 percent
  E. 90 percent

____166. Stimulation of which type of receptor causes peripheral vasoconstriction, mild bronchoconstriction, and increased metabolism?
  A. Alpha$_1$
  B. Alpha$_2$
  C. Beta$_1$
  D. Beta$_2$
  E. Dopaminergic

____167. Stimulation of which of the following receptors increases heart rate, cardiac contractile force, cardiac automaticity, and cardiac conduction?
  A. Alpha$_1$
  B. Alpha$_2$
  C. Beta$_1$
  D. Beta$_2$
  E. Dopaminergic

____168. A type of drug that causes peripheral vasoconstriction is a(n)
  A. beta$_2$ agonist.
  B. beta$_1$ antagonist.
  C. beta$_1$ agonist.
  D. alpha$_1$ antagonist.
  E. alpha$_1$ agonist.

____169. A type of drug that causes increased heart rate, contractility, and conduction is a(n)
  A. beta$_2$ agonist.
  B. beta$_1$ antagonist.
  C. beta$_1$ agonist.
  D. alpha$_1$ antagonist.
  E. alpha$_1$ agonist.

____170. Which of the following is a synthetic catecholamine?
  A. Isoproterenol
  B. Dopamine
  C. Atropine
  D. Propranolol
  E. None of the above

____171. The order in which an electrical impulse travels through the cardiac conduction system is
   A. SA node, internodal pathways, AV node, bundle of His, Purkinje fibers.
   B. AV node, internodal pathways, SA node, bundle of His, Purkinje fibers.
   C. internodal pathways, AV node, SA node, Purkinje fibers, bundle of His.
   D. bundle of His, SA node, AV node, Purkinje fibers, internodal pathways.
   E. bundle of His, SA node, internodal pathways, AV node, Purkinje fibers.

____172. The unique property of myocardial muscle tissue allowing it to transmit an electrical impulse to adjacent cells is
   A. inotropy.
   B. automaticity.
   C. contractility.
   D. conductivity.
   E. depolarization.

____173. Digoxin has which of the following effects on the heart?
   A. Increases the intrinsic firing rate of the SA node
   B. Increases conduction through the AV node
   C. Decreases the ventricular refractory period
   D. Decreases ventricular automaticity
   E. Recharges the firing rate of the Purkinje fibers

____174. The drug of choice for torsade de pointes is
   A. atropine.
   B. bretylium.
   C. magnesium.
   D. digoxin.
   E. adenosine.

____175. Hypertension is a major contributor to all of the following EXCEPT
   A. coronary artery disease.
   B. stroke.
   C. depression.
   D. blindness.
   E. all of the above.

____176. A diuretic is used to
   A. reduce circulating blood volume.
   B. dilate the arterial system.
   C. dilate the venous system.
   D. reduce baroreceptor effectiveness.
   E. increase renal blood flow.

____177. Nitroglycerin rapidly loses its potency when exposed to
   A. humidity.
   B. light.
   C. heat.
   D. cold.
   E. oxygen.

____178. Which of the following statements is true regarding digoxin?
   A. It has a very large therapeutic index.
   B. Individual variability is minor.
   C. Normal use does not cause toxicity in patients.
   D. It may cause the dysrhythmias it is intended to treat.
   E. All of the above are true.

____179. The major side effect of aspirin when it is used to help prevent a heart attack is
   A. stroke.
   B. chest pain.
   C. bleeding.
   D. tachycardia.
   E. metabolic acidosis.

____180. The clotting cascade can be interrupted by
   A. antiplatelets.
   B. anticoagulants.
   C. fibrinolytics.
   D. hemostatic agents.
   E. antifibrinolytics.

____181. Medications that break up blood clots after they have formed are
   A. antiplatelets.
   B. anticoagulants.
   C. fibrinolytics.
   D. hemostatic agents.
   E. analgesics.

_____182. A causative factor for coronary artery disease is
A. low-density lipoproteins (LDLs).
B. very-low-density lipoproteins (VLDLs).
C. high-density lipoproteins (HDLs).
D. intermediate-density lipoproteins (IDLs).
E. all of the above.

_____183. The pathophysiology of asthma has two basic components, which are
A. bronchoconstriction and vasodilation.
B. vasodilation and inflammation.
C. sequestration and inflammation.
D. bronchoconstriction and inflammation.
E. vasodilation and sequestration.

_____184. A nonselective sympathomimetic agent used to treat asthma is
A. terbutaline.
B. albuterol.
C. theophylline.
D. epinephrine.
E. ipratropium.

_____185. Histamine is released during the invasion of an allergen
A. when histaminic cells constrict.
B. as a by-product of antibody-antigen interaction.
C. when mast cells rupture.
D. during the histamine cascade.
E. as a by-product of antigen rupture.

_____186. Histamine plays a significant role in minor and moderate allergic reactions.
A. True
B. False

_____187. A drug that increases the productivity of a cough is a(n)
A. expectorant.
B. mucolytic.
C. antitussive.
D. surfactant.
E. cannabinoid.

_____188. Antacids are antagonists that block the receptors responsible for the production of gastric acids.
A. True
B. False

_____189. A transmitter associated with the vomiting reflex is
A. serotonin.
B. dopamine.
C. acetylcholine.
D. histamine.
E. all of the above.

_____190. An example of an ophthalmic drug used to treat glaucoma is
A. pancreatin.
B. chloramphenicol.
C. dronabinol.
D. timolol.
E. dopamine.

_____191. Oxytocin is produced by the
A. posterior pituitary gland.
B. uterus.
C. adrenal gland.
D. thyroid gland.
E. testes.

_____192. The type of diabetes that typically manifests during adulthood is
A. retrograde.
B. type I.
C. type II.
D. insipidus.
E. none of the above.

_____193. The hormone oxytocin's principal action is to
A. relax the uterine muscles.
B. dilate uterine arterioles.
C. induce labor.
D. cause breast enlargement.
E. none of the above.

____194. Nonsteroidal antiinflammatory drugs (NSAIDs) are used to treat
   A. headache.
   B. fever.
   C. arthritis.
   D. orthopedic injuries.
   E. all of the above.

____195. A solution containing a modified pathogen that stimulates the development of antigens is called a(n)
   A. vaccine.
   B. serum.
   C. immunogen.
   D. rotavirus.
   E. none of the above.

Chapter 4: Intravenous Access and Medication Administration, Part 1

____196. Which of the following is NOT one of the six rights of drug administration?
   A. The right dose
   B. The right person
   C. The right concentration
   D. The right documentation
   E. The right route

____197. Confirmation of a medication order received from medical direction on-line is achieved by
   A. echoing it.
   B. redundancy.
   C. direct duplication.
   D. indirect duplication.
   E. none of the above.

____198. An environment cleaned with material that is toxic to living tissue is
   A. aseptic.
   B. sterile.
   C. medically clean.
   D. disinfected.
   E. none of the above.

____199. A sharps container should be
   A. puncture resistant.
   B. marked as a biohazard container.
   C. a rigid structure.
   D. capable of holding whole needles and preloaded syringes.
   E. all of the above.

____200. One drug commonly administered transdermally is
   A. sodium bicarbonate.
   B. epinephrine.
   C. nitroglycerin.
   D. aspirin.
   E. magnesium.

____201. The route by which a drug is administered into the ear canal is called
   A. transdermal.
   B. sublingual.
   C. buccal.
   D. aural.
   E. none of the above.

____202. When treating an ear infection with medicated gauze, you should pack the gauze firmly into the ear canal.
   A. True
   B. False

____203. The oxygen flow rate associated with nebulizer use is
   A. 5 to 8 liters per minute.
   B. 8 to 10 liters per minute.
   C. 10 to 12 liters per minute.
   D. 12 to 15 liters per minute.
   E. none of the above.

____204. Nebulizers are preferable to metered dose inhalers for patients with respiratory emergencies.
   A. True
   B. False

©2013 Pearson Education, Inc.
Paramedic Care: Principles & Practice, Vol. 2, 4th Ed.

_____205. Endotracheal administration of medications generally requires increasing the drug dosage by
  A. 1 to 1 1/2 times.
  B. 2 to 2 1/2 times.
  C. 3 times.
  D. 5 times.
  E. none of the above.

_____206. Which of the following drugs is NOT administered via the endotracheal route?
  A. Lidocaine
  B. Naloxone
  C. Atropine
  D. Nitroglycerin
  E. Epinephrine

_____207. Which of the following is an advantage of enteral drug administration?
  A. It is convenient.
  B. It is inexpensive.
  C. It requires little equipment.
  D. It requires little training.
  E. All of the above are advantages.

_____208. Drugs absorbed by the stomach and small intestine must pass through the portal system and liver.
  A. True
  B. False

_____209. A drug administered by the oral route should be followed by what volume of water?
  A. 4 to 8 ounces
  B. 8 to 16 ounces
  C. 16 to 32 ounces
  D. 2 cups
  E. No water at all

_____210. Rectal medications should NOT be administered if you note
  A. diarrhea.
  B. rectal bleeding.
  C. hemorrhoids.
  D. severe anal irritation.
  E. any of the above.

_____211. A syringe should be chosen for drug administration that is slightly larger than the volume of drug to be administered.
  A. True
  B. False

_____212. The larger the gauge of a hypodermic needle, the smaller its diameter.
  A. True
  B. False

_____213. The drug container that must be broken to obtain the drug is the
  A. vial.
  B. ampule.
  C. Mix-O-Vial.
  D. preloaded syringe.
  E. medicated solution.

_____214. The total dose of a drug contained in an ampule with 3 mL of a drug in a 0.4-mg/mL concentration is
  A. 0.3 mg.
  B. 1.2 mg.
  C. 4 mg.
  D. 7 mg.
  E. 12 mg.

_____215. Because a vial is vacuum packed, you will have to replace the volume of medication removed with air in order to maintain equilibrium in the vial.
  A. True
  B. False

_____216. The amount of mixing solution you must remove from a vial for mixing with the powered drug with a nonconstituted drug system is
  A. 1 mL.
  B. 2 mL.
  C. $^1/_2$ of the solution.
  D. $^3/_4$ of the solution.
  E. all of the solution.

____217. Which of the following must be screwed together before use?
- **A.** Vial
- **B.** Ampule
- **C.** Mix-O-Vial
- **D.** Preloaded syringe
- **E.** A and C

____218. The administration route in a drug injected just beneath the skin is called
- **A.** intradermal.
- **B.** subcutaneous.
- **C.** intramuscular.
- **D.** intraosseous.
- **E.** none of the above.

____219. The drug administration route that calls for use of a needle with a lumen gauge of 25 to 27 is
- **A.** intradermal.
- **B.** subcutaneous.
- **C.** intramuscular.
- **D.** intraosseous.
- **E.** none of the above.

____220. The drug administration route that requires the needle be inserted at 45° is
- **A.** intradermal.
- **B.** subcutaneous.
- **C.** intramuscular.
- **D.** intraosseous.
- **E.** none of the above.

____221. All of the following are likely to be acceptable sites for intramuscular injection EXCEPT the
- **A.** upper arms.
- **B.** thighs.
- **C.** abdomen.
- **D.** buttocks.
- **E.** deltoids.

____222. At which injection site(s) can you administer more than 1 mL of drug?
- **A.** Intradermal
- **B.** Subcutaneous
- **C.** Intramuscular
- **D.** B and C
- **E.** All of the above

____223. For which intramuscular injection sites can you administer 5 mL or more of the drug?
- **A.** Deltoid
- **B.** Gluteal
- **C.** Vastus lateralis
- **D.** Rectus femoris
- **E.** All except A

____224. When you pull back on the syringe plunger during subcutaneous or intramuscular injection and blood appears, you should
- **A.** inject the drug.
- **B.** inject the drug followed by a small bubble of air.
- **C.** insert the needle 1 cm further.
- **D.** attempt the injection at another site.
- **E.** ignore it because the appearance of blood has no significance.

____225. After injecting heparin intramuscularly, massage the site to enhance systemic absorption.
- **A.** True
- **B.** False

Chapter 4: Intravenous Access and Medication Administration, Part 2

____226. Arterial cannulation presents with fewer hemorrhage control problems but is not used commonly for drug administration because the arteries are difficult to find.
- **A.** True
- **B.** False

____227. Veins of the legs are preferable to those of the arms because they are larger and easier to locate.
- **A.** True
- **B.** False

©2013 Pearson Education, Inc.
Paramedic Care: Principles & Practice, Vol. 2, 4th Ed.

_____ 228. Which of the following are likely to have fragile veins that are hard to cannulate?
   A. Obese patients
   B. Pregnant patients
   C. Geriatric patients
   D. Asthma patients
   E. None of the above

_____ 229. An intravenous fluid that contains electrolytes and water but does not have large proteins is a(n)
   A. colloid.
   B. crystalloid.
   C. isotonic solution.
   D. hypotonic solution.
   E. hypertonic solution.

_____ 230. An intravenous fluid that contains an electrolyte concentration less than that of plasma is a(n)
   A. colloid.
   B. crystalloid.
   C. isotonic solution.
   D. hypotonic solution.
   E. hypertonic solution.

_____ 231. The most desirable replacement for blood lost during trauma is
   A. normal saline.
   B. lactated Ringer's solution.
   C. blood.
   D. 5 percent dextrose in water.
   E. normal Ringer's lactate.

_____ 232. The administration set that is most appropriate when the overall volume of fluid a patient receives must be restricted is a
   A. macrodrip administration set.
   B. microdrip administration set.
   C. measured volume administration set.
   D. blood tubing set.
   E. none of the above.

_____ 233. The most common macrodrip rate equaling 1 mL is
   A. 10 drops.
   B. 25 drops.
   C. 45 drops.
   D. 60 drops.
   E. none of the above.

_____ 234. The administration set most appropriate to administer intravenous solution to a pediatric patient is a
   A. macrodrip administration set.
   B. microdrip administration set.
   C. measured volume administration set.
   D. blood tubing set.
   E. none of the above.

_____ 235. Blood can be administered with fluids like lactated Ringer's because there is little likelihood for coagulation.
   A. True
   B. False

_____ 236. The model of intravenous cannula to use for patients with delicate veins, such as a small child or geriatric patient, is
   A. over-the-needle.
   B. through-the-needle.
   C. hollow needle.
   D. angiocatheter.
   E. A and D.

_____ 237. The lumen of an 18-gauge needle is larger than one of a 22-gauge needle.
   A. True
   B. False

_____ 238. When cleansing the site for intravenous cannulation, you should use a povidone-iodine or alcohol swab and rub firmly, starting from the center and moving outward in expanding circles.
   A. True
   B. False

_____239. Placing a finger over the exterior skin at the point of the tip of the catheter before removing the needle
    A. stops air from entraining into the vessel.
    B. stops blood from flowing out the catheter hub.
    C. prevents the catheter from coming out with the needle.
    D. prevents the catheter tip from becoming an embolism.
    E. A and B.

_____240. The external jugular venous access site is extremely painful for the patient and should be used only for patients with a decreased or complete loss of consciousness.
    A. True
    B. False

_____241. For the measured volume administration set to work properly, you must fill it with at least
    A. 10 mL of fluid.   D. 50 mL of fluid.
    B. 20 mL of fluid.   E. 100 mL of fluid.
    C. 30 mL of fluid.

_____242. Which of the following is a factor that may cause problems with the intravenous flow rates?
    A. Removal of the constricting band
    B. IV solution bag placed above the cannulation site
    C. The cannula tip up against a vein valve
    D. Half-full drip chamber
    E. All of the above

_____243. Which of the following is a complication of peripheral venous access?
    A. Thrombus formation   D. Necrosis
    B. Thrombophlebitis   E. All of the above
    C. Air embolism

_____244. After a bolus of a drug has been administered, you should flush the line with what volume of fluid?
    A. 20 mL   D. 50 mL
    B. 30 mL   E. 100 mL
    C. 40 mL

_____245. An intravenous drug infusion may be administered as either a piggyback or the primary IV line.
    A. True
    B. False

_____246. If you prepare an intravenous drug infusion, the accompanying label must contain all of the following information EXCEPT
    A. the time and date of mixture.
    B. your initials.
    C. the total drug weight mixed in the bag.
    D. the name of the medical direction physician.
    E. the expiration date.

_____247. Which of the following statements is NOT true regarding venous access devices?
    A. They permit repeated access to the central circulation.
    B. They are of stainless steel or plastic construction with a flexible catheter.
    C. They are most often placed in the superior vena cava.
    D. They require a standard 1-inch, 23-gauge catheter.
    E. They present as a raised circle just beneath the skin.

_____248. Blood analysis can determine the concentrations of
    A. gases.   D. cardiac enzymes.
    B. electrolytes.   E. all of the above.
    C. hormones.

©2013 Pearson Education, Inc.
Paramedic Care: Principles & Practice, Vol. 2, 4th Ed.

_____249. Drawing blood and injecting it into the blood tubes in the wrong order may
   A. leave the wrong volume of blood in a tube.
   B. cross-contaminate the blood with anticoagulants.
   C. cause oxidation.
   D. cause precipitation.
   E. dilute the samples.

_____250. The most ideal veins to use to withdraw blood are those of the back of the hand because their infiltration will least affect future venipuncture sites.
   A. True
   B. False

_____251. When drawing blood, completely fill the blood tube, because the anticoagulant is measured for that amount of blood.
   A. True
   B. False

_____252. When drawing blood through a needle that is too small, one possible complication is
   A. hemoconcentration.
   B. hemoagglutination.
   C. hemodilution.
   D. hemolysis.
   E. hemoconiosis.

_____253. Any solution that can be administered by intravenous infusion can be administered by intraosseous infusion.
   A. True
   B. False

_____254. Proper insertion of the intraosseous needle includes
   A. introducing it perpendicular to the puncture site.
   B. inserting it with a twisting motion.
   C. inserting it 2 to 4 mm for entry.
   D. feeling for a "pop" or decreased resistance.
   E. all of the above.

_____255. It is essential to periodically flush the intraosseous needle to keep it patent.
   A. True
   B. False

Chapter 4: Intravenous Access and Medication Administration, Part 3

_____256. A physician orders you to administer 90 mg of acetaminophen to a pediatric patient. The liquid acetaminophen is packaged as a concentration of 500 mg in 8 mL of solution. How much of the medication will you administer?
   A. 0.44 mL   D. 1.44 mL
   B. 1.12 mL   E. 2.44 mL
   C. 1.22 mL

_____257. A physician orders you to give 250 mg of a medication via IV bolus. The multidose vial contains 2 grams of the medication in 10 mL of solution. How much of the medication should you administer?
   A. 0.75 mL   D. 1.5 mL
   B. 1.0 mL   E. 1.75 mL
   C. 1.25 mL

____258. A physician wants you to administer 5 milligrams of medication subcutaneously. The ampule contains 10 mg of the medication in 2 mL of solvent. How much medication should you use?
A. 0.10 mL
B. 0.25 mL
C. 0.50 mL
D. 0.75 mL
E. 1.0 mL

____259. A physician wants you to administer 2 mg per minute of lidocaine to a patient. To prepare the infusion, you mix 2 grams of lidocaine in an IV bag containing 500 milliliters of 5 percent dextrose in water (D_5W). You will use a microdrip administration set (60 drops/mL). What is the infusion rate?
A. 10 drops per minute
B. 20 drops per minute
C. 30 drops per minute
D. 40 drops per minute
E. 50 drops per minute

____260. A physician tells you to administer 500 milliliters of normal saline solution to a patient over 1 hour (60 minutes). The administration tubing is a macrodrip set with a drip factor of 10 drops/mL. At what drip rate would you run this infusion?
A. 0.833 drops per minute
B. 8.33 drops per minute
C. 83.3 drops per minute
D. 833.0 drops per minute
E. None of the above

Chapter 5: Airway Management and Ventilation, Part 1

____261. By the time air reaches the lower airway, it is at body temperature, humidified, and virtually free of airborne particles.
A. True
B. False

____262. The order in which air passes through airway structures during inspiration is
A. trachea, larynx, laryngopharynx, nasopharynx, nares.
B. nares, nasopharynx, trachea, laryngopharynx, larynx.
C. laryngopharynx, nares, nasopharynx, larynx, trachea.
D. nares, nasopharynx, laryngopharynx, larynx, trachea.
E. trachea, nares, laryngopharynx, larynx, nasopharynx.

____263. The location at which the mainstem bronchi and major blood vessels enter the lung is the
A. hilum.
B. parenchyma.
C. vallecula.
D. carina.
E. pleura.

____264. The mainstem bronchus that leaves the trachea at almost a straight angle is the left mainstem bronchus.
A. True
B. False

____265. Parasympathetic receptors cause the bronchioles to
A. constrict.
B. dilate.
C. shorten.
D. stiffen.
E. none of the above.

____266. The narrowest part of the pediatric airway is the
A. cricoid ring.
B. hyoid ring.
C. glottis.
D. carina.
E. tracheal stricture.

©2013 Pearson Education, Inc.
Paramedic Care: Principles & Practice, Vol. 2, 4th Ed.

____267. Which of the following is NOT true regarding the adult and pediatric airway and respiration?
   A. The pediatric airway is smaller in all aspects than that of the adult.
   B. Pediatric ribs are stronger and contribute more to respiration than ribs in adults.
   C. Children rely more on their diaphragms for breathing than adults.
   D. The cricoid cartilage is the narrowest point of the pediatric airway but not of the adult airway.
   E. Children's teeth are softer and more prone to damage than the teeth of adults.

____268. Respiration is the mechanical process that moves air into and out of the lungs.
   A. True.
   B. False.

____269. Ventilation is the exchange of gases between a living organism and its environment.
   A. True.
   B. False.

____270. The active aspect of the respiratory cycle is
   A. inspiration.
   B. expiration.
   C. neither A or B.
   D. both A and B.
   E. the resting stage.

____271. The percentage of carbon dioxide in atmospheric air is approximately
   A. 79 percent.
   B. 4 percent.
   C. 0.4 percent.
   D. 0.04 percent.
   E. 0.10 percent.

____272. The majority of the oxygen carried by the blood is
   A. carried by the hemoglobin.
   B. dissolved in the plasma.
   C. transported as bicarbonate.
   D. found as free gas in the blood.
   E. none of the above.

____273. The reflex that responds to the stretching of the lungs by inhibiting respirations is the
   A. apneustic reflex.
   B. pneumotaxic reflex.
   C. Frank-Starling reflex.
   D. Hering-Breuer reflex.
   E. baroreceptor response.

____274. The primary stimulus that causes respiration to occur is a(n)
   A. increase in pH of the blood.
   B. decrease in pH of the blood.
   C. increase in pH of the cerebrospinal fluid.
   D. decrease in pH of the cerebrospinal fluid.
   E. reduction of oxygen in the blood.

____275. The amount of air in the lung after a maximal inspiration is called the
   A. minute volume.
   B. alveolar air.
   C. tidal volume
   D. dead air space.
   E. total lung capacity.

____276. The normal respiratory rate for a child at rest is
   A. 8 to 12 breaths per minute.
   B. 12 to 20 breaths per minute.
   C. 18 to 24 breaths per minute.
   D. 24 to 32 breaths per minute.
   E. 40 to 60 breaths per minute.

____277. The most common prehospital cause of laryngeal spasm is
   A. aspiration of foreign bodies.
   B. aspiration of blood or vomitus.
   C. overly aggressive intubation.
   D. trauma.
   E. airway edema.

____278. The modified form of respiration that is caused by nasal irritation is the
- **A.** cough.
- **B.** sneeze.
- **C.** hiccup.
- **D.** grunt.
- **E.** sigh.

____279. The respiratory pattern that displays with an increasing rate and depth of respirations alternating gradually with periods of slow, shallow breathing is
- **A.** Kussmaul's respirations.
- **B.** Cheyne-Stokes respirations.
- **C.** Biot's respirations.
- **D.** central neurogenic hyperventilation.
- **E.** agonal respirations.

____280. Snoring is generally related to
- **A.** laryngeal constriction or edema.
- **B.** the tongue blocking the airway.
- **C.** narrowing of the bronchioles.
- **D.** fluids within the airway.
- **E.** foreign bodies in the lower airway.

____281. When using pulse oximetry to guide care, your objective is to achieve an oxygen saturation level of
- **A.** 80 to 85 percent.
- **B.** 85 to 90 percent.
- **C.** 90 to 95 percent.
- **D.** 95 to 99 percent.
- **E.** no less than 100 percent.

____282. Some pulse CO-oximeters use multiple wavelengths of light to detect
- **A.** oxyhemoglobin.
- **B.** carboxyhemoglobin.
- **C.** methemoglobin.
- **D.** total hemoglobin.
- **E.** all of the above.

____283. Capnography is a valuable assessment tool for which of the following?
- **A.** To ensure proper initial endotracheal tube placement
- **B.** To assess systemic metabolism
- **C.** To ensure proper continued endotracheal tube placement
- **D.** To assess status of circulation and ventilation
- **E.** All of the above

____284. Which of the following occurs in pulmonary embolism and similar conditions that increase dead space ventilation causing a decrease in ETCO$_2$ levels throughout the respiratory cycle?
- **A.** Curare cleft
- **B.** Chronic obstructive pulmonary disease
- **C.** Ventilation/perfusion mismatch
- **D.** Hyperventilation
- **E.** Endotracheal circuit leak

____285. Peak expiratory flow testing can be used as a crude measure of respiratory efficacy. Improving measurements can indicate poor response to treatment of acute respiratory illness.
- **A.** True
- **B.** False

Chapter 5: Airway Management and Ventilation, Part 2

____286. Unconscious patients who require airway and ventilation interventions, such as BVM ventilation or intubation, are usually best maintained in an ear-to-sternal-notch position, in which the supine patient's head is elevated to the point where the ear and the sternal notch are horizontally aligned.
- **A.** True
- **B.** False

____287. The obese patient needing BVM ventilation should be placed in the
- **A.** recovery position.
- **B.** ramped position.
- **C.** Fowler's position.
- **D.** sniffing position.
- **E.** Trendelenburg position.

_____288. Which of the following oxygen delivery devices provides 40 to 60 percent oxygen at 10 L/min?
    A. Nasal cannula   **D.** Partial rebreather mask
    B. Venturi mask   **E.** Nonrebreather mask
    C. Simple face mask

_____289. Which of the following devices maintains a steady level of pressure during both inhalation and exhalation?
    A. BiPAP device   **D.** CPAP device
    B. High-pressure regulator   **E.** None of the above
    C. Therapy regulator

_____290. The nasopharyngeal airway should be inserted into the largest nare unless there is resistance to its insertion or the septum is deviated.
    A. True
    B. False

_____291. The preferred technique of insertion for the oropharyngeal airway in pediatric patients calls for partially inserting the airway, rotating the device 180°, then continuing the insertion.
    A. True
    B. False

_____292. Adult bag-valve masks do not have pop-off valves because patients with poor lung compliance would likely activate the valves before effective ventilation is achieved.
    A. True
    B. False

_____293. Cricoid pressure maneuver is performed by
    A. displacing the thyroid cartilage upward.
    B. displacing the tongue forward.
    C. depressing the cricoid cartilage posteriorly.
    D. squeezing the trachea between the fingers.
    E. placing pressure on the abdomen to expel air.

_____294. The percentage of oxygen delivered to the patient when using the demand valve device is about
    A. 40 percent.   **D.** 90 percent.
    B. 50 percent.   **E.** 100 percent.
    C. 75 percent.

_____295. Mouth-to-mouth/mouth-to-nose ventilation provides limited oxygen delivery, as expired air contains only
    A. 13 percent oxygen.   **D.** 19 percent oxygen.
    B. 15 percent oxygen.   **E.** 21 percent oxygen.
    C. 17 percent oxygen.

Chapter 5: Airway Management and Ventilation, Part 3

_____296. Esophageal Tracheal Combitubes (ETCs) come in two sizes for patients over
    A. 2 feet tall.
    B. 3 feet tall.
    C. 4 feet tall
    D. 5 feet tall.
    E. none of the above—there is no minimum height.

_____297. The PtL airway is inserted in a patient suspected of cervical spine injury
    A. using the nasal route.
    B. using a neutral position.
    C. with one cuff preinflated.
    D. with the head and neck flexed.
    E. all of the above.

_____298. All of the following are considered supraglottic airway devices EXCEPT

    A. Laryngeal Mask Airway.

    B. CookGas AirQ airway.

    C. S.A.L.T. airway

    D. Ambu Laryngeal Mask airway.

    E. King LT airway.

_____299. Indications for endotracheal intubation include all of the following EXCEPT

    A. respiratory arrest.

    B. epiglottitis.

    C. inability to protect the airway.

    D. obstruction due to foreign object, swelling, or burns.

    E. anaphylaxis with respiratory difficulty.

_____300. The tip of the straight laryngoscope blade is designed to

    A. engage the nasopharynx.

    B. just enter the glottic opening.

    C. fit into the vallecula.

    D. fit into arytenoid fossa.

    E. fit under the epiglottis.

_____301. Paramedics should learn to listen for air leakage and place only enough air in the cuff to inflate it without causing a leak.

    A. True

    B. False

_____302. When using the stylet for intubation, the tip of the device

    A. should extend 3 mm beyond the end of the endotracheal tube.

    B. should be even with the end of the endotracheal tube.

    C. should stop just short of the distal end.

    D. is moved in or out during the intubation attempt as needed.

    E. none of the above.

_____303. The straight, semirigid device with a distal bent tip that is covered with a protective resin used to facilitate endotracheal intubations when only the epiglottis may be visualized is called the

    A. Magill introducer.

    B. esophageal detector.

    C. endotracheal tube introducer.

    D. malleable stylet.

    E. none of the above.

_____304. All of the following are complications to the patient associated with endotracheal intubation EXCEPT

    A. damage to teeth.

    B. soft-tissue damage to the oropharynx.

    C. patient hypoxia during intubation attempts.

    D. endobronchial intubation.

    E. hyperkalemia.

_____305. Which of the following is NOT an indication of esophageal intubation?

    A. Absence of chest rise with ventilation

    B. Condensation on the endotracheal tube

    C. A falling pulse oximetry reading

    D. Increasing abdominal distension

    E. Absent waveform on capnography

_____306. Which of the following is NOT true regarding endotracheal intubation?

    A. The laryngoscope is held in the right hand.

    B. The laryngoscope is inserted into the right side of the mouth.

    C. The straight blade lifts the epiglottis.

    D. The curved blade fits into the vallecula.

    E. You should advance the ET tube into the glottis, 1 to 2 cm beyond the tube cuff.

©2013 Pearson Education, Inc.
Paramedic Care: Principles & Practice, Vol. 2, 4th Ed.

_____307. Which of the following is NOT used to confirm proper endotracheal tube placement?
   A. Visualization of the tube passing through the glottis
   B. Rapid return noted on EDD
   C. Changing color on an $ETCO_2$ detector
   D. Condensation on the endotracheal tube with exhalation
   E. The presence of phonation

_____308. When the endotracheal tube is in the esophagus, the esophageal detector device will be difficult to withdraw because the esophagus will seal shut.
   A. True
   B. False

_____309. Nasotracheal intubation may be the best or only option in the patient with trismus or with an anticipated difficult laryngoscopy.
   A. True
   B. False

_____310. Nasotracheal intubation is contraindicated for a
   A. patient with a potential spine injury.
   B. patient not in arrest or deeply comatose.
   C. patient with a fractured jaw.
   D. severely obese patient.
   E. patient with nasal fractures.

_____311. Which of the following is NOT a disadvantage associated with nasotracheal intubation?
   A. BNTI is often more difficult and time consuming than orotracheal intubation.
   B. There is significant risk of epistaxis.
   C. It cannot be used if the patient has trismus or an anticipated difficult laryngoscopy.
   D. There is a significant risk of sinusitis.
   E. Smaller diameter tubes must be used.

_____312. In attempting digital intubation, the fingers of the rescuer must reach to the
   A. epiglottis.   D. laryngeal opening.
   B. posterior nares.   E. cricoid cartilage.
   C. back of the tongue.

_____313. The use of a laryngoscope and the passage of an endotracheal tube may cause a child's heart rate to drop dramatically, which may reduce cardiac output and blood pressure.
   A. True
   B. False

_____314. Relative contraindications to performing cricothyrotomy in the field include inability to identify anatomical landmarks, crush injury to the larynx, suspected tracheal transection, and underlying anatomical abnormalities such as tumor or subglottic stenosis.
   A. True
   B. False

_____315. Which of the following is NOT a complication of needle cricothyrotomy?
   A. Barotrauma from overinflation
   B. Excessive bleeding due to improper catheter placement
   C. Hypoventilation from improper equipment
   D. Prevention of passage of a subsequent endotracheal tube
   E. Tracheal compression from hemorrhage or subcutaneous emphysema

_____316. When performing a surgical or open cricothyrotomy, you first make a small vertical incision through the skin, then a vertical incision through the cricothyroid membrane.
   A. True
   B. False

_____317. MAI techniques give you the option of managing airways that you could not otherwise manage because the patient is too awake or has trismus, and they do it early in the clinical course when the procedure may be easier and the patient has more reserve to tolerate complications.
   A. True
   B. False

_____318. The major difference between succinylcholine and vecuronium as paralytics in prehospital care is that vecuronium
   A. causes fasciculations.
   B. has a shorter time to onset.
   C. has a much longer duration.
   D. increases intracranial pressure.
   E. all of the above.

_____319. It is essential that a pediatric patient be premedicated with vecuronium before the administration of succinylcholine, because fasciculations are otherwise likely to cause musculoskeletal trauma.
   A. True
   B. False

_____320. If possible, the patient receiving rapid sequence intubation should be preoxygenated using a non-rebreather mask with high-concentration oxygen for at least 3 minutes.
   A. True
   B. False

Chapter 5: Airway Management and Ventilation, Part 4

_____321. Potential problems with patients who have a stoma include
   A. respiratory distress.
   B. bleeding internally or externally.
   C. clogged tracheostomy tube.
   D. dislodged tracheostomy tube.
   E. all of the above.

_____322. Generally, suctioning attempts should be limited to no longer than
   A. 10 seconds.
   B. 30 seconds.
   C. 45 seconds.
   D. 60 seconds.
   E. as long as needed to clear the airway.

_____323. When no contraindication exists, the nasogastric tube is preferred for gastric decompression.
   A. True
   B. False

_____324. Simple transport ventilations have a pop-off valve that opens when airway pressure exceeds
   A. 30 cm/H_2O.
   B. 40 cm/H_2O.
   C. 50 cm/H_2O.
   D. 60 cm/H_2O.
   E. 70 cm/H_2O.

_____325. A significant percentage of claims and lawsuits that are filed against prehospital providers involve airway issues, and often these cases are won or lost based on the field documentation.
   A. True
   B. False

©2013 Pearson Education, Inc.
Paramedic Care: Principles & Practice, Vol. 2, 4th Ed.

WORKBOOK ANSWER KEY

Note: Throughout Answer Key, textbook page references are shown in italic.

CHAPTER 1

PART 1

MULTIPLE CHOICE

1.	D	*p. 6*	**6.**	A	*p. 9*	**11.**	A	*p. 9*
2.	D	*p. 7*	**7.**	E	*p. 9*	**12.**	E	*p. 9*
3.	B	*p. 8*	**8.**	B	*p. 9*	**13.**	C	*p. 9*
4.	B	*p. 9*	**9.**	C	*p. 9*	**14.**	B	*p. 9*
5.	B	*p. 9*	**10.**	E	*p. 9*	**15.**	D	*p. 10*

SPECIAL PROJECT

MATCHING

1.	K	*p. 10*	**6.**	H	*pp. 9–10*	**11.**	B	*p. 9*
2.	G	*p. 9*	**7.**	I	*p. 10*	**12.**	J	*p. 10*
3.	D	*p. 9*	**8.**	E	*p. 9*	**13.**	E	*p. 9*
4.	F	*p. 9*	**9.**	C	*p. 9*	**14.**	A	*p. 9*
5.	L	*p. 10*	**10.**	A	*p. 9*	**15.**	B	*p. 9*

PART 2

MULTIPLE CHOICE

1.	A	*p. 12*	**6.**	D	*pp. 16–17*	**11.**	C	*p. 22*
2.	E	*p. 13*	**7.**	C	*p. 18*	**12.**	A	*p. 25*
3.	C	*p. 14*	**8.**	B	*p. 19*	**13.**	B	*p. 25*
4.	A	*p. 15*	**9.**	B	*p. 20*	**14.**	C	*p. 27*
5.	A	*p. 15*	**10.**	E	*pp. 21–22*	**15.**	C	*pp. 28–30*

SPECIAL PROJECT

MATCHING

1.	B	*pp. 28–30*	**5.**	B	*pp. 28–30*
2.	A	*pp. 28–30*	**6.**	C	*pp. 28–30*
3.	D	*pp. 28–30*	**7.**	A	*pp. 28–30*
4.	C	*pp. 28–30*	**8.**	D	*pp. 28–30*

PART 3

MULTIPLE CHOICE

1.	D	*p. 30*	**9.**	B	*pp. 45–46*
2.	B	*pp. 31–33*	**10.**	E	*p. 50*
3.	E	*p. 33*	**11.**	C.	*p. 54*
4.	A	*p. 34*	**12.**	B	*p. 55*
5.	D	*p. 37*	**13.**	B	*p. 56*
6.	C	*pp. 40–41*	**14.**	B	*p. 56*
7.	A	*p. 43*	**15.**	C	*pp. 57–58*
8.	C	*p. 44*			

SPECIAL PROJECT

LABELING

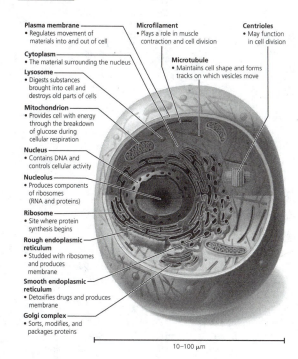

Plasma membrane —
• Regulates movement of materials into and out of cell

Cytoplasm —
• The material surrounding the nucleus

Lysosome —
• Digests substances brought into cell and destroys old parts of cells

Mitochondrion —
• Provides cell with energy through the breakdown of glucose during cellular respiration

Nucleus —
• Contains DNA and controls cellular activity

Nucleolus —
• Produces components of ribosomes (RNA and proteins)

Ribosome —
• Site where protein synthesis begins

Rough endoplasmic reticulum —
• Studded with ribosomes and produces membrane

Smooth endoplasmic reticulum —
• Detoxifies drugs and produces membrane

Golgi complex —
• Sorts, modifies, and packages proteins

Microfilament —
• Plays a role in muscle contraction and cell division

Microtubule —
• Maintains cell shape and forms tracks on which vesicles move

Centrioles —
• May function in cell division

10–100 μm

PART 4

MULTIPLE CHOICE

1.	A	*p. 59*	**9.**	B	*p. 62*
2.	C	*pp. 59–60*	**10.**	E	*p. 63*
3.	A	*p. 60*	**11.**	D	*pp. 64–65*
4.	D	*p. 60*	**12.**	A	*p. 65*
5.	E	*p. 60*	**13.**	C	*p. 65*
6.	C	*p. 60*	**14.**	D	*p. 66*
7.	C	*pp. 60–61*	**15.**	A	*p. 68*
8.	B	*pp. 61–62*			

SPECIAL PROJECT

MATCHING

1.	Q.	*p. 62*	**11.**	A.	*p. 62*
2.	B.	*p. 62*	**12.**	F.	*p. 62*
3.	R.	*p. 64*	**13.**	C.	*p. 62*
4.	M.	*p. 65*	**14.**	J.	*p. 64*
5.	E.	*p. 62*	**15.**	J.	*p. 64*
6.	K.	*p. 64*	**16.**	N.	*p. 65*
7.	T.	*p. 62*	**17.**	O.	*p. 65*
8.	H.	*p. 64*	**18.**	P.	*p. 65*
9.	D.	*p. 62*	**19.**	G.	*p. 64*
10.	I.	*p. 64*	**20.**	S.	*p. 64*

## PART 5

MULTIPLE CHOICE

1.	E	*p. 69*	14.	B	*p. 75*
2.	C	*p. 69*	15.	B	*p. 75*
3.	B	*pp. 69–70*	16.	C	*p. 76*
4.	C	*p. 70*	17.	D	*p. 77*
5.	A	*p. 70*	18.	A	*p. 79*
6.	B	*p. 71*	19.	D	*p. 79*
7.	D	*p. 71*	20.	B	*p. 82*
8.	D	*p. 71*	21.	E	*p. 82*
9.	B	*p. 72*	22.	D	*p. 84*
10.	B	*p. 73*	23.	A	*pp. 84–85*
11.	E	*p. 73*	24.	B	*p. 85*
12.	C	*p. 73*	25.	E	*p. 86*
13.	C	*p. 73*			

SPECIAL PROJECT

MATCHING

1.	A	*p. 81*	6.	D	*p. 84*
2.	C	*p. 82*	7.	B	*pp. 81–82*
3.	E	*p. 83*	8.	E	*p. 83*
4.	D	*p. 84*	9.	C	*p. 82*
5.	E	*p. 83*	10.	B	*pp. 81–82*

PART 6

MULTIPLE CHOICE

1.	B	*p. 86*	12.	C	*p. 92*
2.	C	*p. 86*	13.	B	*pp. 93–94*
3.	C	*p. 87*	14.	A	*p. 95*
4.	B	*p. 88*	15.	B	*p. 95*
5.	C	*p. 88*	16.	C	*p. 97*
6.	A	*p. 88*	17.	E	*p. 99*
7.	C	*p. 88*	18.	D	*p. 99*
8.	A	*p. 89*	19.	B	*pp. 106–107*
9.	B	*p. 89*	20.	D	*p. 107*
10.	E	*p. 90*	21.	E	*pp. 107–108*
11.	A	*p. 91*	22.	D	*p. 112*

SPECIAL PROJECT

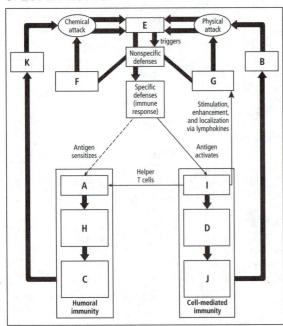

CHAPTER 2

MULTIPLE CHOICE

1.	D	*p. 123*	14.	C	*p. 128*
2.	B	*p. 123*	15.	C	*p. 129*
3.	E	*p. 123*	16.	A	*p. 129*
4.	A	*p. 123*	17.	D	*p. 130*
5.	B	*p. 123*	18.	A	*p. 130*
6.	B	*pp. 123–124*	19.	E	*p. 131*
7.	E	*p. 124*	20.	A	*p. 131*
8.	A	*p. 125*	21.	E	*p. 132*
9.	C	*p. 125*	22.	B	*p. 132*
10.	C	*p. 126*	23.	E	*p. 132*
11.	A	*p. 127*	24.	A	*p. 132–133*
12.	D	*p. 127*	25.	A	*p. 133*
13.	B	*p. 127*			

MATCHING

26.	F	*p. 131*	31.	H	*p. 132*
27.	G	*p. 131*	32.	D	*p. 128*
28.	A	*p. 125*	33.	B	*p. 126*
29.	E	*p. 129*	34.	C	*p. 127*
30.	D	*p. 128*	35.	A	*p. 125*

SPECIAL PROJECT

NORMAL VITAL SIGNS

See Table 2-1 on text p. 123.

CHAPTER 3

PART 1

MULTIPLE CHOICE

1.	D	*p. 139*	21.	D	*p. 147*
2.	A	*p. 139*	22.	A	*p. 149*
3.	B	*p. 140*	23.	D	*pp. 150–151*
4.	A	*p. 140*	24.	B	*p. 151*
5.	B	*p. 140*	25.	D	*p. 151*
6.	B	*p. 140*	26.	B	*p. 151*
7.	C	*p. 141*	27.	C	*p. 151*
8.	C	*p. 141*	28.	C	*p. 152*
9.	E	*p. 142*	29.	E	*p. 152*
10.	B	*p. 142*	30.	C	*p. 152*
11.	E	*p. 142*	31.	C	*p. 152*
12.	E	*pp. 144–145*	32.	B	*p. 152*
13.	A	*p. 144*	33.	D	*pp. 152–153*
14.	B	*pp. 145–146*	34.	B	*p. 153*
15.	E	*p. 145*	35.	A	*p. 153*
16.	D	*p. 146*	36.	C	*p. 153*
17.	D	*p. 146*	37.	A	*p. 154*
18.	A	*p. 146*	38.	D	*p. 154*
19.	C	*p. 146*	39.	E	*p. 154*
20.	B	*p. 146*	40.	C	*pp. 154–155*

SPECIAL PROJECT: CROSSWORD PUZZLE

Crossword answers (across and down):
FILTRATION · ACTIVE · SYNTHETIC · SYRUP · BIOASSAY · MINERAL · NASAL · SPIRIT · ORAL · EFFICACY · AGONIST · BIOEQUIVALENT · ANIMAL · EXTRACT · TABLET · RECEPTOR

PART 2

MULTIPLE CHOICE

#	Ans	Page		#	Ans	Page
1.	E	p. 156		41.	D	p. 183
2.	B	p. 156		42.	E	p. 183
3.	E	p. 156		43.	B	p. 182–183
4.	A	p. 156		44.	E	p. 182–183
5.	D	p. 156		45.	B	p. 183
6.	C	p. 156		46.	A	p. 183
7.	B	p. 157		47.	D	p. 186
8.	C	p. 159		48.	D	p. 186
9.	C	p. 159		49.	D	p. 187
10.	A	p. 159		50.	B	p. 187
11.	D	p. 159		51.	B	p. 187
12.	B	p. 159		52.	A	p. 193
13.	B	p. 163		53.	B	p. 193
14.	B	p. 164		54.	C	p. 194
15.	A	p. 164		55.	D	p. 195
16.	B	p. 167		56.	C	p. 195
17.	A	p. 167		57.	C	p. 197
18.	C	p. 167		58.	C	p. 197
19.	D	p. 168		59.	A	p. 198
20.	D	p. 168		60.	D	p. 198
21.	D	p. 170		61.	E	p. 198
22.	B	p. 170		62.	E	p. 200
23.	B	p. 171		63.	B	p. 200
24.	B	p. 171		64.	B	p. 200
25.	A	p. 171		65.	D	p. 200
26.	B	p. 171		66.	C	p. 201
27.	B	p. 172		67.	E	p. 201
28.	B	p. 172		68.	C	p. 201
29.	A	p. 172		69.	A	p. 201
30.	A	p. 172		70.	C	p. 203
31.	D	p. 173		71.	B	p. 203
32.	D	p. 173		72.	A	p. 203
33.	C	p. 174		73.	C	p. 203
34.	B	p. 174		74.	E	p. 205
35.	D	p. 177		75.	E	p. 206
36.	B	p. 177		76.	A	p. 208
37.	D	p. 177, 180		77.	E	p. 208
38.	D	p. 180		78.	A	p. 208
39.	A	p. 181		79.	C	p. 209
40.	B	p. 183		80.	C	p. 210

#	Ans	Page		#	Ans	Page
81.	B	p. 210		86.	B	p. 213
82.	B	p. 210		87.	E	p. 215
83.	A	p. 210		88.	B	p. 216
84.	D	p. 211		89.	B	p. 216
85.	A	p. 212		90.	A	p. 216

SPECIAL PROJECT

This is an exercise that does not require an answer key.

CHAPTER 4

PART 1

MULTIPLE CHOICE

#	Ans	Page		#	Ans	Page
1.	A	pp. 229–230		24.	B	p. 238
2.	B	p. 230		25.	A	p. 238
3.	D	p. 230		26.	B	p. 239
4.	E	p. 230		27.	C	p. 239
5.	A	p. 230		28.	B	p. 240
6.	A	p. 231		29.	D	p. 242
7.	C	pp. 231–232		30.	B	p. 243
8.	D	p. 232		31.	B	p. 243
9.	A	p. 232		32.	B	p. 244
10.	C	pp. 232–233		33.	A	p. 244
11.	E	p. 233		34.	A	p. 245
12.	D	p. 234		35.	E	pp. 245, 247
13.	C	p. 234		36.	A	p. 249
14.	C	p. 234		37.	D	p. 249
15.	E	p. 235		38.	B	pp. 249, 251
16.	D	p. 235		39.	C	p. 251
17.	A	p. 235		40.	A	p. 251
18.	B	p. 236		41.	D	pp. 251, 253
19.	A	pp. 236–237		42.	C	p. 253
20.	C	p. 238		43.	D	pp. 249–250, 253
21.	A	p. 238		44.	D	p. 253
22.	E	p. 238		45.	B	p. 254
23.	A	p. 238				

SPECIAL PROJECT

MATCHING

#	Ans	Page		#	Ans	Page
1.	D	p. 247		9.	C	p. 238
2.	A	p. 234		10.	C	p. 240
3.	B	p. 238		11.	A	p. 233
4.	D	p. 247		12.	D	p. 247
5.	A	p. 235		13.	A	p. 234
6.	A	p. 236		14.	D	p. 247
7.	D	p. 247		15.	B	p. 237
8.	B	p. 236				

PART 2

MULTIPLE CHOICE

#	Ans	Page		#	Ans	Page
1.	E	p. 255		11.	A	p. 258
2.	E	p. 255		12.	E	p. 258
3.	D	p. 255		13.	D	p. 258
4.	B	pp. 255–256		14.	C	p. 259
5.	A	p. 256		15.	A	pp. 259–260
6.	C	p. 256		16.	A	p. 260
7.	E	p. 256		17.	A	p. 260
8.	D	p. 257		18.	A	p. 261
9.	E	p. 257		19.	B	p. 261
10.	E	p. 257		20.	B	p. 261

21.	D	*p. 261*	36.	A	*p. 272*
22.	B	*p. 262*	37.	B	*p. 274*
23.	B	*p. 262*	38.	E	*p. 275*
24.	B	*p. 262*	39.	A	*p. 275*
25.	A	*p. 262*	40.	B	*p. 276*
26.	C	*p. 265*	41.	C	*p. 276*
27.	C	*p. 265*	42.	B	*p. 276*
28.	E	*p. 265*	43.	C	*p. 276*
29.	E	*pp. 265–266*	44.	A	*p. 277*
30.	D	*p. 268*	45.	C	*p. 277*
31.	D	*p. 268*	46.	A	*p. 277*
32.	B	*p. 268*	47.	A	*p. 278*
33.	D	*p. 268*	48.	C	*p. 279*
34.	C	*pp. 268–269*	49.	C	*p. 283*
35.	A	*p. 269*	50.	D	*p. 283*

SPECIAL PROJECT

MEDICATION ADMINISTRATION: PERSONAL BENCHMARKING

This is an exercise that does not require an answer key.

PART 3

MULTIPLE CHOICE

1.	D	*p. 284*	6.	A	*p. 285*
2.	A	*p. 284*	7.	E	*p. 285*
3.	C	*p. 284*	8.	D	*p. 286*
4.	D	*p. 284*	9.	A	*p. 286*
5.	A	*p. 285*	10.	A	*p. 290*

SPECIAL PROJECT

DRIP MATH WORKSHEET 1

1. $R = 5\ 15$ drops/min $\lim\limits_{x \to \infty}$

$V = ?$
$T = 25$ min
$D = 60$ drops/mL
$V = R \times T = 15$ drops/min $\times\ 25$ min

$V = \dfrac{15\ drops \times 25\ min}{min}$

$V = 375$ drops/D

$= \dfrac{375\ drops \times mL}{60\ drops} = \dfrac{375\ mL}{60} = 6.25$

2. $R = V/T = 250$ mL/60 min
$V = 250$ mL
$T = 6$ min
$D_1 = 60$ drops/mL
$D_2 = 60$ drops/mL

A. $R = V/T$

$= \dfrac{250\ mL}{60\ min} = \dfrac{4.17\ mL}{min}$

$= \dfrac{4.17\ mL \times 60\ drops}{min \times mL} = \dfrac{250\ drops}{min}$

B. $R = V/T$

$= \dfrac{250\ mL}{60\ min} = \dfrac{4.17\ mL}{min}$

$= \dfrac{4.17\ mL \times 10\ drops}{min \times mL} = \dfrac{41.7\ drops}{min}$

3. $R = 32$ drops/min
$V = 50$ mL
$T = ?$
$D = 45$ drops/mL
$R(mL) = R(min) \times D$
$R(mL) = 32$ drops/min $\times\ 45$ drops/mL

$R(mL) = \dfrac{32\ drops \times mL}{45\ drops \times min} = \dfrac{32\ mL}{45\ min}$

$= 0.71$ mL/min

$T = V/R = \dfrac{50\ mL \times min}{0.71\ mL} = 70$ min

4. $R = 4$ drops/sec $\times\ 60$ sec/min

$= \dfrac{4\ drops \times 60\ sec}{sec \times min} = 240\,|drops\,/\,min$

$V = ?$
$T = 45$ min
$D = 10$ drops/mL
$V = R \times T = 240$ drops/min $\times\ 45$ min

$= \dfrac{240\ drops \times 45\ min}{min} = 10,800\ drops$

$V = 10,800\ drops\ /\ D = \dfrac{10,800\ mL}{10\ drops}$

$= \dfrac{10,800\ mL}{10} = 1,080$ mL

5. $R = ?$
$V = 1.5$ mL/min
$T = 1$ min
$D_1 = 60$ drops/mL
$D_2 = 45$ drops/mL
$D_3 = 10$ drops/mL

A. $R = V/T = \dfrac{1.5\ mL}{1\ min} = \dfrac{1.5\ mL \times D_1}{1\ min}$

$= \dfrac{1.5\ mL \times 60\ drops}{min \times mL} = 90\ drops/min$

B. $R = V/T = \dfrac{1.5\ mL}{1\ min} = \dfrac{1.5\ mL \times D_2}{1\ min}$

$= \dfrac{1.5\ mL \times 45\ drops}{min \times mL} = 67.5\ drops/min$

C. $R = V/T = \dfrac{1.5\ mL}{1\ min} = \dfrac{1.5\ mL \times D_3}{1\ min}$

$= \dfrac{1.5\ mL \times 10\ drops}{min \times mL} = 15\ drops/min$

DRUG MATH WORKSHEET 2

1. $Dh = 1$ mg
   $Vh = 5$ mL
   $Dd = 0.5$ mg
   $Va = ?$

   $$Va = \frac{Vh \times Dd}{Dh} = \frac{5\,mL \times 0.5\,mg}{1\,mg}$$

   $$= \frac{2.5\,mL}{1} = 2.5\,mL$$

2. $Dh = 80$ mg
   $Vh = 4$ mL
   $Dd = 40$ mg
   $Va = ?$

   $$Va = \frac{Vh \times Dd}{Dh} = \frac{4\,mL \times 40\,mg}{80\,mg}$$

   $$= \frac{160 \times mL}{80} = 2\,mL$$

3. **A.** $Dh = 1$ g (1,000 mg)
   $Vh = 1,000$ mL
   $Dd = 1$ mg
   $Va = ?$

   $$Va = \frac{Vh \times Dd}{Dh} = \frac{1,000\,mL \times 1\,mg}{1\,g}$$

   $$= \frac{1,000\,mL \times 1\,mg}{1,000\,mg} = \frac{1\,mL}{1} = 1\,mL$$

   B. $Dh = 1$ g (1,000 mg)
   $Vh = 1,000$ mL
   $Dd = 1$ mg
   $Va = ?$

   $$Va = \frac{Vh \times Dd}{Dh} = \frac{10,000\,mL \times 1\,mg}{1\,g}$$

   $$= \frac{10,000\,mL \times 1\,mg}{1,000\,mg} = \frac{10\,mL}{1} = 10\,mL$$

4. Desired Dose = Patient Weight × 0.2 mg/kg

   $$= \frac{6\,Kg \times 0.2\,mg}{Kg} = 1.2\,mg$$

   $Dh = 6$ mg
   $Vh = 2$ mL
   $Dd = 1.2$ mg
   $Va = ?$

   $$Va = \frac{Vh \times Dd}{Dh} = \frac{2\,mL \times 1.2\,mg}{6\,mg}$$

   $$= \frac{2.4\,mL}{6} = 0.4\,mL$$

CHAPTER 5

PART 1

MULTIPLE CHOICE

1.	A	*p. 298*	21.	A	*p. 306*
2.	B	*p. 298–299*	22.	E	*p. 306*
3.	C	*p. 299*	23.	C	*p. 307*
4.	A	*p. 299*	24.	C	*p. 307*
5.	C	*p. 298–301*	25.	A	*p. 308*
6.	C	*p. 300*	26.	C	*p. 309*
7.	E	*p. 300*	27.	B	*p. 309*
8.	D	*p. 301*	28.	B	*p. 309*
9.	A	*p. 301*	29.	B	*p. 311*
10.	B	*p. 301*	30.	E	*p. 311*
11.	E	*p. 302*	31.	D	*p. 311*
12.	D	*p. 300, 302*	32.	A	*p. 312*
13.	A	*p. 303*	33.	C	*p. 312*
14.	B	*p. 303*	34.	B	*p. 313*
15.	C	*p. 304*	35.	B	*p. 314*
16.	A	*p. 305*	36.	C	*p. 316*
17.	E	*p. 305*	37.	D	*p. 316*
18.	C	*p. 305*	38.	A	*p. 316*
19.	C	*pp. 305–306*	39.	A	*p. 320*
20.	B	*p. 306*	40.	E	*pp. 318–320*

SPECIAL PROJECT

LABEL THE DIAGRAM

A. Tonsil
B. Tongue
C. Vallecula
D. Epiglottis
E. Vocal cords
F. Trachea
G. Cricoid cartilage
H. Esophagus

AIRWAY OBSTRUCTION

1. The tongue. In the absence of muscle tone, the relaxed tongue drops back in the larynx, blocking the airway.
2. Foreign body. An object, usually food, becomes lodged in the laryngopharynx and blocks the airway.
3. Trauma. Trauma may disrupt the integrity of the airway, thereby allowing it to collapse or physically blocking the airway. Additionally, loose teeth or blood clots may obstruct the airway.
4. Laryngeal edema or spasm. Swelling of the laryngeal tissue may occlude the airway, or spasm of the vocal cords may occur secondary to intubation attempts.
5. Aspiration. The inhalation of teeth, dentures, blood, food, or vomitus may obstruct the airway.

NORMAL RESPIRATORY VALUES

% Oxygen:	21% in inspired air; 14% in expired air
PaO_2:	80–100 torr
% Carbon Dioxide:	0.04% in inspired air; 5% in expired air
$PaCP_2$:	35–45 torr

NORMAL RESPIRATORY RATES/VOLUMES

Infant:	40 to 60
Child:	18 to 24
Adult:	12 to 20

Tidal volume:	500 mL
Alveolar volume:	350 mL
Dead space volume:	150 mL
Minute volume:	3,000 to 5,000 mL

PART 2

MULTIPLE CHOICE

1.	A	*p. 321*	9.	D	*pp. 326–327*
2.	D	*p. 321*	10.	A	*p. 327*
3.	A	*p. 322*	11.	C	*p. 327*
4.	B	*p. 323*	12.	E	*p. 328*
5.	B	*p. 324*	13.	B	*p. 328*
6.	E	*p. 325*	14.	A	*pp. 328–329*
7.	B	*pp. 325–326*	15.	D	*p. 329*
8.	D	*p. 326*			

SPECIAL PROJECT

TABLE 5–5 | Basic Rules of Capnography	
Symptom	**Possible Cause**
Sudden drop of $ETCO_2$ to zero	• Esophageal intubation • Ventilator disconnection or defect in ventilator • Defect in CO_2 analyzer
Sudden decrease of $ETCO_2$ (not to zero)	• Leak in ventilator system; obstruction • Partial disconnect in ventilator circuit • Partial airway obstruction (secretions)
Exponential decrease of $ETCO_2$	• Pulmonary embolism • Cardiac arrest • Hypotension (sudden) • Severe hyperventilation
Change in CO_2 baseline	• Calibration error • Water droplet in analyzer • Mechanical failure (ventilator)
Sudden increase in $ETCO_2$	• Accessing an area of lung previously obstructed • Release of tourniquet • Sudden increase in blood pressure
Gradual lowering of $ETCO_2$	• Hypovolemia • Decreasing cardiac output • Decreasing body temperature; hypothermia; drop in metabolism
Gradual increase in $ETCO_2$	• Rising body temperature • Hypoventilation • CO_2 absorption • Partial airway obstruction (foreign body); reactive airway disease

PART 3

MULTIPLE CHOICE

1.	D	*p. 330*	19.	B	*p. 342*
2.	B	*pp. 330–331*	20.	D	*p. 342*
3.	C	*p. 331*	21.	A	*p. 342*
4.	E	*p. 333*	22.	B	*p. 345–346*
5.	A	*p. 334*	23.	B	*p. 349–350*
6.	D	*p. 334*	24.	C	*p. 351*
7.	E	*p. 336*	25.	C	*p. 359*
8.	B	*p. 337*	26.	A	*p. 359*
9.	C	*p. 337*	27.	B	*p. 362*
10.	C	*p. 338*	28.	A	*p. 362*
11.	C	*p. 338*	29.	A	*p. 365*
12.	B	*p. 338*	30.	E	*p. 365*
13.	A	*pp. 338–339*	31.	B	*pp. 367–368*
14.	A	*p. 339*	32.	D	*p. 368*
15.	A	*p. 339*	33.	A	*p. 368*
16.	B	*p. 339*	34.	B	*p. 370*
17.	E	*p. 341*	35.	D	*p. 371*
18.	B	*p. 341*			

SPECIAL PROJECT

PROBLEM SOLVING: AIRWAY MAINTENANCE

1. suction, laryngoscope, stylet, tape, stethoscope, endotracheal tube, 10-mL syringe, water-soluble gel, Magill forceps, Standard Precautions
2. Laryngoscope: Check blade—bright white and nonflickering light. Tube cuff: Inflate with 10 mL of air using syringe. Does cuff hold air? Endotracheal tube: Have one larger and one smaller tube available.
3. Ventilate the patient.
4. Fill syringe with 10 to 15 mL of air. Position the patient's head. Grasp the laryngoscope handle in the left hand. Insert blade in the right side of the patient's mouth. Displace tongue to left. Insert blade to the epiglottis. Lift laryngoscope along axis of handle. Visualize the vocal folds and glottis. Grasp tube and pass it between the cords. Inflate the cuff and auscultate.
5. Visualize with the laryngoscope the tube passing through the cords. Check the depth of the tube against the mouth. Auscultate all lung fields for bilaterally equal breath sounds. Auscultate the epigastrium for gurgling sounds. Employ capnography; observe for chest rise.
6. If the tube is placed in the esophagus, remove it, ventilate the patient, and attempt to place another tube in the trachea. Re-auscultate and assure the new tube is properly placed.

PART 4

MULTIPLE CHOICE

1.	D	*p. 374*	6.	B	*p. 377*
2.	E	*p. 374*	7.	C	*p. 377*
3.	B	*p. 375*	8.	C	*p. 377*
4.	D	*p. 376*	9.	E	*p. 379*
5.	A	*pp. 376–377*	10.	A	*p. 380*

Paramedic Care: Principles & Practice, Vol. 2, 4th Ed.

TABLE 5–15 | Advantages and Disadvantages of Various Suction Types

Type	Advantages	Disadvantages
Hand-powered	Lightweight, portable, inexpensive, simple to operate	Limited volume, manually powered, fluid contact components are not disposable
Oxygen-powered	Small, lightweight	Limited suction power, uses a lot of oxygen
Battery-operated	Lightweight, portable, excellent suction power, simple to operate and troubleshoot in the field	Battery memory decreases with time; mechanically more complicated than hand-powered, some fluid contact components are not disposable
Mounted	Strong suction, adjustable vacuum power, disposable fluid contact components	Not portable, cannot be serviced in the field, no substitute power source

CONTENT REVIEW ANSWER KEY

Chapter 1: Pathophysiology, Part 1

1. A *p. 6*
2. E *p. 8*
3. D *p. 8*
4. E *p. 9*
5. A *p. 11*

Chapter 1: Pathophysiology, Part 2

6.	D	*p. 15*	11.	A	*p. 26*
7.	B	*p. 23*	12.	B	*p. 28*
8.	D	*p. 23*	13.	A	*p. 29*
9.	B	*p. 26*	14.	A	*p. 29*
10.	C	*p. 26*	15.	C	*p. 26*

Chapter 1: Pathophysiology, Part 3

16.	A	*p. 31*	31.	C	*p. 44*
17.	E	*p. 35*	32.	D	*p. 44*
18.	D	*p. 37*	33.	E	*p. 45*
19.	B	*p. 37*	34.	A	*p. 45*
20.	E	*p. 38*	35.	E	*pp. 45–46*
21.	A	*p. 38*	36.	B	*p. 46*
22.	D	*p. 39*	37.	C	*p. 46*
23.	A	*p. 40*	38.	C	*p. 46*
24.	C	*pp. 40–41*	39.	D	*p. 46*
25.	B	*p. 41*	40.	E	*pp. 47–50*
26.	A	*pp. 41–42*	41.	A	*p. 50*
27.	D	*p. 42*	42.	C	*p. 55*
28.	C	*p. 43*	43.	C	*p. 55*
29.	D	*p. 43*	44.	A	*p. 56*
30.	C	*p. 44*	45.	A	*p. 56*

Chapter 1: Pathophysiology, Part 4

46. B *p. 61*
47. B *p. 61*
48. D *pp. 63–65*
49. B *p. 65*
50. C *p. 65*

Chapter 1: Pathophysiology, Part 5

51.	A	*p. 70*	58.	A	*p. 75*
52.	B	*p. 70*	59.	A	*p. 76*
53.	E	*p. 71*	60.	C	*p. 76*
54.	E	*p. 72*	61.	E	*p. 77*
55.	E	*p. 73*	62.	E	*p. 77*
56.	A	*p. 73*	63.	D	*p. 79*
57.	A	*p. 74*	64.	A	*p. 79*

65.	A	*p. 80*	68.	D	*p. 84*
66.	B	*p. 81*	69.	A	*p. 85*
67.	C	*p. 82*	70.	C	*p. 86*

Chapter 1: Pathophysiology, Part 6

71.	D	*p. 87*	86.	C	*p. 99*
72.	E	*p. 87*	87.	B	*p. 102*
73.	B	*p. 88*	88.	A	*p. 103*
74.	A	*p. 88*	89.	E	*pp. 103–104*
75.	B	*p. 88*	90.	C	*p. 105*
76.	E	*pp. 88–89*	91.	A	*p. 105*
77.	A	*p. 89*	92.	A	*pp. 106–107*
78.	A	*p. 89*	93.	C	*p. 107*
79.	D	*p. 90*	94.	C	*p. 109*
80.	B	*p. 91*	95.	B	*p. 110*
81.	D	*p. 92*	96.	E	*p. 112*
82.	B	*p. 92*	97.	E	*p. 113*
83.	B	*pp. 98–99*	98.	B	*p. 114*
84.	A	*p. 99*	99.	A	*p. 114*
85.	A	*p. 99*	100.	A	*p. 114*

Chapter 2: Human Life Span Development

101.	C	*p. 122*	109.	A	*p. 127*
102.	A	*p. 122*	110.	E	*p. 128*
103.	A	*p. 123*	111.	C	*p. 129*
104.	B	*p. 123*	112.	C	*p. 130*
105.	C	*pp. 123,124*	113.	D	*p. 130*
106.	C	*p. 125*	114.	E	*pp. 131–132*
107.	A	*pp. 125–126*	115.	E	*p. 131*
108.	B	*p. 127*			

Chapter 3: Emergency Pharmacology, Part 1

116.	D	*pp. 139–140*	131.	B	*p. 151*
117.	C	*pp. 139–140*	132.	B	*p. 151*
118.	E	*p. 140*	133.	B	*p. 151*
119.	C	*p. 140*	134.	D	*p. 151*
120.	D	*p. 141*	135.	B	*p. 151*
121.	D	*p. 142*	136.	D	*p. 152*
122.	A	*p. 142*	137.	E	*p. 152*
123.	E	*p. 144*	138.	A	*p. 152*
124.	B	*p. 145*	139.	C	*p. 152–153*
125.	B	*p. 146*	140.	A	*pp. 153*
126.	D	*p. 146*	141.	E	*p. 153*
127.	E	*p. 147*	142.	B	*p. 154*
128.	C	*p. 147*	143.	E	*p. 154*
129.	B	*p. 150*	144.	A	*p. 154*
130.	E	*pp. 150–151*	145.	D	*p. 155*

Chapter 3: Emergency Pharmacology, Part 2

146.	A	*p. 156*	171.	A	*pp. 187–188*
147.	B	*p. 156*	172.	D	*p. 188*
148.	C	*p. 156*	173.	C	*p. 193*
149.	A	*p. 159*	174.	C	*p. 194*
150.	A	*p. 159*	175.	C	*p. 194*
151.	E	*p. 164*	176.	A	*p. 194*
152.	A	*p. 167*	177.	B	*p. 198*
153.	E	*p. 168*	178.	D	*p. 198*
154.	C	*p. 168*	179.	C	*p. 200*
155.	A	*p. 168*	180.	B	*p. 200*
156.	C	*p. 170*	181.	C	*p. 200*
157.	A	*p. 171*	182.	A	*p. 200*
158.	E	*p. 172*	183.	D	*p. 201*
159.	C	*p. 172*	184.	D	*p. 202*
160.	A	*p. 173*	185.	C	*p. 203*
161.	D	*p. 173*	186.	A	*p. 203*
162.	C	*p. 173*	187.	A	*p. 205*
163.	D	*p. 174*	188.	B	*p. 205*
164.	E	*p. 177*	189.	E	*p. 206*
165.	D	*p. 181*	190.	D	*p. 208*
166.	A	*p. 181*	191.	A	*p. 210*
167.	C	*p. 182*	192.	C	*p. 210*
168.	E	*pp. 181–182*	193.	C	*p. 212*
169.	C	*p. 182*	194.	E	*p. 215*
170.	A	*p. 186*	195.	A	*p. 216*

Chapter 4: Intravenous Access and Medication Administration, Part 1

196.	C	*p. 230*	211.	A	*p. 243*
197.	A	*p. 230*	212.	A	*p. 243*
198.	D	*p. 232*	213.	B	*p. 244*
199.	E	*p. 232*	214.	B	*p. 244*
200.	C	*p. 233*	215.	A	*p. 245*
201.	D	*p. 236*	216.	E	*p. 247*
202.	B	*p. 236*	217.	D	*p. 247*
203.	A	*p. 237*	218.	B	*p. 249*
204.	A	*p. 238*	219.	A	*p. 249*
205.	B	*p. 238*	220.	B	*p. 251*
206.	D	*p. 238*	221.	C	*pp. 251–252*
207.	E	*p. 238*	222.	C	*pp. 251–252*
208.	A	*p. 238*	223.	E	*pp. 251–252*
209.	A	*p. 240*	224.	D	*pp. 251–253*
210.	E	*p. 242*	225.	B	*p. 254*

Chapter 4: Intravenous Access and Medication Administration, Part 2

226.	B	*pp. 254–255*	239.	E	*p. 262*
227.	B	*p. 255*	240.	A	*pp. 262–263*
228.	C	*p. 255*	241.	A	*p. 265*
229.	B	*p. 256*	242.	C	*pp. 265–266*
230.	D	*p. 256*	243.	E	*pp. 267–268*
231.	C	*p. 257*	244.	A	*p. 269*
232.	B	*p. 258*	245.	B	*p. 269*
233.	A	*p. 258*	246.	D	*p. 269*
234.	C	*p. 259*	247.	D	*p. 273*
235.	B	*p. 260*	248.	E	*p. 275*
236.	C	*p. 261*	249.	B	*p. 276*
237.	A	*p. 261*	250.	B	*p. 276*
238.	A	*p. 262*	251.	A	*p. 276*

252.	D	*p. 277*	254.	E	*pp. 280–283*
253.	A	*p. 277*	255.	A	*p. 283*

Chapter 4: Intravenous Access and Medication Administration, Part 3

256.	D	*p. 287*
257.	C	*pp. 287–288*
258.	E	*p. 288*
259.	C	*p. 289*
260.	C	*p. 290*

Chapter 5: Airway Management and Ventilation, Part 1

261.	A	*p. 299*	274.	D	*p. 306*
262.	D	*pp. 298–302*	275.	E	*p. 307*
263.	A	*p. 301*	276.	C	*p. 307*
264.	B	*p. 301*	277.	C	*p. 309*
265.	A	*p. 301*	278.	B	*p. 311*
266.	A	*p. 302*	279.	B	*p. 311*
267.	B	*p. 302*	280.	B	*p. 312*
268.	B	*p. 303*	281.	D	*p. 314*
269.	B	*p. 303*	282.	E	*pp. 314–315*
270.	A	*p. 303*	283.	E	*p. 315*
271.	D	*p. 305*	284.	C	*pp. 318–319*
272.	A	*p. 305*	285.	B	*p. 320*
273.	D	*p. 306*			

Chapter 5: Airway Management and Ventilation, Part 2

286.	A	*p. 321*	291.	B	*pp. 326–327*
287.	B	*p. 321*	292.	A	*p. 328*
288.	C	*pp. 323–324*	293.	C	*p. 328*
289.	D	*p. 324*	294.	E	*p. 329*
290.	A	*p. 325*	295.	C	*p. 327*

Chapter 5: Airway Management and Ventilation, Part 3

296.	C	*p. 330*	309.	A	*p. 349*
297.	B	*p. 333*	310.	E	*pp. 349–350*
298.	E	*pp. 333–334*	311.	C	*pp. 349–350*
299.	B	*p. 336*	312.	A	*p. 352*
300.	E	*p. 337*	313.	A	*p. 356*
301.	A	*p. 339*	314.	A	*p. 359*
302.	C	*p. 339*	315.	D	*pp. 359–360*
303.	C	*pp. 339–340*	316.	B	*p. 362*
304.	E	*pp. 341–342*	317.	A	*p. 364*
305.	B	*p. 342*	318.	C	*p. 368*
306.	A	*pp. 342–345*	319.	B	*p. 368*
307.	E	*pp. 345–346*	320.	A	*p. 369*
308.	A	*p. 346*			

Chapter 5: Airway Management and Ventilation, Part 4

321.	E	*p. 374*
322.	A	*p. 375*
323.	A	*p. 377*
324.	D	*p. 379*
325.	A	*p. 380*

©2013 Pearson Education, Inc.
Paramedic Care: Principles & Practice, Vol. 2, 4th Ed.

EMERGENCY DRUG CARDS

The following pages contain prepared cards. Each card represents one of the drugs commonly used by the paramedic. They identify the name and class of the drug, provide a brief description, and note its indications, contraindications, precautions, common dosages, and routes of administration.

Detach and cut out the cards and review each one in detail. Be sure that your instructor identifies which drugs are used in your system and which cards need to be modified to indicate your system's specific indications, contraindications, precautions, doses, and methods of administration. You may also wish to prepare cards for the drugs used in your system that are not included in this card set. Two card templates are included to assist you.

Once your cards are prepared, begin to familiarize yourself with all of the information contained on the card when presented with the drug name. You will notice that the drug name appears on the back of each card. Working on just a few cards each week and then reviewing them as your course progresses will help you commit to memory the essential information you must know about each drug.

Name/Class: ACE INHIBITORS (Enalapril, Captopril, Lisinopril, Ramipril)/Angiotensin-converting enzyme inhibitors.

Description: ACE inhibitors interfere with the development of angiotension, reducing peripheral vascular resistance, blood pressure, and cardiac afterload.

Indications: AMI or heart failure without hypotension; hypertension.

Contraindications: Pregnancy, hypersensitivity to the drug, elevated serum potassium, hypotension (<100 SBP), or hypovolemia; IV form is contraindicated in STEMI.

Precautions: Renal failure.

Dosage/Route: Enalapril—2.5 mg PO, 1.25 mg IV over 5 min (IV form contraindicated in STEMI); Captopril—6.25 mg PO; Lisinopril—5 mg PO; Ramipril—2.5 mg PO.

Name/Class: ACETAMINOPHEN (Tylenol, Anacin-3)/Analgesic, Antipyretic

Description: Acetaminophen is a clinically proven analgesic/antipyretic with little effect on platelet function.

Indications: For mild to moderate pain and fever when aspirin is otherwise not tolerated.

Contraindications: Hypersensitivity, children under 3 years.

Precautions: Patients with hepatic disease, children under 12 years with arthritic conditions, alcoholism, malnutrition, thrombocytopenia.

Dosage/Route: 325 to 650 mg. PO every 4 to 6 hours. 650 mg PR every 4 to 6 hours.

Name/Class: ACTIVATED CHARCOAL (Actidose)/Adsorbent

Description: Activated charcoal is a specially prepared charcoal that will adsorb and bind toxins from the gastrointestinal tract.

Indications: Acute ingested poisoning.

Contraindications: An airway that cannot be controlled; ingestion of cyanide, mineral acids, caustic alkalis, organic solvents, iron, ethanol, methanol.

Precautions: Administer only after emesis or in those cases where emesis is contraindicated.

Dosage/Route: 1 g/kg mixed with at least 6 to 8 oz of water, then PO or via an NG tube.

ACE INHIBITORS

ACETAMINOPHEN

ACTIVATED CHARCOAL

Name/Class: ADENOSINE (Adenocard)/Antidysrhythmic

Description: Adenosine is a naturally occurring agent that can "chemically cardiovert" PSVT to a normal sinus rhythm. It has a half-life of 10 seconds and does not cause hypotension.

Indications: Narrow, complex supraventricular tachycardia refractory to vagal maneuvers.

Contraindications: Hypersensitivity, 2nd- and 3rd-degree heart block, sinus node disease, asthma.

Precautions: It may cause transient dysrhythmias; COPD.

Dosage/Route: 6 mg rapidly (over 1 to 3 sec) IV, then flush the line rapidly with saline. If ineffective, 12 mg in 1 to 2 min, may be repeated. Ped: 0.1 mg/kg to a maximum of 6 mg. (rapidly) IV followed by rapid saline flush, then 0.2 mg/kg in 1 to 2 min to max 2nd dose of 12 mg.

Name/Class: ALBUTEROL (Proventil, Ventolin)/Sympathomimetic Bronchodilator

Description: Albuterol is a synthetic sympathomimetic that causes bronchodilatation with less cardiac effect than epinephrine and reduces mucus secretion, pulmonary capillary leaking, and edema in the lungs during allergic reactions.

Indications: Bronchospasm and asthma in COPD.

Contraindications: Hypersensitivity to the drug.

Precautions: The patient may experience tachycardia, anxiety, nausea, cough, wheezing, and/or dizziness. Vital signs and breath sounds must be monitored; use caution with elderly, cardiac, or hypertensive patients.

Dosage/Route: Two inhalations (90 mcg) via metered dose inhaler (2 sprays) or 2.5 mg in 2.5 to 3 mL NS via nebulizer, repeat as needed. The duration of effect is 3 to 6 hours. Ped: 0.15 mg/kg in 2.5 to 3 mL NS via nebulizer, repeat as needed.

Name/Class: ALTEPLASE RECOMBINANT (tPA) (Activase)/Thrombolytic

Description: Recombinant DNA–derived form of human tPA promotes thrombolysis by forming plasmin. Plasmin, in turn, degrades fibrin and fibrinogen and, ultimately, the clot.

Indications: To thrombolyse in acute myocardial infarction, acute ischemic stroke, and pulmonary embolism.

Contraindications: Active internal bleeding, suspected aortic dissection, traumatic CPR, recent hemorrhagic stroke (6 mo), intracranial or intraspinal surgery or trauma (2 mo), pregnancy, uncontrolled hypertension, hypersensitivity to thrombolytics.

Precautions: Recent major surgery, cerebral vascular disease, recent GI or GU bleeding, recent trauma, hypertension, patient > 75 years, current oral anticoagulants, hemorrhagic ophthalmic conditions.

Dosage/Route: *MI*: 15 mg IV, then 0.75 mg/kg (up to 50 mg) over 30 min, then 0.5 mg/kg (up to 35 mg) over 60 min up to 100 mg. *Stroke*: 0.09 mg/kg over 1 min. then 0.91 mg/kg (up to 90 mg) over next 60 min.

Pulmonary embolism: 100 mg IV infusion over 2 hours.

ADENOSINE

ALBUTEROL

ALTEPLASE RECOMBINANT

Name/Class: AMINOPHYLLINE (Aminophylline, Somophyllin)/Methylxanthine Bronchodilator

Description: Aminophylline is a methylxanthine that prolongs bronchodilation and decreased mucus production and has mild cardiac and CNS stimulating effects.

Indications: Bronchospasm in asthma and COPD refractory to sympathomimetics and other bronchodilators and in CHF.

Contraindications: Hypersensitivity to methylxanthines or uncontrolled cardiac dysrhythmias.

Precautions: Cardiovascular disease, hypertension or taking theophylline, hepatic impairment, diabetes, hyperthyroidism, young children, glaucoma, peptic ulcers, acute influenza or influenza immunization, the elderly. Watch for PVCs or tachycardia. May cause hypotension.

Dosage/Route: 250 to 500 mg IV over 20 to 30 min. Ped: 6 mg/kg over 20 to 30 min. Max 12 mg/kg/day.

Name/Class: AMIODARONE (Cordarone, Pacerone)/Antidysrhythmic

Description: Amiodarone is an antidysrhythmic that prolongs the duration of the action potential and refractory period and relaxes smooth muscles, reducing peripheral vascular resistance and increasing coronary blood flow.

Indications: Life-threatening recurrent ventricular and supraventricular dysrhythmias that have not responded to other antidysrhythmic agents.

Contraindications: Hypersensitivity, cardiogenic shock, severe sinus bradycardia, advanced heart block.

Precautions: Hepatic impairment, pregnancy, nursing mothers, children.

Dosage/Route: *Ventricular fibrillation:* 300 mg IV push, then repeat dose of 150 mg IV push if **needed.** Ped: 5 mg/kg IV/IO, then repeat up to total dose of 15 mg/kg. *Ventricular tachycardia:* 150 to 300 mg IV over 10 min, then 1 mg/min over next 6 hours. Ped: 5 mg/kg IV/IO over 20 to 60 min, then repeat up to total dose of 15 mg/kg.

Name/Class: AMYL NITRITE (Amyl Nitrite)/Vasodilator

Description: Amyl nitrite is a short-acting vasodilator similar to nitroglycerin. Binds with hemoglobin to help biodegrade cyanide.

Indications: Acute cyanide poisoning.

Contraindications: None for acute cyanide poisoning.

Precautions: None.

Dosage/Route: 1 to 2 inhalants. Ped: same as adult.

AMINOPHYLLINE

AMIODARONE

AMYL NITRITE

Name/Class: ANISTREPLASE (APSAC) (Eminase)/Thrombolytic

Description: Anistreplase causes thrombolysis by converting plasminogen into plasmin, which then dissolves the fibrin and fibrinogen of the clot.

Indications: To reduce infarct size in acute MI.

Contraindications: Active internal bleeding, suspected aortic dissection, traumatic CPR, recent hemorrhagic stroke, intracranial or intraspinal surgery or trauma, tumors, pregnancy, hypertension, hypersensitivity to anistreplase or streptokinase.

Precautions: Recent major surgery, cerebral vascular disease, recent GI or GU bleeding, recent trauma, hypertension, patients over 75 years, current oral anticoagulants, hemorrhagic ophthalmic conditions.

Dosage/Route: 30 units IV over 2 to 5 min.

Name/Class: ASPIRIN (Acetylsalicylic Acid) (Alka-Seltzer, Bayer, Empirin, St. Joseph Children's)/Analgesic, Antipyretic, Platelet Inhibitor, Anti-inflammatory

Description: Aspirin inhibits agents that cause the production of inflammation, pain, and fever. It relieves mild to moderate pain by acting on the peripheral nervous system, lowers body temperature in fever, and powerfully inhibits platelet aggregation.

Indications: Chest pain suggestive of an MI.

Contraindications: Hypersensitivity to salicylates, active ulcer disease, asthma.

Precautions: Allergies to other NSAIDs, bleeding disorders, children or teenagers with varicella or influenza-like symptoms.

Dosage/Route: 160 to 325 mg PO (chewable, non-enteric-coated).

Name/Class: ATENOLOL (Tenormin)/Antidysrhythmic, Antihypertensive

Description: Atenolol is a selective beta blocker that reduces the rate and force of cardiac contraction and lowers cardiac output and blood pressure.

Indications: Non-Q-wave MI and unstable angina.

Contraindications: Sinus bradycardia, 2nd- or 3rd-degree heart block, CHF, cardiogenic failure or shock.

Precautions: Asthma, COPD, CHF controlled by digitalis and diuretics.

Dosage/Route: 5 mg slow IV every 5 min. to 15 mg. Ped: 0.8 to 1.5 mg/kg/day PO (max 2 mg/kg/day).

ANISTREPLASE (APSAC)

ASPIRIN

ATENOLOL

Name/Class: ATRACURIUM (Tracrium)/Nondepolarizing Neuromuscular Blocker

Description: Atracurium is a synthetic skeletal muscle relaxant that produces a short-duration neuromuscular blockade.

Indications: To produce skeletal muscle relaxation to facilitate endotracheal intubation and IPPV.

Contraindications: Myasthenia gravis.

Precautions: Asthma, anaphylaxis, cardiovascular or neuromuscular disease, electrolyte or acid-base imbalance, dehydration, pulmonary impairment.

Dosage/Route: 0.4 to 0.5 mg/kg IV. Ped: < 2 years 0.3 to 0.4 mg/kg, otherwise same as adult.

Name/Class: ATROPINE/Parasympatholytic

Description: Atropine blocks the parasympathetic nervous system, specifically the vagal effects on heart rate. It does not increase contractility but may increase myocardial oxygen demand. Decreases airway secretions.

Indications: Hemodynamically significant bradycardia and organophosphate poisoning.

Contraindications: None in the emergency setting.

Precautions: AMI, glaucoma, hypothermic bradycardia.

Dosage/Route: *Symptomatic bradycardia*:
0.5 mg IV. Repeat 3 to 5 min to 3 mg. Ped: 0.02 mg/kg IV, 0.04 to 0.06 mg/kg ET, may repeat IV dose once up to 1 mg for child or 3 mg for adolescent. Organophosphate poisoning: 2 to 5 mg IV/IM/IO/10 to 15 min. Ped: 0.05 mg/kg IV/IM/IO/ 10 to 15 min.

Organophosphate poisoning: 2 to 4 mg IV/IO or higher may be needed. Ped: <12 years_0.02–0.05 mg/kg IV/IO, may repeat every 20 to 30 minutes as needed. >12 years—2 mg IV/IO, may repeat 1to 2 mg IV/IO every 20 to 30 minutes as needed.

Name/Class: BUMETANIDE (Bumex)/Loop Diuretic

Description: Bumetanide is related to furosemide, though it has a faster rate of onset, a greater diuretic potency (40 times), shorter duration, and produces only mild hypotension.

Indications: To promote diuresis in CHF and pulmonary edema.

Contraindications: Hypersensitivity to bumetanide and other sulfonamides.

Precautions: Pregnancy (use only for life-threatening conditions).

Dosage/Route: 0.5 to 1 mg IM/IV over 1 to 2 min, repeat in 2 to 3 hours as needed.

ATRACURIUM

ATROPINE

BUMETANIDE

Name/Class: BUTORPHANOL (Stadol)/Synthetic Narcotic Analgesic

Description: Butorphanol is a centrally acting synthetic narcotic analgesic about 5 times more potent than morphine. A schedule IV narcotic.

Indications: Moderate to severe pain.

Contraindications: Hypersensitivity, head injury, undiagnosed abdominal pain.

Precautions: May cause withdrawal in narcotic-dependent patients.

Dosage/Route: 1 mg IV or 3 to 4 mg IM over 3 to 4 hours.

Name/Class: CALCIUM CHLORIDE (Calcium Chloride)/Electrolyte

Description: Calcium chloride increases myocardial contractile force and increases ventricular automaticity.

Indications: Hyperkalemia, hypocalcemia, hypermagnesemia, calcium channel blocker toxicity.

Contraindications: Ventricular fibrillation, hypercalcemia, possible digitalis toxicity.

Precautions: It may precipitate toxicity in patients taking digoxin. Ensure the IV line is in a large vein and flushed before using and after calcium.

Dosage/Route: 500 to 1,000 mg IV (5 to 10 mL of 10% solution) as needed. Ped: 20 mg/kg IV/IO, as needed.

Name/Class: CALCIUM GLUCONATE (Kalcinate)/Electrolyte

Description: Calcium gluconate increases myocardial contractile force and increases ventricular automaticity. It is more potent than calcium chloride.

Indications: Hyperkalemia, hypermagnesemia, calcium channel blocker toxicity.

Contraindications: Ventricular fibrillation.

Precautions: It may precipitate toxicity in patients taking digitalis, with renal or cardiac insufficiency, and immobilized patients.

Dosage/Route: 15 to 30 mL of 10% solution, repeated as necessary. Ped: 60 to 100 mg/kg (0.61 mL) slow IV/IO push, may repeat.

BUTORPHANOL

CALCIUM CHLORIDE

CALCIUM GLUCONATE

Name/Class: CHLORDIAZEPOXIDE (Librium)/Sedative, Hypnotic

Description: Chlordiazepoxide is a benzodiazepine derivative that produces mild sedation and anticonvulsant, skeletal muscle relaxant, and prolonged hypnotic effects.

Indications: Severe anxiety and tension, acute alcohol withdrawal symptoms (DTs).

Contraindications: Hypersensitivity to benzodiazepines, pregnant and nursing mothers, children under 6.

Precautions: Primary depressive disorders or psychoses, acute alcohol intoxication.

Dosage/Route: 50 to 100 mg IV/IM.

Name/Class: CHLORPROMAZINE (Thorazine)/Tranquilizer, Antipsychotic

Description: Chlorpromazine is a phenothiazine derivative used to manage psychotic episodes by providing strong sedation and moderate extrapyramidal symptoms. Produces reduced initiative, interest, and affect.

Indications: Acute psychotic episode, intractable hiccups, nausea/vomiting.

Contraindications: Hypersensitivity to phenothiazines, coma, sedative overdose, acute alcohol withdrawal, children < 6 months.

Precautions: Agitated states with depression, seizure disorders, respiratory infection or COPD, glaucoma, diabetes, hypertension, peptic ulcer, prostatic hypertrophy, breast cancer, thyroid impairment, cardiovascular impairment, hepatic impairment, patients exposed to extreme heat or organophosphates.

Dosage/Route: 25 to 50 mg IM. Ped: 0.5 mg/kg IM or 1 mg/kg PR.

Name/Class: CLOPIDOGREL (Plavix)/Anti-platelet agent

Description: Clopidogrel inhibits platelet aggregation and prolongs clotting time.

Indications: ST segment depression MI (Non-STEMI) and dynamic T wave inversion and for MI and stroke patients who cannot tolerate aspirin.

Contraindications: Hypersensitivity to the drug, pathologic bleeding or bleeding risk.

Precautions: Liver disease, pregnancy.

Dosage/Route: 300 to 600 mg PO.

CHLORDIAZEPOXIDE

CHLORPROMAZINE

CLOPIDOGREL

Name/Class: DEXAMETHASONE (Decadron)/Steroid

Description: Dexamethasone is a long-acting synthetic adrenocorticoid with intense anti-inflammatory activity. It prevents the accumulation of inflammation generating cells at the sites of infection or injury.

Indications: Anaphylaxis, asthma, COPD, spinal cord edema.

Contraindications: No absolute contraindications in the emergency setting. Relative contraindications: systemic fungal infections, acute infections, tuberculosis, varicella, vaccine or live virus vaccinations.

Precautions: Herpes simplex, keratitis, myasthenia gravis, hepatic or renal impairment, diabetes, CHF, seizures, psychic disorders, hypothyroidism, GI ulceration.

Dosage/Route: 4 to 24 mg IV/IM. Ped: 0.5 to 1 mg/kg.

Name/Class: DEXTROSE 50% IN WATER (D$_{50}$W)/Carbohydrate

Description: Dextrose is a simple sugar that the body can rapidly metabolize to create energy.

Indications: Hypoglycemia.

Contraindications: None in hypoglycemia.

Precautions: Increased ICP. Determine blood glucose level before administration. Ensure good venous access.

Dosage/Route: 25g D$_{50}$W (50 mL) IV. Ped: 2 to 4 mL/kg of a 25% solution IV.

Name/Class: DIAZEPAM (Valium)/Antianxiety, Hypnotic, Anticonvulsant, Sedative

Description: Diazepam is a benzodiazepine sedative and skeletal muscle relaxant that reduces tremors, induces amnesia, and reduces the incidence and recurrence of seizures. It relaxes muscle spasms in orthopedic injuries and produces amnesia for painful procedures (cardioversion).

Indications: Major motor seizures, status epilepticus, premedication before cardioversion, muscle tremors due to injury, acute anxiety.

Contraindications: Hypersensitivity to the drug, shock, coma, acute alcoholism, depressed vital signs, obstetric patients, neonates.

Precautions: Psychoses, depression, myasthenia gravis, hepatic or renal impairment, addiction, elderly or very ill patients, COPD. Due to a short half-life of the drug, seizure activity may recur.

Dosage/Route: *Seizures*: 5 to 10 mg IV/IM. Ped: 0.5 to 2 mg IV/IM.

Acute anxiety: 2 to 5 mg IV/IM. Ped: 0.5 to 2 mg IM.

Premedication: 5 to 15 mg IV. Ped: 0.2 to 0.5 mg/kg IV.

DEXAMETHASONE

DEXTROSE 50% IN WATER (D$_{50}$W)

DIAZEPAM

Name/Class: DIAZOXIDE (Hyperstat)/Antihypertensive

Description: Diazoxide is a rapid-acting thiazide nondiuretic hypotensive and hyperglycemia agent that reduces BP and peripheral vascular resistance.

Indications: Rapidly decreases BP in hypertensive crisis.

Contraindications: Hypersensitivity to thiazides, cerebral bleeding, eclampsia, significant coronary artery disease.

Precautions: Diabetes, impaired cerebral or cardiac circulation, renal impairment, corticosteroid or progesterone therapy, gout, uremia.

Dosage/Route: 1 to 3 mg/kg IV up to 150 mg, repeated/5 to 15 min, as needed. Ped: same as adult.

Name/Class: DIGOXIN (Digoxin, Lanoxin)/Cardiac Glycoside

Description: Digoxin is a rapid-acting cardiac glycoside used in the treatment of CHF and rapid atrial dysrhythmias. It increases the force and velocity of myocardial contraction and cardiac output. It also decreases conduction through the AV node, thus decreasing heart rate.

Indications: Increase cardiac output in CHF and to stabilize supraventricular tachydysrhythmias.

Contraindications: Hypersensitivity, ventricular fibrillation, ventricular tachycardia except due to CHF.

Precautions: Reduce dosage if digitoxin taken within 2 weeks. Toxicity potentiated by an MI and with hypokalemia, hypocalcemia, advanced heart disease, incomplete heart block, cor pulmonale, hyperthyroidism, respiratory impairment, children, elderly or debilitated patients, hypomagnesemia.

Dosage/Route: 0.004 to 0.006 mg/kg (4 to 6 mcg/kg) over 5 min.

Name/Class: DIGOXIN IMMUNE FAB (Digibind)/Antidote

Description: Digoxin immune FAB is comprised of fragments of antibodies specific for digoxin (and effective for digitoxin) and prevents the drug from binding to receptor sites.

Indications: Life-threatening digoxin or digitoxin toxicity.

Contraindications: Hypersensitivity to sheep products and renal or cardiac failure.

Precautions: Patients with prior sheep or bovine antibody fragments, renal impairment, allergies.

Dosage/Route: Dose dependent upon patient digoxin or digitoxin levels.

DIAZOXIDE

DIGOXIN

DIGOXIN IMMUNE FAB

Name/Class: DILTIAZEM (Cardizem)/Calcium Channel Blocker

Description: Diltiazem is a slow calcium channel blocker similar to verapamil. It dilates coronary and peripheral arteries and arterioles, thus increasing circulation to the heart and reducing peripheral vascular resistance.

Indications: Supraventricular tachydysrhythmias (atrial fibrillation, atrial flutter, and PSVT refractory to adenosine) and to increase coronary artery perfusion in angina.

Contraindications: Hypersensitivity, sick sinus syndrome, 2nd- or 3rd-degree heart block, systolic BP < 90, diastolic BP < 60, wide-complex tachycardia and WPW.

Precautions: CHF (especially with beta blockers), conduction abnormalities, renal or hepatic impairment, the elderly, nursing mothers.

Dosage/Route: 0.25 mg/kg (15 to 20 mg) IV over 2 min, may repeat in 15 min with 0.35 mg/kg (20 to 25 mg) over 2 min.

Name/Class: DIMENHYDRINATE (Dramamine)/Antihistamine

Description: Dimenhydrinate is related to diphenhydramine though it is most frequently used for the prevention and treatment of motion sickness and vertigo rather than any antihistamine properties.

Indications: To relieve nausea/vomiting associated with motion sickness and narcotic use.

Contraindications: None in the emergency setting.

Precautions: Seizure disorders and asthma.

Dosage/Route: 12.5 to 25 mg IV; 50 mg IM/4 hours as needed. Ped: 1.25 mg/kg/4 hours up to 300 mg/day.

Name/Class: DIMERCAPROL (BAL in Oil)/Antidote

Description: Dimercaprol is a dithiol compound that combines with the ions of various heavy metals to form nontoxic compounds that can be excreted.

Indications: Antidote for acute arsenic, mercury, lead, and gold poisoning.

Contraindications: Hepatic and severe renal impairment and poisonings due to cadmium, iron, selenium, and uranium.

Precautions: Hypertensive patients.

Dosage/Route: *Gold and arsenic:* 2.5 to 3 mg/kg IM. Ped: same as adult.

Mercury: 5 mg/kg IM. Ped: same as adult.

Lead: 4 mg/kg IM. Ped: same as adult.

DILTIAZEM

DIMENHYDRINATE

DIMERCAPROL

Name/Class: DIPENHYDRAMINE (Benadryl)/Antihistamine

Description: Diphenhydramine blocks histamine release, thereby reducing bronchoconstriction, vasodilation, and edema.

Indications: Anaphylaxis, allergic reactions, and dystonic reactions.

Contraindications: Asthma and other lower respiratory diseases.

Precautions: May induce hypotension, headache, palpitations, tachycardia, sedation, drowsiness, and/or disturbed coordination.

Dosage/Route: 25 to 50 mg IV/IM. Ped: 2 to 5 mg/kg.

Name/Class: DOBUTAMINE (Dobutrex)/Sympathomimetic

Description: Dobutamine is a synthetic catecholamine and beta agent that increases the strength of cardiac contraction without appreciably increasing rate.

Indications: To increase cardiac output in congestive heart failure/cardiogenic shock.

Contraindications: Hypersensitivity to sympathomimetic amines, ventricular tachycardia, hypovolemia without fluid resuscitation.

Precautions: Atrial fibrillation or preexisting hypertension.

Dosage/Route: 2 to 20 mcg/kg/min IV titrated to effect. Ped: same as adult.

Name/Class: DOPAMINE (Intropin)/Sympathomimetic

Description: Dopamine is a naturally occurring catecholamine that increases cardiac output without appreciably increasing myocardial oxygen consumption. It maintains renal and mesenteric blood flow while inducing vasoconstriction and increasing systolic blood pressure.

Indications: Nonhypovolemic hypotension (70 to 100 mmHg) and cardiogenic shock.

Contraindications: Hypovolemic hypotension without aggressive fluid resuscitation, tachydysrhythmias, ventricular fibrillation, pheochromocytoma.

Precautions: Occlusive vascular disease, cold injury, arterial embolism. Ensure adequate fluid resuscitation of the hypovolemic patient.

Dosage/Route: 2 to 20 mcg/kg/min, IV, titrated to effect. Ped: same as adult.

DIPHENHYDRAMINE

DOBUTAMINE

DOPAMINE

Name/Class: DROPERIDOL (Inapsine)/Antiemetic

Description: Droperidol is related to haloperidol and antagonizes the emetic properties of morphine-like analgesics. It may also produce hypotension and mild sedation.

Indications: Nausea and vomiting (second line), to produce a tranquilizing effect, and in some cases as an antipsychotic.

Contraindications: Intolerance.

Precautions: Elderly and debilitated patients; hypotension; hepatic, renal, or cardiac impairment; Parkinson's disease.

Dosage/Route: 2.5 to 10 mg IV. Ped: 0.088 to 0.165 mg/kg IV.

Name/Class: ENOXAPARIN (Lovenox)/Anticoagulant

Description: Enoxaparin is a heparin derivative that prevents the conversion of fibrinogen to fibrin.

Indications: To inhibit clot formation in unstable angina and non-Q-wave myocardial infarction.

Contraindications: Hypersensitivity to the drug, pork products, or heparin; major active bleeding; thrombocytopenia.

Precautions:

Dosage/Route: *Unstable angina and non-Q-wave MI:* 1 mg/kg subcutaneously.

Pulmonary embolism: 0.5 mg/kg IV.

Name/Class: EPINEPHRINE (Adrenalin)/Sympathomimetic

Description: Epinephrine is a naturally occurring catecholamine that increases heart rate, cardiac contractile force myocardial electrical activity, systemic vascular resistance, and systolic blood pressure and decreases overall airway resistance and automaticity. It also, through bronchial artery constriction, may reduce pulmonary congestion and increase tidal volume and vital capacity.

Indications: To restore rhythm in cardiac arrest and severe allergic reactions.

Contraindications: Hypersensitivity to sympathomimetic amines, narrow-angle glaucoma; hemorrhagic, traumatic, or cardiac shock; coronary insufficiency; dysrhythmias; organic brain or heart disease; during labor.

Precautions: Elderly or debilitated patients, hypertension, diabetes, hyperthyroidism, Parkinson's disease, tuberculosis, asthma, emphysema, children < 6 years.

Dosage/Route: *Arrest:* 1 mg of 1:10,000 IV every 3 to 5 min (ET: 2 to 2.5 mg diluted in 10 mL NS). Ped: 0.01 mg/kg (0.1 mL/kg) 1:10,000 IV/IO every 3 to 5 min. (ET: 0.1 mg/kg 1:1,000). *Allergic reactions:* 0.3 to 0.5 mg of 1:1,000 SQ/IM every 5 to 15 min as needed or 0.5 to 1 mg of 1:10,000 IV if subcutaneous dose ineffective or severe reaction. Ped: 0.01 mg/kg of 1:1,000 subcutaneously every 10 to 15 min or 0.01 mg/kg of 1:10,000 IV if subcutaneous dose ineffective or severe.

DROPERIDOL

ENOXAPARIN

EPINEPHRINE

Name/Class: ESMOLOL (Brevibloc)/Beta Blocker

Description: Esmolol is an ultra-short-acting cardioselective beta blocker that inhibits the actions of the catecholamines.

Indications: Supraventricular tachycardias with rapid ventricular responses.

Contraindications: Cardiac failure, 2nd- and 3rd-degree block, sinus bradycardia, cardiogenic shock.

Precautions: Allergies or bronchial asthma, emphysema, CHF, diabetes, renal impairment.

Dosage/Route: 20 to 100 mcg/kg/min IV for 1 min, loading dose, then 50 mcg/kg/min over 4 min. If unsuccessful, repeat loading dose over 4 min, then 100 mcg/kg/min over 4 min.

Name/Class: ETOMIDATE (Amidate)/Hypnotic

Description: Etomidate is an ultra-short-acting nonbarbiturate hypnotic with no analgesic effects and limited cardiovascular and respiratory effects.

Indications: Induce sedation for rapid sequence intubation.

Contraindications: Hypersensitivity.

Precautions: Marked hypotension, severe asthma, severe cardiovascular disease.

Dosage/Route: 0.1 to 0.3 mg/kg IV over 15 to 30 sec. Ped: 0.2 to 0.4 mg/kg IV/IO over 30 to 60 sec. Max 20 mg.

Name/Class: FENTANYL (Sublimaze)/Narcotic Analgesic

Description: Fentanyl is a potent synthetic narcotic analgesic similar to morphine and meperidine but with a more rapid and less-prolonged action.

Indications: Induce sedation for endotracheal intubation/moderate to severe pain.

Contraindications: MAO inhibitors within 14 days, myasthenia gravis.

Precautions: Increased intracranial pressure, elderly, debilitated, COPD, respiratory problems, hepatic and renal insufficiency.

Dosage/Route: 25 to 100 mcg slowly IV (2 to 3 min). Ped: 2 mcg/kg slow IV/IM.

Name/Class: FLECAINIDE (Tambocor)/Antidysrhythmic

Description: Flecainide is a local anesthetic and antidysrhythmic that slows myocardial conduction and effectively suppresses PVCs and a variety of atrial and ventricular dysrhythmias.

Indications: Atrial flutter, atrial fibrillation, AV re-entrant tachycardia, or SVT associated with WPW syndrome.

Contraindications: Hypersensitivity, 2nd- or 3rd-degree heart block, right bundle branch block with left hemiblock, cardiogenic shock, significant hepatic impairment.

Precautions: CHF, sick sinus syndrome, renal impairment.

Dosage/Route: 100 mg PO/12 hour or 2 mg/kg IV at 10 mg/min. Ped: 1 to 3 mg/kg/day PO in three equal doses (max 8 mg/kg/day).

Name/Class: FLUMAZENIL (Romazicon)/Benzodiazepine Antagonist

Description: Flumazenil is a benzodiazepine antagonist used to reverse the sedative, recall, and psychomotor effects of diazepam, midazolam, and the other benzodiazepines.

Indications: Respiratory depression secondary to the benzodiazepines.

Contraindications: Hypersensitivity to flumazenil or benzodiazepines; those patients who take flumazenil for status epilepticus or seizures; seizure-prone patients during labor and delivery; tricyclic antidepressant overdose.

Precautions: Hepatic impairment, elderly, pregnancy, nursing mothers, head injury, alcohol and drug dependency, physical dependence on benzodiazepines.

Dosage/Route: 0.2 mg IV over 15 sec repeated at 0.3 mg over 30 sec. if no response, then 0.5 mg over 30 sec. every minute to affect or 3 mg.

Name/Class: FOSPHENYTOIN (Cerebyx)/Anticonvulsant

Description: Fosphenytoin is a drug that, once administered, is converted to phenytoin and causes the anticonvulsant properties associated with that drug.

Indications: Seizure control and status epilepticus.

Contraindications: Hypersensitivity, seizures due to hypoglycemia, sinus bradycardia, heart block, Stokes-Adams syndrome, late pregnancy, lactating mothers.

Precautions: Hepatic or renal impairment, alcoholism, hypotension, bradycardia, heart block, severe CAD, diabetes, hyperglycemia, respiratory depression.

Dosage/Route: 15 to 20 mg PE/kg IV given at 100 to 150 mg PE/min (PE = phenytoin equivalent).

FLECAINIDE

FLUMAZENIL

FOSPHENYTOIN

Name/Class: FUROSEMIDE (Lasix)/Diuretic

Description: Furosemide is a rapid-acting, potent diuretic and antihypertensive that inhibits sodium reabsorption by the kidney. Its vasodilating effects reduce venous return and cardiac workload.

Indications: Congestive heart failure and pulmonary edema.

Contraindications: Hypersensitivity to furosemide or the sulfonamides, fluid and electrolyte depletion states, heptic coma, pregnancy (except in life-threatening circumstances).

Precautions: Infants, elderly, hepatic impairment, nephrotic syndrome, cardiogenic shock associated with acute MI, gout, patients receiving digitalis or potassium-depleting steroids.

Dosage/Route: 0.5 to 1.0 mg/kg slowly over 1 to 2 min, if no response give 2 mg/kg slowly over 1 to 2 min.

Name/Class: GLUCAGON (GlucaGen)/Hormone, Antihypoglycemic

Description: Glucagon is a protein secreted by pancreatic cells that causes a breakdown of stored glycogen into glucose and inhibits the synthesis of glycogen from glucose.

Indications: Hypoglycemia without IV access and to reverse beta-blocker overdose.

Contraindications: Hypersensitivity to glucagon or protein compounds.

Precautions: Cardiovascular or renal impairment. Effective only if there are sufficient stores of glycogen in the liver.

Dosage/Route: *Hypoglycemia:* 1 mg IM/SQ repeat every 5 to 20 min. Ped: 0.03 mg/kg IM/SQ.

Beta-blocker overdose: 3 mg IV over 1 min. Ped: 50 to 150 mcg/kg IV over 1 min.

Name/Class: GLYCOPROTEIN IIb/IIIa INHIBITORS: Abciximab (ReoPro), Eptifibatide (Integrilin), Tirofiban (Aggrastat)/Glycoprotein IIb/IIIa Inhibitors

Description: These drugs inhibit glycoprotein receptors on the platelet membrane, inhibiting their aggregation.

Indications: Unstable angina and NSTEMI.

Contraindications: Active bleeding within 30 days or bleeding disorder, intracranial hemorrhage.

Precautions: Current glycoprotein IIb/IIIa inhibitor use.

Dosage/Route: Abciximab 0.25 mg/kg IV; Eptifibatide 180 mcg/kg IV over 1 to 2 minutes; Tirofiban 0.4 mcg/kg per minute for 30 min.

FUROSEMIDE

GLUCAGON

GLYCOPROTEIN IIb/IIIa INHIBITORS

Name/Class: HALOPERIDOL (Haldol)/Antipsychotic

Description: Haloperidol is believed to block dopamine receptors in the brain associated with mood and behavior, is a potent antiemetic, and impairs temperature regulation.

Indications: Acute psychotic episodes.

Contraindications: Parkinson's disease, seizure disorders, coma, alcohol depression, CNS depression, thyrotoxicosis, with other sedatives.

Precautions: Elderly or debilitated patients; urinary retention; glaucoma; severe cardiovascular disease; anticonvulsant, anticoagulant, or lithium therapy.

Dosage/Route: 2 to 10 mg IM. Ped: Children > 3 years, 0.015 to 0.15 mg/kg/day PO in 2 or 3 divided doses.

Name/Class: HEPARIN (Heparin)/Anticoagulant

Description: Heparin is a rapid-onset anticoagulant, enhancing the effects of antithrombin III and blocking the conversion of prothrombin to thrombin and fibrinogen to fibrin.

Indications: To prevent thrombus formation in acute MI.

Contraindications: Hypersensitivity; active bleeding or bleeding tendencies; recent eye, brain, or spinal surgery; shock.

Precautions: Alcoholism, elderly, allergies, indwelling catheters, menstruation, pregnancy, cerebral embolism.

Dosage/Route: 60 IU/kg (max bolus 4,000 IU).

Name/Class: HYDRALAZINE (Apresoline)/Antihypertensive

Description: Hydralazine reduces blood pressure by arterial vasodilation, increasing cardiac output and renal and cerebral blood flow.

Indications: Hypertensive crisis and preeclampsia.

Contraindications: Hypersensitivity, coronary artery or mitral valve disease, AMI, tachydysrhythmias.

Precautions: CVA, renal impairment, and MAO inhibitor use.

Dosage/Route: 20 to 40 mg IV/IM repeated in 4 to 6 hours. Ped: 0.1 to 0.5 mg/kg/day IV/IM.

HALOPERIDOL

HEPARIN

HYDRALAZINE

Name/Class: HYDROCORTISONE (Solu-Cortef)/Steroid

Description: Hydrocortisone is a short-acting synthetic steroid that inhibits histamine formation, storage, and release from mast cells, reducing allergic response.

Indications: Inflammation during allergic reactions, severe anaphylaxis, asthma, COPD.

Contraindications: Hypersensitivity to glucocorticoids.

Precautions: Limited precautions in acute care.

Dosage/Route: 40 to 250 mg IV/IM. Ped: 4 to 8 mg/kg IV/IM divided over 24 hours.

Name/Class: HYDROXYZINE (Vistaril)/Antihistamine

Description: Hydroxyzine is an antihistamine with depressive, sedative, antiemetic, and bronchodilator properties.

Indications: Acute anxiety, nausea/vomiting.

Contraindications: Hypersensitivity.

Precautions: Elderly.

Dosage/Route: *Anxiety*: 50 to 100 mg deep IM. Ped: 1 mg/kg deep IM.

Nausea/vomiting: 25 to 50 mg deep IM. Ped: 1 mg/kg deep IM.

Name/Class: IBUPROFEN (Advil, Motrin, Nuprin, Excedrin IB)/Nonsteroidal Anti-inflammatory Drug (NSAID)

Description: Ibuprofen is the prototype NSAID with significant analgesic and antipyretic properties. It also inhibits platelet aggregation and increases bleeding time.

Indications: Reduce fever and relieve minor to moderate pain.

Contraindications: Sensitivity to aspirin or other NSAIDs, active peptic ulcer, bleeding abnormalities.

Precautions: Hypertension, GI ulceration, hepatic or renal impairment, cardiac decompensation.

Dosage/Route: 200 to 800 mg PO every 4 to 6 hours up to 1,200 mg/day. Ped: 5 to 10 mg/kg PO/4 to 6 hours up to 40 mg/kg/day.

HYDROCORTISONE

HYDROXYZINE

IBUPROFEN

Name/Class: IBUTILIDE (Corvert)/Antidysrhythmic

Description: Ibutilide is a short-acting antidysrhythmic that may convert atrial flutter and fibrillation or may assist with electrical cardioversion.

Indications: Recent onset atrial flutter and fibrillation.

Contraindications: Hypersensitivity, hypokalemia, hypomagnesemia.

Precautions: CHF, low ejection fraction, recent MI, prolonged QT intervals, hepatic impairment, cardiovascular disorder other than atrial dysrhythmias, or drugs that prolong the QT interval, lactation.

Dosage/Route: 1 mg over 10 min IV. Patients < 60 kg, 0.01 mg/kg IV over 10 min., may repeat in 10 min as needed.

Name/Class: INAMRINONE (Inocor)/Cardiac Inotrope

Description: Inamrinone enhances myocardial contractility, increasing output, and reduces systemic vascular resistance.

Indications: To increase cardiac output in CHF or children in septic shock or myocardial dysfunction.

Contraindications: Hypersensitivity to amrinone or bisulfites.

Precautions: CHF immediately after MI (may cause ischemia).

Dosage/Route: CHF: 0.75 mg/kg IV over 2 to 3 min, then drip at 5 to 15 mcg/kg/min titrated to hemodynamic response (may repeat bolus at 30 min).

Septic shock or CHF in peds: 0.75 to 1 mg/kg IV over 5 min, repeated up to 2 times to 3 mg/kg.

Name/Class: INSULIN (Regular Insulin, Humulin, NovoLog, Novolin)/Hormone

Description: Insulin is a naturally occurring protein that promotes the uptake of glucose by the cells.

Indications: Hyperglycemia and diabetic coma.

Contraindications: Hypersensitivity and hypoglycemia.

Precautions:

Dosage/Route: 5 to 10 units IV/IM/SC. Ped: 2 to 4 units IV/IM/SC.

IBUTILIDE

INAMRINONE

INSULIN

Name/Class: IPECAC SYRUP/Emetic

Description: Ipecac syrup is a gastric irritant and acts on the emetic centers of the medulla to induce vomiting. Emesis usually occurs within 5 to 10 minutes.

Indications: Poisoning and overdose.

Contraindications: Reduced level of consciousness, corrosive ingestion, petroleum distillate ingestion, alkali ingestion, antiemetic ingestion (especially phenothiazine).

Precautions: Monitor the airway and have suction ready. Administer activated charcoal only after emesis. Caution with heart disease patients.

Dosage/Route: 30 mL PO, followed by 1 to 2 glasses of water, repeat in 20 min as needed. Ped: 15 mL PO followed by 1 to 2 glasses of water, repeat in 20 min as needed.

Name/Class: IPRATROPIUM (Atrovent)/Anticholinergic

Description: Ipratropium is a bronchodilator used in the treatment of respiratory emergencies that causes bronchial dilation and dries respiratory tract secretions by blocking acetylcholine receptors.

Indications: Bronchospasm associated with asthma, COPD, inhaled irritants.

Contraindications: Hypersensitivity to atropine or its derivatives, or as a primary treatment for acute bronchospasm.

Precautions: Elderly, cardiovascular disease, hypertension.

Dosage/Route: 500 mcg in 2.5 to 3 mL NS via nebulizer or 2 sprays from a metered dose inhaler. Ped: 125 to 250 mcg in 2.5 to 3 mL NS via nebulizer, or 1 or 2 sprays of a metered dose inhaler.

Name/Class: ISOETHARINE (Bronkosol)/Sympathomimetic Bronchodilator

Description: Isoetharine is a synthetic sympathomimetic with rapid onset and prolonged duration that relaxes the bronchial smooth muscles, decreasing airway resistance and helping clear secretions.

Indications: Bronchospasm in asthma and COPD.

Contraindications: Hypersensitivity to or use of sympathomimetic amines, pre-existing tachydysrhythmias, allergy to sodium bisulfite agents.

Precautions: Elderly, hypertension, acute coronary artery disease, CHF, hyperthyroidism, diabetes, tuberculosis, seizures.

Dosage/Route: 1 or 2 sprays via metered dose inhaler, 0.5 mL in 2 to 3 mL saline via nebulizer.

Ped: 0.01 mL/kg of 1% solution (max 0.5 mL) diluted in 2 to 3 mL saline by nebulizer.

IPECAC SYRUP

IPRATROPIUM

ISOETHARINE

Name/Class: KETAMINE (Ketalar)/ Sedative/Hypnotic and Analgesic

Description: Ketamine is a phencyclidine derivative that is unique among sedative, hypnotic, and analgesic agents. It is used as an induction agent for RSI and for sedation. Ketamine has strong amnestic properties.

Indications: Induction agent for rapid sequence induction.

Contraindications: Patients with hypersensitivity to the drug. Significantly elevated blood pressure.

Precautions: Precautions: Hallucinations can occur with emergency, particularly on emergence. Emergency airway and resuscitative equipment and drugs must be available.

Dosage/Route: 1.0 to 4.5 mf/kg IV over 1 min or 0.5 to 13 mg/kg IM one time. Ped: 1.5 mg/kg IV over 1 min. or 4 to 5 mg/kg IM.

Name/Class: KETOROLAC (Toradol)/Nonsteroidal Anti-inflammatory Drug (NSAID)

Description: Ketorolac is an injectable NSAID that exhibits analgesic, anti-inflammatory, and antipyretic properties without sedative effects.

Indications: Mild or moderate pain.

Contraindications: Hypersensitivity to ketorolac, aspirin, or other NSAIDs; asthma.

Precautions: Peptic ulcers, renal or hepatic impairment, elderly.

Dosage/Route: 30 mg IV/IM (15 mg > 65 years or weighs < 50 kg)

Name/Class: LABETALOL (Trandate, Normodyne)/Beta Blocker

Description: Labetalol is a beta blocker with some alpha blocker characteristics. It induces vasodilation, reduces peripheral vascular resistance, and lowers blood pressure.

Indications: Acute hypertensive crisis.

Contraindications: Asthma, CHF, 2nd- and 3rd-degree heart block, severe bradycardia, cardiogenic shock.

Precautions: COPD, heart failure, hepatic impairment, diabetes, peripheral vascular disease.

Dosage/Route: 10 mg slow IV, then 20 to 40 mg/10 min as needed, up to 150 mg OR a bolus of 10 mg, then continuous drip of 2–8 mg/min.

KETAMINE

KETOROLAC

LABETALOL

Name/Class: LIDOCAINE (Xylocaine)/Antidysrhythmic

Description: Lidocaine is an antidysrhythmic that suppresses automaticity and raises stimulation threshold of the ventricles. It also causes sedation, anticonvulsant, and analgesic effects.

Indications: Pulseless ventricular tachycardia, ventricular fibrillation, ventricular tachycardia (w/pulse).

Contraindications: Hypersensitivity to amide-type local anesthetics, supraventricular dysrhythmias, Stokes-Adams syndrome, 2nd- and 3rd-degree heart block, bradycardias.

Precautions: Hepatic or renal impairment, CHF, hypoxia, respiratory depression, hypovolemia, myasthenia gravis, shock, debilitated patients, elderly, family history of malignant hypothermia.

Dosage/Route: *Cardiac arrest:* 1 to 1.5 mg/kg IV/IO repeated at 0.5 to 0.75 every 5 to 10 min up to 3 mg/kg, follow conversion with a drip of 1 to 4 mg/min. Ped: 1 mg/kg IV/IO, to 100 mg, follow conversion with a drip of 20 to 50 mcg/kg/min.

Ventricular tachycardia (w/pulse): 0.5 to 1.5 mg/kg slow IV/IO. May repeat at one-half dose every 5 to 10 min until conversion up to 3 mg/kg. Follow conversion with an infusion of 1 to 4 mg/min. Ped: 1 mg/kg IV/IO, followed by a drip at 20 to 50 mcg/kg/min.

Name/Class: LORAZEPAM (Ativan)/Sedative

Description: Lorazepam is the most potent benzodiazepine available. It has strong antianxiety, sedative, hypnotic, and skeletal muscle relaxant properties, and a relatively short half-life.

Indications: Sedation for cardioversion and status epilepticus.

Contraindications: Sensitivity to benzodiazepines.

Precautions: Narrow-angle glaucoma, depression or psychosis, coma, shock, acute alcohol intoxication, renal or hepatic impairment, organic brain syndrome, myasthenia gravis, GI disorders, elderly, debilitated, limited pulmonary reserve.

Dosage/Route: *Sedation:* 1 to 4 mg IM, 0.5 to 2 mg IV. Ped: 0.03 to 0.5 mg/kg IV/IM/PR up to 4 mg.

Status epilepticus: 2 mg slow IV/PR (2 mg/min). Ped: 0.1 mg/kg slow IV/PR (2 to 5 min).

Name/Class: MAGNESIUM SULFATE (Magnesium)/Electrolyte

Description: Magnesium sulfate is an electrolyte that acts as a calcium channel blocker, acting as a CNS depressant and anticonvulsant. It also depresses the function of smooth, skeletal, and cardiac muscles.

Indications: Torsade de Pointes, eclamptic seizures. In children for status asthmaticus nonresponsive to beta agents.

Contraindications: Heart block, myocardial damage, shock, persistent hypertension, hypocalcemia.

Precautions: Renal impairment, digitalized patients, other CNS depressants, neuromuscular blocking agents.

Dosage/Route: Cardiac Arrest: 1 to 2 g d diluted in 10 mL of D_5W IV/IO. Ped: 25 to 50 mg/kg IV/IO, max dose 2 g.

Torsades: 1 to 2 g diluted in 50 to 100 mL of D_5W over 5 to 60 minutes. Follow with 0.5 to 1. g per hour IV titrated to effect. Ped: 25 to 50 mg/kg IV/IO (max dose 2 g) over 15 to 20 min.

Status Asthmaticus (pediatric only): 25 to 50 mg/kg IV/IO over 15 to 30 min. Max dose 2 g.

Eclampsia: 2 to 4 g IV/IM.

Name/Class: MANNITOL (Osmitrol)/Osmotic Diuretic

Description: Mannitol is an osmotic diuretic that draws water into the intravascular space through its hypertonic effects, then causes diuresis.

Indications: Cerebral edema.

Contraindications: Hypersensitivity, pulmonary edema, CHF, organic CNS disease, intracranial bleeding, shock, renal failure, severe dehydration.

Precautions:

Dosage/Route: 0.5 to 1 g/kg over 5 to 10 min IV. Ped: 50 mcg/kg over 10 to 60 min.

Name/Class: MEPERIDINE (Demerol)/Narcotic Analgesic

Description: Meperidine is a synthetic narcotic with sedative and analgesic properties comparable to morphine but without hemodynamic side effects.

Indications: Moderate to severe pain.

Contraindications: Hypersensitivity, seizure disorders, acute abdomen prior to diagnosis.

Precautions: Increased intracranial pressure, asthma or other respiratory conditions, supraventricular tachycardias, prostatic hypertrophy, urethral stricture, glaucoma, elderly or debilitated patients, renal or hepatic impairment, hypothyroidism, Addison's disease.

Dosage/Route: 25 to 100 mg IV, 50 to 100 mg IM. Ped: 1 mg/kg IV/IM.

Name/Class: METAPROTERENOL (Alupent)/Sympathomimetic Bronchodilator

Description: Metaproterenol is a synthetic sympathomimetic amine, similar to isoproterenol that causes smooth muscle relaxation of the bronchial tree, decreasing airway resistance, facilitating mucus drainage, and increasing vital capacity.

Indications: Bronchospasm, as in asthma and COPD.

Contraindications: Hypersensitivity to sympathomimetic agents, tachydysrhythmias, hyperthyroidism.

Precautions: Elderly, hypertension, coronary artery disease, diabetes.

Dosage/Route: 0.65 mg via metered dose inhaler (2 sprays); 0.2 to 0.3 mL in 2.5 to 3 mL NS via nebulizer. Ped: 0.1 to 0.2 mL/kg (5% solution) in 2.5 to 3 mL NS via nebulizer.

MANNITOL

MEPERIDINE

METAPROTERENOL

Name/Class: METARAMINOL (Aramine)/Sympathomimetic

Description: Metaraminol is a sympathomimetic similar to norepinephrine but less potent, with gradual onset and longer duration. It causes systemic vasoconstriction and increased cardiac contraction strength, increasing blood pressure and reducing flow to the kidneys.

Indications: Hypotension in a normovolemic patient.

Contraindications: Hypovolemia; MAO inhibitor therapy; peripheral or mesenteric thrombosis; pulmonary edema; cardiac arrest; untreated hypoxia, hypercapnia, and acidosis.

Precautions: Digitalized patients, hypertension, thyroid disease, diabetes, hepatic impairment, malaria.

Dosage/Route: 100 mg/500 mL D_5W or NS, titrated to blood pressure: 5 to 10 mg IM.

Name/Class: METHYLPREDNISOLONE (Solu-Medrol)/Corticosteroid, Anti-inflammatory

Description: Methylprednisolone is a synthetic adrenal corticosteroid, effective as an anti-inflammatory and used in the management of allergic reactions and in some cases of shock. It is sometimes used in the treatment of spinal cord injury.

Indications: Spinal cord injury, asthma, severe anaphylaxis, COPD.

Contraindications: No major contraindications in the emergency setting.

Precautions: Only a single dose should be given in the prehospital setting.

Dosage/Route: *Asthma/COPD/anaphylaxis:* 125 to 250 mg IV/IM. Ped: 1 to 2 mg/kg/dose IV/IM.

Spinal cord injury: 30 mg/kg IV over 15 min, after 45 min an infusion of 5.4 mg/kg/hr.

Name/Class: METOCLOPRAMIDE (Reglan)/Antiemetic

Description: Metoclopramide is a dopamine antagonist similar to procainamide but with few antidysrhythmic or anesthetic properties. Its antiemetic properties stem from rapid gastric emptying and desensitization of the vomiting reflex.

Indications: Nausea and vomiting.

Contraindications: Hypersensitivity, allergy to sulfite agents, seizure disorders, pheochromocytoma, mechanical GI obstruction or perforation, breast cancer.

Precautions: CHF, hypokalemia, renal impairment, GI hemorrhage, intermittent porphyria.

Dosage/Route: 10 to 20 mg IM; 10 mg slow IV (over 1 to 2 min). Ped: 1 to 2 mg/kg/dose.

Name/Class: METOPROLOL (Lopressor)/Beta Blocker

Description: Metroprolol is a beta-adrenergic blocking agent that reduces heart rate, cardiac output, and blood pressure.

Indications: AMI.

Contraindications: Cardiogenic shock, sinus bradycardia < 45, 2nd- or 3rd-degree heart block, PR interval > 0.24, cor pulmonale, asthma, COPD.

Precautions: Hypersensitivity, hepatic or renal impairment, cardiomegaly, CHF controlled by digitalis and diuretics, AV conduction defects, thyrotoxicosis, diabetes, peripheral vascular disease.

Dosage/Route: 5 mg slow IV/5 min up to 3 times.

Name/Class: MIDAZOLAM (Versed)/Sedative

Description: Midazolam is a short-acting benzodiazepine with CNS depressant, muscle relaxant, anticonvulsant, and anterograde amnestic effects.

Indications: To induce sedation before cardioversion or intubation.

Contraindications: Hypersensitivity to benzodiazepines, narrow-angle glaucoma, shock, coma, acute alcohol intoxication.

Precautions: COPD, renal impairment, CHF, elderly.

Dosage/Route: 1 to 5.0 mg slow IV; 0.07 to 0.08 mg/kg IM (usually 5 mg). Ped: 0.05 to 0.2 mg/kg IV: 0.1 to 0.15 mg/kg IM; 3 mg intranasal.

Name/Class: MILRINONE (Primacor)/Cardiac Inotrope, Vasodilator

Description: Milrinone is related to amrinone and increases the strength of cardiac contraction without increasing rate, increasing cardiac output without increasing oxygen demand.

Indications: CHF or pediatric septic shock.

Contraindications: Hypersensitivity.

Precautions: Elderly, pregnancy, nursing mothers.

Dosage/Route: *CHF:* 50 mcg/kg IV over 10 min, then a drip of 0.375 to 0.75 mcg/kg/min IV.

Ped: (septic shock) 50 mcg/kg IV/IO over 10 to 60 min., then a drip of 0.25 to 0.75 mcg/kg/min.

METOPROLOL

MIDAZOLAM

MILRINONE

Name/Class: MORPHINE SULFATE (Morphine, Duramorph)/Narcotic Analgesic

Description: Morphine sulfate is a potent analgesic and sedative that causes some vasodilation, reducing venous return, and reduced myocardial oxygen demand.

Indications: Moderate to severe pain and in MI and to reduce venous return in pulmonary edema.

Contraindications: Hypersensitivity to opiates, undiagnosed head or abdominal injury, hypotension or volume depletion, acute bronchial asthma, COPD, severe respiratory depression, pulmonary edema due to chemical inhalation.

Precautions: Elderly, children, debilitated patients. Naloxone should be readily available to counteract the effects of morphine.

Dosage/Route: *MI:* 2 to 4 mg IV/IO every 5 to 15 min *Pain:* 2 to 15 mg IV; 5 to 20 mg.

IM/subcutaneous. Ped: 0.05 to 0.1 mg/kg IV; 0.1 to 0.2 mg/kg IM/subcutaneous.

Name/Class: NALBUPHINE (Nubain)/Narcotic Analgesic

Description: Nalbuphine is a synthetic narcotic analgesic equivalent to morphine, though its respiratory depression does not increase with higher doses.

Indications: Moderate to severe pain.

Contraindications: Hypersensitivity, undiagnosed head or abdominal injury.

Precautions: Impaired respirations, narcotic dependency.

Dosage/Route: 0.4 to 2 mg IV/IO/IM (2 to 2.5 times the dose ET), repeated/2 to 3 min as needed up to 10 mg.

Ped: 0.1 to 2.0 mg/kg IV/IO.

Name/Class: NALOXONE (Narcan)/Narcotic Antagonist

Description: Naloxone is a pure narcotic antagonist that blocks the effects of both natural and synthetic narcotics and may reverse respiratory depression.

Indications: Narcotic and synthetic narcotic overdose, coma of unknown origin.

Contraindications: Hypersensitivity to the drug, non-narcotic-induced respiratory depression.

Precautions: Possible dependency (including newborns). It also has a half-life that is shorter than that of most narcotics; hence the patient may return to the overdose state.

Dosage/Route: 0.4 to 0.4 mg IV/IM (2 to 2.5 times the dose ET) or 0.4 to 0.8 mg IM/SQ repeated every 2 as needed up to 10 mg. Ped: 0.1 mg IV/IM (2 to 2.5 times the dose ET) repeated every 2 min as needed. Max dose 2 mg.

MORPHINE SULFATE

NALBUPHINE

NALOXONE

Name/Class: NIFEDIPINE (Procardia, Adalat)/Calcium Channel Blocker

Description: Nifedipine is a calcium channel blocker that reduces coronary artery spasm in angina. It also decreases peripheral vascular resistance, blood pressure, and cardiac workload.

Indications: Severe hypertension and angina.

Contraindications: Hypersensitivity or hypotension.

Precautions: Monitor blood pressure carefully, since it can drop significantly with nifedipine use.

Dosage/Route: One 10 to 20 mg capsule SL/PO.

Name/Class: NITROGLYCERIN (Nitrostat)/Nitrate

Description: Nitroglycerin is a rapid smooth muscle relaxant that reduces peripheral vascular resistance, blood pressure, venous return, and cardiac workload.

Indications: Chest pain associated with angina and acute myocardial infarction, acute pulmonary edema.

Contraindications: Hypersensitivity, tolerance to nitrates, severe anemia, head trauma, hypotension, increased ICP, patients taking sildenafil, glaucoma, shock.

Precautions: May induce headache that is sometimes severe. Nitroglycerin is light sensitive and will lose potency when exposed to the air.

Dosage/Route: 1 tablet (0.4 mg) 3 tablets, or ½ to 1 inch of topical ointment, or 0.4 mg (one spray)SL up to 3 sprays in 15 min.

Name/Class: NITROUS OXIDE (Nitronox)/Analgesic (gas)

Description: Nitrous oxide is a self-administered analgesic gas composed of 50% oxygen and 50% nitrous oxide. Its effects last only 2 to 5 minutes after administration ceases.

Indications: Musculoskeletal, burn, and ischemic chest pain; severe anxiety (including hyperventilation).

Contraindications: Possible bowel obstruction, pneumothorax or tension pneumothorax, COPD, head injury, impaired mental status, drug intoxication.

Precautions: Use in well-ventilated area. It may cause nausea and vomiting.

Dosage/Route: It is self-administered inhalation until the pain is relieved or the patient drops the mask.

NIFEDIPINE

NITROGLYCERIN

NITROUS OXIDE

Name/Class: NOREPINEPHRINE (Levophed)/Sympathomimetic Agent

Description: Norepinephrine is a naturally occurring catecholamine and causes vasoconstriction, cardiac stimulation, and increased blood pressure, myocardial oxygen demand, and coronary blood flow.

Indications: Refractory hypotension and neurogenic shock.

Contraindications: Hypotension due to hypovolemia.

Precautions: Hypertension, hyperthyroidism, severe heart disease, elderly, MAO inhibitor therapy, patients receiving tricyclic antidepressants. Monitor blood pressure frequently and infuse the drug through the largest vein available as it may cause tissue necrosis.

Dosage/Route: 0.1 to 0.5 mcg/kg/min IV/IO, titrated to response. Ped: 0.1 to 2 mcg/kg/min titrated to BP (rarely used).

Name/Class: ONDANSETRON (Zofran)/Antiemetic

Description: Ondansetron is a selective serotonin receptor antagonist preventing nausea and vomiting.

Indications: Nausea and vomiting.

Contraindications: Hypersensitivity to the drug.

Precautions: Pregnancy, nursing mothers, and children under 3 years.

Dosage: 4 to 8 mg over 1 to 5 min IV

Name/Class: OXYGEN/Oxidizing Agent (Gas)

Description: Oxygen is an odorless, colorless, tasteless gas, essential for life. It is one of the most important emergency drugs.

Indications: Hypoxia or anticipated hypoxia, or in any medical or trauma patient to improve respiratory efficiency.

Contraindications: There are no contraindications to oxygen therapy.

Precautions: Chronic obstructive pulmonary disease and very prolonged administration of high concentrations in the newborn.

Dosage/Route: Hypoxia: 100% by inhalation or IPPV.

Name/Class: OXYTOCIN (Pitocin)/Hormone

Description: Oxytocin is a naturally occurring hormone that causes the uterus to contract, thereby inducing labor, encouraging delivery of the placenta, and controlling postpartum hemorrhage.

Indications: Severe postpartum hemorrhage.

Contraindications: Hypersensitivity, prehospital administration before delivery of the infant or infants.

Precautions: Before delivery may induce uterine rupture and fetal dysrhythmias, hypertension, intracranial bleeding, asphyxia. Uterine tone, ECG, and vital signs should be monitored during administration.

Dosage/Route: 3 to 10 units IM after delivery of the placenta. 10 to 20 units in 500 mL of D_5W or NS IV titrated to effect.

Name/Class: PANCURONIUM (Pavulon)/Nondepolarizing Neuromuscular Blocker

Description: Pancuronium is a nondepolarizing neuromuscular blocker that causes paralysis without bronchospasm or hypotension; it does not cause the fasciculations associated with polarizing agents.

Indications: To facilitate endotracheal intubation.

Contraindications: Hypersensitivity to pancuronium or bromides, or tachycardia.

Precautions: Debilitated patients; myasthenia gravis; pulmonary, hepatic, or renal disease; fluid or electrolyte imbalance.

Dosage/Route: 0.04 to 0.1 mg/kg IV. Ped: same as adult.

Name/Class: PHENOBARBITAL (Luminal)/Anticonvulsant

Description: Phenobarbital is a long-acting barbiturate anticonvulsant with sedative and hypnotic effects that limits the spread of seizure activity.

Indications: Seizures, status epilepticus, acute anxiety.

Contraindications: Hypersensitivity to barbiturates.

Precautions: Hepatic, renal, cardiac, or respiratory impairment; allergies; elderly or debilitated patients; fever; hyperthyroidism; diabetes; severe anemia; hypoadrenal function; during labor, delivery, and lactation.

Dosage/Route: 100 to 300 mg slow IV/IM. Ped: 6 to 10 mg/kg slow IV/IM.

Name/Class: PHENYTOIN (Dilantin)/Anticonvulsant

Description: Phenytoin is a derivative related to phenobarbital that reduces the spread of electrical discharges in the motor cortex and inhibits seizures. It also has antidysrhythmic properties that **could depress spontaneous ventricular depolarization.**

Description: Phenytoin is a derivative related to phenobarbital that reduces the spread of electrical discharges in the motor cortex and inhibits seizures. It also has antidysrhythmic properties that counteract the effects of digitalis.

Indications: Seizures, status epilepticus, cardiac dysrhythmias secondary to digitalis toxicity.

Contraindications: Hypersensitivity to hydantoin products, seizures due to hypoglycemia, sinus bradycardia, heart block, Adams-Stokes syndrome.

Precautions: Hepatic or renal impairment, alcoholism, cardiogenic shock, elderly or debilitated patients, diabetes, hyperglycemia, bradycardia, heart block, respiratory depression.

Dosage/Route: *Seizures, status epilepticus:* 15 to 18 mg/kg slow IV. Ped: 8 to 10 mg/kg slow IV.

Dysrhythmias: 100 mg slow IV (over 5 min) to a maximum 1,000 mg. Ped: 3 to 5 mg/kg slow IV.

Name/Class: PHYSOSTIGMINE (Antilirium)/Parasympathomimetic

Description: Physostigmine inhibits the breakdown of acetylcholine, resulting in prolonged parasympathetic effects. It is sometimes used as an antidote for anticholinergic (e.g., atropine) and tricyclic antidepressant overdoses.

Indications: Tricyclic antidepressant (CNS and cardiac effects) and anticholinergic overdose.

Contraindications: Asthma, diabetes, gangrene, cardiovascular disease, narrow-angle glaucoma.

Precautions: Reduce dose (or administer atropine) if increased salivation, emesis, or bradycardia develop.

Dosage/Route: 0.5 to 3 mg IV (not faster than 1 mg min), repeat as needed. Ped: 0.01 to 0.03 mg/kg/ 15 to 20 min to max 2 mg.

Name/Class: PRALIDOXIME (2-PAM)/Cholinesterase Reactivator

Description: Pralidoxime reactivates cholinesterase and reinstitutes the degrading of acetylcholine and restores normal neuromuscular transmission. It is used to reverse severe organophosphate poisoning.

Indications: Organophosphate poisoning.

Contraindications: Carbamate insecticides (Sevin), inorganic phosphates, and organophosphates having no anticholinesterase activity, asthma, peptic ulcer disease, severe cardiac disease, or patients receiving aminophylline, theophylline, morphine, succinylcholine, reserpine, or phenothiazines.

Precautions: Rapid administration may result in tachycardia, laryngospasm, and muscle rigidity. Excited or manic behavior may be noted after regaining consciousness.

Dosage/Route: 1 to 2 g in 250 to 500 mL NS infused over 30 min; or 1 to 2 g IM/SQ if IV not feasible. Ped: 20 to 40 mg/kg IV/IM subcutaneous.

Name/Class: PROCAINAMIDE (Pronestyl)/Antiarrhythmic

Description: Procainamide prolongs ventricular repolarization, slows conduction, and decreases myocardial excitability.

Indications: Ventricular fibrillation and pulseless ventricular tachycardia refractory to lidocaine.

Contraindications: Hypersensitivity to procainamide or procaine, myasthenia gravis, 2nd- or 3rd-degree heart block.

Precautions: Hypotension, cardiac enlargement, CHF, AMI, ventricular dysrhythmias from digitalis, hepatic or renal impairment, electrolyte imbalance, bronchial asthma.

Dosage/Route: 20 mg/min IV drip up to 17 mg/kg to effect, then 1 to 4 mg/min. Ped: 15 mg/kg IV/IO over 30 to 60 min.

Name/Class: PROCHLORPERAZINE (Compazine)/Antiemetic

Description: Prochlorperazine is a phenothiazine derivative similar to chlorpromazine with potent antiemetic properties and fewer sedative, hypotensive, and anticholinergic effects.

Indications: Severe nausea and vomiting or acute psychosis.

Contraindications: Hypersensitivity to phenothiazines, coma, depression.

Precautions: Breast cancer, children with acute illness or dehydration.

Dosage/Route: 5 to 10 mg IV/IM. Ped: 0.13 mg/kg IV/IM/PR if > 10 kg or > 2 years.

Name/Class: PROMETHAZINE (Phenergan)/Antiemetic

Description: Promethazine is an anticholinergic agent that enhances the effects of analgesics and is a potent antiemetic.

Indications: Nausea and vomiting, motion sickness, to enhance the effects of analgesics, to induce sedation.

Contraindications: Hypersensitivity to phenothiazines.

Precautions: Hepatic, respiratory, or cardiac impairment; asthma; hypertension; elderly or debilitated patients.

Dosage/Route: 12.5 to 25 mg IV/IM/PR. Ped: 0.5 mg/kg IV/IM/PR.

PROCAINAMIDE

PROCHLORPERAZINE

PROMETHAZINE

Name/Class: PROPAFANONE (Rythmol)/Antidysrhythmic

Description: Propafanone is an antidysrhythmic that stabilizes the myocardial membranes, reduces automaticity and the rate of single and multiple PVCs, and suppresses ventricular tachycardia.

Indications: Ventricular and supraventricular dysrhythmias.

Contraindications: Hypersensitivity, uncontrolled CHF, cardiogenic shock, sick sinus syndrome, AV block, bradycardia, hypotension, bronchospastic disorders, electrolyte imbalances, non-life-threatening dysrhythmias, COPD, nursing mothers.

Precautions: CHF, AV block, hepatic or renal impairment, elderly, pregnancy.

Dosage/Route: 150 to 300 mg PO/8 hours or 1 to 2 mg/kg IV at 10 mg/min.

Name/Class: PROPRANOLOL (Inderal)/Beta Blocker

Description: Propranolol is a nonselective beta blocker affecting both bronchial and cardiac sites. It reduces heart rate, myocardial irritability, contraction force, cardiac output, and blood pressure.

Indications: Ventricular fibrillation and pulseless ventricular tachycardia refractory to lidocaine and bretylium and selected SVTs.

Contraindications: 2nd- and 3rd-degree heart blocks, CHF, cor pulmonale, sinus bradycardia, cardiac impairment, cardiogenic shock, bronchospasm or bronchial asthma, COPD, adrenergic-augmenting psychotropic, MAO inhibitors.

Precautions: Peripheral vascular disease, bee sting allergy, mild COPD, renal or hepatic impairment, diabetes, hypoglycemia, myasthenia gravis, WPW syndrome, major surgery.

Dosage/Route: 0.1 mg/kg divided into three equal doses given every 2 to 3 min, slow IV (do not exceed 1 mg/min). May repeat in 2 min.

Name/Class: PROSTAGLANDIN E_1 (Prostin VR Pediatric)/Vasodilator

Description: Prostaglandin E_1 is derived from fatty acids and causes vasodilation, inhibits platelet aggregation, and stimulates intestinal and uterine smooth muscles. It also helps maintain ductus arteriosus patency in newborn infants.

Indications: Infant cyanotic heart disease.

Contraindications:

Precautions: Constant respiratory monitoring is required.

Dosage/Route: Infant: 0.05 to 0.1 mcg/kg/min IV/IO.

PROPAFANONE

PROPRANOLOL

PROSTAGLANDIN E$_1$

Name/Class: RACEMIC EPINEPHRINE (microNefrin, Vaponefrin)/Sympathomimetic Agonist

Description: Racemic epinephrine is a variation of epinephrine used only for inhalation to induce bronchodilation and to reduce laryngeal edema and mucus secretion.

Indications: Croup (laryngotracheobronchitis).

Contraindications: Hypersensitivity, hypertension, epiglottitis.

Precautions: May result in tachycardia and other dysrhythmias. Patient vital signs and ECG should be monitored.

Dosage/Route: 0.25 to 0.75 mL of a 2.5 n% solution in 2 mL NS once by nebulizer. Ped: same as adult.

Name/Class: RETEPLACE RECOMBINANT (Retivase)/Thrombolytic

Description: Recombinant DNA–derived form of human tPA promotes thrombolysis by forming plasmin. Plasmin, in turn, degrades fibrin and fibrinogen and, ultimately, the clot.

Indications: To thrombolyze in acute myocardial infarction and pulmonary embolism.

Contraindications: Active internal bleeding, suspected aortic dissection, traumatic CPR, recent hemorrhagic stroke (6 mo), intracranial or intraspinal surgery or trauma (2 mo), pregnancy, uncontrolled hypertension, hypersensitivity to thrombolytics.

Precautions: Recent major surgery, cerebral vascular disease, recent GI or GU bleeding, recent trauma, hypertension, patient > 75 years, current oral anticoagulants, hemorrhagic ophthalmic conditions.

Dosage/Route: AMI: 10 units IV over 2 min. Repeat in 30 min.

Name/Class: SODIUM BICARBONATE (NaHCO$_3$)/Alkalizing Agent

Description: Sodium bicarbonate provides vascular bicarbonate to assist the buffer system in reducing the effects of metabolic acidosis and in the treatment of some overdoses.

Indications: Tricyclic antidepressant and barbiturate overdose, refractory acidosis, hyperkalemia.

Contraindications: None when used in severe hypoxia or late cardiac arrest.

Precautions: May cause alkalosis if given in too large a quantity. It may also deactivate vasopressors and may precipitate with calcium chloride.

Dosage/Route: 1 mEq/kg IV/IO Ped: 1 mEq/kg IV/IO (4.2% concentration recommended for use in infants < 1 month old.

RACEMIC EPINEPHRINE

RETEPLACE RECOMBINANT

SODIUM BICARBONATE

Name/Class: SODIUM NITROPRUSSIDE (Nipride, Nitropress)/Nitrate

Description: Sodium nitroprusside is a rapid-acting hypotensive agent producing peripheral vasodilation and a mild increase in heart rate, a decrease in cardiac output, and a slight decrease in peripheral vascular resistance.

Indications: Hypertensive crisis CHF and pulmonary edema.

Contraindications: Compensatory hypertension or impaired cerebral circulation (head injury, stroke), hypotension, hypovolemia, use of ED medications.

Precautions: Hepatic or renal impairment, hyponatremia, hypothyroidism.

Dosage/Route: 0.1 mcg/kg/min gradually titrated to effect or 10 mg/kg/min. (50 to 100 mg/250 ml D_5W). Ped: 0.3 to 1 mcg/kg/min. Titrate up to 8 mcg/kg/min as needed.

E

Name/Class: SOTALOL (Betapace)/Beta Blocker, Antidysrhythmic

Description: Sotalol is a nonselective beta blocker that slows heart rate and decreases AV conduction and irritability.

Indications: Ventricular and supraventricular dysrhythmias.

Contraindications: Hypersensitivity, bronchial asthma, sinus bradycardia, 2nd- and 3rd-degree heart block, long QT syndromes, cardiogenic shock, uncontrolled CHF, COPD.

Precautions: CHF, electrolyte disturbances, recent MI, diabetes, sick sinus rhythms, renal impairment.

Dosage/Route: 1 to 1.5 mg/kg IV/IO.

Name/Class: STREPTOKINASE (Streptase)/Fibrinolytic

Description: Streptokinase is a fibrinolytic that acts by activating the process that converts plasminogen to plasmin and results in the degradation of fibrin and fibrinogen and decreases erythrocyte aggregation.

Indications: AMI, deep vein thrombosis (DVT), pulmonary embolism.

Contraindications: Active internal bleeding, aortic dissection, traumatic CPR, recent stroke, intracranial or intraspinal surgery or trauma (within 2 months), intracranial tumors, uncontrolled hypertension, pregnancy, hypersensitivity to anistreplase or streptokinase.

Precautions: Recent major surgery (10 days), patients > 75 years, cerebral vascular disease, GI or GU bleeding, recent trauma, hypertension, hemorrhagic conditions, ophthalmic conditions, oral anticoagulant use.

Dosage/Route: *AMI:* 1.5 million units IV over 1 hour.

DVT and pulmonary emboli: 250,000 units IV over 30 min, then 100,000 units/hr.

SODIUM NITROPRUSSIDE

SOTALOL

STREPTOKINASE

Name/Class: SUCCINYLCHOLINE (Anectine)/Depolarizing Neuromuscular Blocker

Description: Succinylcholine is an ultra-short-acting depolarizing neuromuscular blocker.

Indications: Facilitated endotracheal intubation.

Contraindications: Hypersensitivity, family history of malignant hyperthermia, penetrating eye injury, narrow-angle glaucoma.

Precautions: Severe burn or crush injury; electrolyte imbalances; hepatic, renal, cardiac, or pulmonary impairment; fractures; spinal cord injury; dehydration; severe anemia; porphyria.

Dosage/Route: 1 to 2 mg/kg IV/IO. Ped: 1 to 2 mg/kg IV/IO.

Name/Class: TENECTEPLASE (TNKase)/Thrombolytic

Description: Recombinant DNA–derived form of human tPA promotes thrombolysis by forming plasmin. Plasmin, in turn, degrades fibrin and fibrinogen and, ultimately, the clot.

Indications: To thrombolyze in acute myocardial infarction and pulmonary embolism.

Contraindications: Active internal bleeding, suspected aortic dissection, traumatic CPR, recent hemorrhagic stroke (6 mo), intracranial or intraspinal surgery or trauma (2 mo), pregnancy, uncontrolled hypertension, hypersensitivity to thrombolytics.

Precautions: Recent major surgery, cerebral vascular disease, recent GI or GU bleeding, recent trauma, hypertension, patient > 75 years, current oral anticoagulants, hemorrhagic ophthalmic conditions.

Dosage/Route: AMI: 30 to 50 mg. IV, weight adjusted, over 5 seconds.

Name/Class: TERBUTALINE (Brethine, Bricanyl)/Sympathetic Agonist

Description: Terbutaline is a synthetic sympathomimetic that causes bronchodilatation with less cardiac effect than epinephrine.

Indications: Bronchial asthma and bronchospasm in COPD.

Contraindications: Hypersensitivity to the drug.

Precautions: The patient may experience palpitations, anxiety, nausea, and/or dizziness. Vital signs and breath sounds must be monitored; use caution with cardiac or hypertensive patients.

Dosage/Route: Two inhalations with a metered dose inhaler, repeated once in 1 min or 0.25 mg SQ repeated in 15 to 30 min.

SUCCINYLCHOLINE

TENECTEPLASE

TERBUTALINE

Name/Class: THIAMINE/Vitamin

Description: Thiamine is vitamin B_1, which is required to convert glucose into energy. It is not manufactured by the body and must be constantly provided from ingested foods.

Indications: Coma of unknown origin, chronic alcoholism with associated coma, delirium tremens.

Contraindications: None.

Precautions: Known hypersensitivity to the drug.

Dosage/Route: 50 to 100 mg IV/IM. Ped: 10 to 25 mg IV/IM.

Name/Class: VASOPRESSIN (Pitressin)/Hormone, Vasopressor

Description: Vasopressin is a hormone with strong vasopressive and antidiuretic properties but that may precipitate angina and/or AMI.

Indications: To increase peripheral vascular resistance in arrest (CPR) or to control bleeding from esophageal varices.

Contraindications: Chronic nephritis with nitrogen retention, ischemic heart disease, PVCs, advanced arteriosclerosis, 1st stage of labor.

Precautions: Epilepsy, migraine, heart failure, angina, vascular disease, hepatic impairment, elderly, children.

Dosage/Route: *Arrest:* 40 units IV/IO. Ped: 0.4 to 1 unit/kg IV/IO

Esophageal varices: 0.02 to 0.04 units/min IV drip.

Name/Class: VECURONIUM (Norcuron)/Nondepolarizing Skeletal Muscle Relaxant

Description: Vecuronium is a nondepolarizing skeletal muscle relaxant similar to pancuronium with minimal cardiovascular effects.

Indications: Facilitated endotracheal intubation.

Contraindications: Hypersensitivity.

Precautions: Hepatic or renal impairment, impaired fluid and electrolyte or acid-base balance, severe obesity, myasthenia gravis, elderly or debilitated patients, malignant hyperthermia.

Dosage/Route: 0.1 to 0.15 mg/kg IV. Ped: same as adult.

THIAMINE

VASOPRESSIN

VECURONIUM

Name/Class: VERAPAMIL (Isoptin, Calan)/Calcium Channel Blocker

Description: Verapamil is a calcium channel blocker that slows AV conduction, suppresses re-entry dysrhythmias such as PSVT, and slows ventricular responses to atrial tachydysrhythmias. Verapamil also dilates coronary arteries and reduces myocardial oxygen demand.

Indications: PSVT refractory to adenosine, atrial flutter, and atrial fibrillation with rapid ventricular response.

Contraindications: Severe hypotension, cardiogenic shock, 2nd- or 3rd-degree heart block, CHF, sinus node disease, accessory AV pathways, WPW syndrome. It should not be administered to persons taking beta blockers.

Precautions: Hepatic and renal impairment, MI with coronary artery occlusion, myocardial stenosis.

Dosage/Route: 2.5 to 5 mg IV bolus over 2 to 3 min, then 5 to 10 mg after 15 to 30 min to a max of 20 mg. Ped: newborn—0.1 to 0.2 mg/kg (not to exceed 2 mg), age 1 to 15—0.1 to 0.3 mg/kg (not to exceed 5 mg).

Name/Class:

Description:

Indications:

Contraindications:

Precautions:

Dosage/Route:

Name/Class:

Description:

Indications:

Contraindications:

Precautions:

Dosage/Route:

VERAPAMIL

DRUG NAME

DRUG NAME